General Symptoms

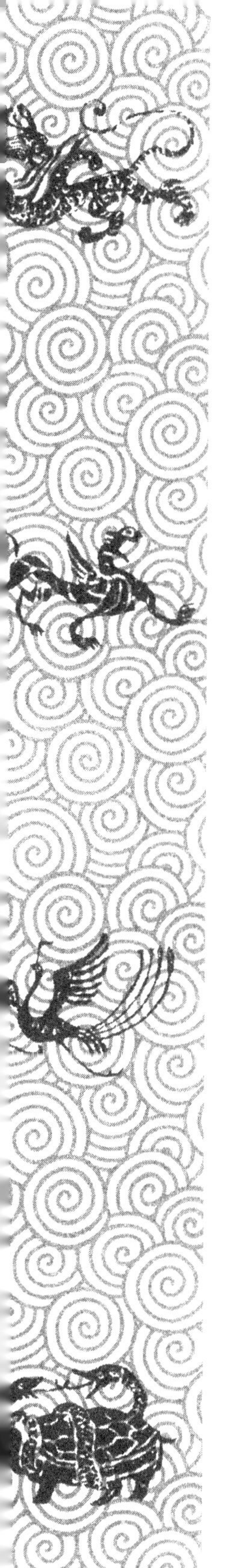

The Treatment of Disease in TCM

VOLUME 7:

General Symptoms

by Philippe Sionneau
& Lü Gang

BLUE POPPY PRESS

Published by:

BLUE POPPY PRESS
A Division of Blue Poppy Enterprises, Inc.
4804 SE 69th Avenue
Portland, OR 97206

First Edition, March 2000
Second Printing, May, 2009
Third Printing, November, 2010
Fourth Printing, November, 2011
Fifth Printing, January, 2013
Sixth Printing, January, 2014
Seventh Printing, January, 2015
Eighth Printing, November, 2015
Ninth Printing, July, 2017
Tenth Printing, September, 2018
Eleventh Printing, September, 2020
Twelfth Printing, September, 2021

ISBN 1-891845-14-4
ISBN 978-1-891845-14-7
Library of Congress #91-83249

The information in this book is given in good faith. However, the translators and the publishers cannot be held responsible for any error or omission. Nor can they be held in any way responsible for treatment given on the basis of information contained in this book. The publishers make this information available to English language readers for scholarly and research purposes only.

The publishers do not advocate nor endorse self-medication by laypersons. Chinese medicine is a professional medicine. Laypersons interested in availing themselves of the treatments described in this book should seek out a qualified professional practitioner of Chinese medicine.

COMP Designation: Original work using a standard translational terminology

Cover design by Jeff Fuller, Crescent Moon

Printed at Frederic Printing, Aurora, CO

16 15 14 13 12

Table of Contents

Aversion to Wind & Cold *(Wei Wu Feng Han)*

Aversion to wind and cold refers to a chilly feeling which is not improved by obtaining warmth. Patients with this symptom may only experience aversion to wind as though they were undressed or a slight chilly shivering feeling. This condition is often a manifestation of the fight between evil and righteous qi.

Disease causes, disease mechanisms:

"One *fen* (*i.e.*, one tenth) of aversion to cold suggests one *fen* of exterior condition." This saying implies that aversion to wind and cold is an important symptom of exterior patterns, and this is most often true. However, aversion to cold may also be seen in some non-exterior patterns where the righteous qi fights forcefully against evils and this fight causes disharmony between the constructive and defensive qi.

1. Contraction of the external evils

When external evils invade the body, they start in the exterior of the body where the defensive yang keeps guard to defend the body. When such evils invade, the defensive yang swiftly arises to fight against the invading evils. If the defensive yang wins, the evils will be expelled. However, if the evils overcome the defensive yang, the defensive yang will become depressed and blocked. Because defensive yang is also responsible for warming the exterior, if the defensive yang becomes depressed and blocked, it is not able to warm the exterior. Thus there will be aversion to wind and cold. The external evils most often causing this condition are wind, cold, heat, dampness, and summerheat, and only sometimes dryness. For more details, please refer to Chapter 4 below.

2. Exterior cold & interior heat

This disease mechanism is usually seen in patients who are already suffering from internal heat and then contract external cold evils. As stated above, because the defensive qi is responsible for both defending and warming the exterior, such cold evils may fetter and deprive the exterior of the body of warming yang qi, thus leading to aversion to wind and cold regardless of the fact that there is concomitant internal heat.

3. Sore toxins

What Chinese medicine refers to as sores usually develop from external contraction of fire heat evils, excessive consumption of fatty, sweet foods, or from external injury. Within such sores there is putrid flesh and vanquished blood. These are recognized as evils by the body's righteous qi which struggles against them. If these evils are rampant and overcome the righteous qi, causing disharmony between the constructive and defensive, there will be aversion to wind and cold.

4. Invasion of malaria evils

This disease mechanism often occurs in individuals with habitual yang vacuity. Malaria evils tend to lodge in the shao yang. The shao yang is the pivot which is halfway between the exterior and interior. If malaria evils invade and lodge in the shao yang, the defensive qi will be inhibited or blocked. Once again, because the defensive qi cannot warm the exterior, there is aversion to wind and cold.

Treatment based on pattern discrimination:

1. Wind evils assailing the exterior

Symptoms: Aversion to wind, slight fever,[1] headache and distention, dizziness, slight body aching, slight sweating, thin, white tongue fur, and a floating pulse

Therapeutic principles: Course wind and resolve the exterior

Acupuncture & moxibustion:

Feng Men (Bl 12)	Together, these points course wind and resolve
Feng Chi (GB 20)	the exterior when needled with draining method.
He Gu (LI 4)	These points free and disinhibit the yang ming and
Wai Guan (TB 5)	the triple burner respectively. Together, they dispel
	the evils when needled with draining method.

Additions & subtractions: For itchy throat, prick *Shao Shang* (Lu 11) to bleed. For nasal congestion and discharge, add *Ying Xiang* (LI 20).

---

[1] In Chinese, what we are translating as fever is "emission of heat." Fever is actually a Western medical concept which was not a part of traditional Chinese medicine until only after China's contact with Western medicine.

Chinese medicinal formula: *Gui Zhi Tang* (Cinnamon Twig Decoction)

Ingredients: Uncooked Ramulus Cinnamomi Cassiae (*Gui Zhi*), 9g, uncooked Radix Albus Paeoniae Lactiflorae (*Bai Shao*), 9g, mix-fried Radix Glycyrrhizae (*Gan Cao*), 6g, uncooked Rhizoma Zingiberis (*Sheng Jiang*), 9g, Fructus Zizyphi Jujubae (*Da Zao*), 3 pieces

Additions & subtractions: For coughing and/or panting, add ginger mix-fried Cortex Magnoliae Officinalis (*Hou Po*), 9g, and Semen Pruni Armeniacae (*Xing Ren*), 9g. For severe body aching, add uncooked Radix Puerariae (*Ge Gen*), 9g. For incessant sweating, add Radix Lateralis Praeparatus Aconiti Carmichaeli (*Fu Zi*), 6g. For habitual bodily qi vacuity, add Radix Codonopsitis Pilosulae (*Dang Shen*), 12g, or Radix Panacis Ginseng (*Ren Shen*), 6g. For habitual bodily yin vacuity, add Rhizoma Polygonati Odorati (*Yu Zhu*), 12g.

Remarks: This pattern is often seen in clinical practice at the very beginning of exterior conditions when evils are not strong. At that time, it may be difficult to make a clear discrimination between cold and heat. A single day's powerful, individualized treatment is often sufficient to treat this condition. For this, heavy moxibustion on *Da Zhui* (GV 14) followed by *Gui Zhi Tang* (Cinnamon Twig Decoction) is usually effective. However, after taking *Gui Zhi Tang,* one must also eat a bowl of a fresh ginger and rice porridge. Then the patient should rest covered in bed to induce sweating.

2. Cold evils fettering the exterior

Symptoms: Severe aversion to wind and cold, headache, nasal congestion, nasal discharge, slight fever but frequent shivering, body aches, rigidity and pain in the nape of the neck and upper back, thin, white tongue fur, and a floating, tight pulse

Therapeutic principles: Resolve the exterior and scatter cold

Acupuncture & moxibustion:

Da Zhui (GV 14)	Together, these points resolve the exterior and
Feng Men (Bl 12)	disperse cold when moxaed and needled with
Feng Chi (GB 20)	draining method.
He Gu (LI 4)	Together, these points promote sweating when
Fu Liu (Ki 7)	needled with draining and supplementing method
	respectively.

Additions and subtractions: For headache, add *Tou Wei* (St 8). For coughing, add *Fei Shu* (Bl 13).

Chinese medicinal formula: *Ma Huang Tang* (Ephedra Decoction)

Ingredients: Uncooked Herba Ephedrae (*Ma Huang*), 9g, uncooked Ramulus Cinnamomi Cassiae (*Gui Zhi*), 6g, Semen Pruni Armeniacae (*Xing Ren*), 12g, Radix Glycyrrhizae (*Gan Cao*), 3g

Additions & subtractions: For only slight cold, subtract Cinnamon. For concomitant interior heat with vexatious thirst and a higher fever, add uncooked Gypsum Fibrosum (*Shi Gao*), 20g. For coughing and/or panting, subtract Cinnamon and add Fructus Perillae Frutescentis (*Su Zi*), 9g, and Cortex Radicis Mori Albi (*Sang Bai Pi*), 9g. For severe pain in the nape of the neck and upper back, add uncooked Radix Puerariae (*Ge Gen*), 9g.

3. Summerheat dampness damaging the defensive qi

Symptoms: Slight aversion to cold, high fever, head distention, chest oppression, nausea and vomiting, sweating, thirst, short voidings of dark-colored urine, slimy, yellow tongue fur, and a soggy, rapid pulse

Therapeutic principles: Eliminate summerheat, clear heat and transform dampness

Acupuncture & moxibustion:

Da Zhui (GV 14) *Zhi Gou* (TB 6) *He Gu* (LI 4)	Together, these points eliminate summerheat and clear heat when needled with draining method.
Zhong Wan (CV 12) *Zu San Li* (St 36)	Together, these points transform dampness and harmonize the center when needled with even draining and even supplementing method.

Additions & subtractions: For heart vexation, add *Jian Shi* (Per 5). For coughing, add *Fei Shu* (Bl 13). For severe head distention, add *Ben Shen* (GB 13). For glomus in the stomach, add *Jian Li* (CV 1).

Chinese medicinal formula: *Xin Jia Xiang Ru Yin* (New Additions Elsholtzia Drink)

Ingredients: Herba Elsholtziae Seu Moslae (*Xiang Ru*), 6g, Flos Lonicerae Japonicae (*Jin Yin Hua*), 9g, Flos Dolichoris Lablabis (*Bian Dou Hua*), 9g, ginger mix-fried Cortex Magnoliae Officinalis (*Hou Po*), 6g, Fructus Forsythiae Suspensae (*Lian Qiao*), 9g

Additions & subtractions: For severe aversion to wind and cold, add Herba Agastachis Seu Pogostemi (*Huo Xiang*), 9g, and uncooked Rhizoma Zingiberis (*Sheng Jiang*), 9g.

4. Wind heat invading the lungs

Symptoms: Aversion to wind and cold, fever, fever is more prominent than aversion to cold, slight sweating, headache, red throat, dry mouth, coughing, thin, yellow tongue fur, and a floating, rapid pulse

Therapeutic principles: Resolve the exterior, clear heat and diffuse the lungs

Acupuncture & moxibustion:

Da Zhui (GV 14) *Feng Chi* (GB 20) *Wai Guan* (TB 5) *Qu Chi* (LI 11)	Together, these points course wind, clear heat, and resolve the exterior when needled with draining method.
Yu Ji (Lu 10)	Clears lung heat and stops coughing when needled with draining method

Additions & subtractions: For sore throat, prick *Shao Shang* (Lu 11) to bleed. For symptoms due to heat toxins, prick *Shi Xuan* (EX-UE-11). For cough with profuse phlegm, add *Fei Shu* (Bl 13). For high fever, prick *Wei Zhong* (Bl 40) to bleed.

Chinese medicinal formula: *Yin Qiao San* (Lonicera & Forsythia Powder)

Ingredients: Flos Lonicerae Japonicae (*Yin Hua*), 9g, Fructus Forsythiae Suspensae (*Lian Qiao*), 9g, Herba Menthae Haplocalycis (*Bo He*), 6g, Semen Praeparatus Sojae (*Dan Dou Chi*), 6g, Radix Platycodi Grandiflori (*Jie Geng*), 6g, Herba Schizonepetae Tenuifoliae (*Jing Jie*), 6g, Rhizoma Phragmitis Communis (*Lu Gen*), 10g, Folium Bambusae (*Zhu Ye*), 6g, Fructus Arctii Lappae (*Niu Bang Zi*), 9g, Radix Glycyrrhizae (*Gan Cao*), 6g

Additions & subtractions: For severe headache, add Folium Mori Albi (*Sang Ye*), 9g, and yellow Flos Chrysanthemi Morifolii (*Ju Hua*), 15g. For coughing and/or panting, add Semen Pruni Armeniacae (*Xing Ren*), 12g. For interior heat with vexatious thirst and red urine, add Fructus Gardeniae Jasminoidis

(*Zhi Zi*), 6g, Rhizoma Anemarrhenae Asphodeloidis (*Zhi Mu*), 9g, and Radix Scutellariae Baicalensis (*Huang Qin*), 6g. For severe thirst, add Tuber Ophiopogonis Japonici (*Mai Men Dong*), 9g, and uncooked Radix Rehmanniae (*Sheng Di*), 9g. For painful throat, add Fructificatio Lasiosphaerae Seu Calvatiae (*Ma Bo*), 9g, Radix Scrophulariae Ningpoensis (*Xuan Shen*), 9g, and Rhizoma Belamcandae Chinensis (*She Gan*), 9g.

Remarks: In Western countries, *Yin Qiao Pian (i.e., Yin Qiao Jie Du Pian)* is often prescribed for this pattern. This is a good patent medicine but is often erroneously used. For real efficacy, the dosage must be 3-5 times more than the stated dosage of the manufacturer, and treatment must last at least three days even if the symptoms disappear after the first day. To further increase this medicine's efficacy and avoid side effects such as abdominal distention, loose stools, and poor appetite, the patient must swallow the pills with a decoction of fresh ginger.

5. Dry evils damaging the lungs

Symptoms: Aversion to wind and cold, slight fever, headache, no sweating, nasal congestion with clear discharge at the same time as a dry nose, dry throat, dry, cracked lips, dry cough with scanty phlegm, a red tongue with white fur, and a fine, rapid pulse

Therapeutic principles: Diffuse the lungs, resolve the exterior, and moisten dryness

Acupuncture & moxibustion:

He Gu (LI 4) *Lie Que* (Lu 7)	Combining the exterior and interior, together, these points course the exterior and scatter cold when needled with draining method.
Feng Men (Bl 12) *Feng Chi* (GB 20)	Together, these points dispel wind and clear dryness when needled with draining method.
Chi Ze (Lu 5) *Fei Shu* (Bl 13)	Together, these points moisten the lungs when needled with supplementing method.

Additions & subtractions: For warm dryness manifested by predominant fever, slight aversion to cold, headache, slight sweating, coughing of scanty sticky phlegm, dry nose and throat, thirst, a red tongue with white fur, and a large pulse on the right side, subtract *Feng Men* and *Feng Chi*, but add *Qu Chi* (LI 11), *Da Zhui* (GV 14), and *San Yin Jiao* (Sp 6).

Chinese medicinal formula: Modified *Xing Su San* (Apricot & Perilla Powder)

Ingredients: Folium Perillae Frutescentis (*Zi Su Ye*), 6g, Semen Pruni Armeniacae (*Xing Ren*), 6g, Bulbus Fritillariae Cirrhosae (*Chuan Bei Mu*), 6g, Sclerotium Poriae Cocos (*Fu Ling*), 6g, Radix Peucedani (*Qian Hu*), 6g, Radix Platycodi Grandiflori (*Jie Geng*), 6g, Fructus Citri Aurantii (*Zhi Ke*), 6g, Radix Glycyrrhizae (*Gan Cao*), 6g, uncooked Pericarpium Citri Reticulatae (*Chen Pi*), 6g, uncooked Rhizoma Zingiberis (*Sheng Jiang*), 3g, Fructus Zizyphi Jujubae (*Da Zao*), 2 pieces

Additions & subtractions: For dry evils damaging fluids and transforming into heat, subtract Poria and Aurantium and add Fructus Forsythiae Suspensae (*Lian Qiao*), 9g, Fructus Gardeniae Jasminoidis (*Zhi Zi*), 9g, and Bulbus Lilii (*Bai He*), 9g.

6. Cold dampness fettering the exterior

Symptoms: Aversion to wind and cold, slight fever which mainly occurs in the afternoon, no sweating, head distention as if the head were swathed, heavy limbs, vexatious pain in the joints, slimy, white tongue fur, and a floating, tight or slow pulse

Therapeutic principles: Scatter cold, expel dampness, and resolve the exterior

Acupuncture & moxibustion:

Feng Men (Bl 12)	Together, these points warm and scatter cold evils
Wai Guan (TB 5)	and promote sweating to resolve the exterior when
He Gu (LI 4)	needled with moxibustion on the needle heads.

Qing Leng Yuan (TB 11)	Together, these points expel dampness when
Yin Ling Quan (Sp 9)	needled with draining method.

Additions & subtractions: For coughing with hoarse voice, add *Lie Que* (Lu 7). For glomus in the stomach and slimy tongue fur, add *Zhong Wan* (CV 12). For inhibited sweating, add *Shang Wan* (CV 13).

Chinese medicinal formula: *Huo Xiang Zheng Qi San* (Agastaches Correct the Qi Powder)

Ingredients: Herba Agastachis Seu Pogostemi (*Huo Xiang*), 9g, Folium Perillae Frutescentis (*Zi Su Ye*), 9g, Radix Angelicae Dahuricae (*Bai Zhi*), 6g, Pericarpium Arecae Catechu (*Da Fu Pi*), 6g, Sclerotium Poriae Cocos (*Fu Ling*), 9g, stir-fried Rhizoma Atractylodis Macrocephalae (*Bai Zhu*), 9g, clear Rhizoma Pinelliae Ternatae (*Ban Xia*), 6g, stir-fried Pericarpium Citri Reticulatae (*Chen Pi*), 6g, ginger mix-fried Cortex Magnoliae Officinalis (*Hou Po*), 6g, Radix Platycodi Grandiflori (*Jie Geng*), 6g, mix-fried Radix Glycyrrhizae (*Gan Cao*), 3g

Additions & subtractions: For severe aversion to cold and fever, add Radix Ledebouriellae Divaricatae (*Fang Feng*), 9g, and Herba Schizonepetae Tenuifoliae (*Jing Jie*), 9g. For cold dampness transforming into damp heat with agitation, thirst, and slimy, yellow tongue fur, subtract Magnolia and Atractylodes and add Rhizoma Coptidis Chinensis (*Huang Lian*), 6g, Herba Eupatorii Fortunei (*Pei Lan*), 9g, and Folium Nelumbinis Nuciferae (*He Ye*), 6g.

7. Exterior cold & interior heat

Symptoms: Aversion to wind cold, fever, vexatious pain in the joints, nasal congestion, hoarse voice, vexatious thirst, sore throat, cough with yellow phlegm, dark-colored urine, white or yellow tongue fur, and a floating, rapid pulse

Therapeutic principles: Course wind, scatter cold, and clear heat

Acupuncture & moxibustion:

Da Zhui (GV 14) *Wai Guan* (TB 5) *He Gu* (LI 4)	Together, these points course wind, scatter cold, and resolve the exterior when needled with draining method.
Chi Ze (Lu 5) *Qu Chi* (LI 11) *Fei Shu* (Bl 13)	Together, these points clear heat when needled with draining method.

Additions & subtractions: For severe coughing, add *Yu Ji* (Lu 10). For predominant exterior cold, subtract *Fei Shu* but needle *Feng Men* (Bl 12) with moxi-bustion on the heads of the needle. For predominant interior heat with constipation and thirst, add *Nei Ting* (St 44) and *Tian Shu* (St 25).

Chinese medicinal formula: *Da Qing Long Tang* (Major Blue Dragon Decoction)

Ingredients: Uncooked Herba Ephedrae (*Ma Huang*), 9g, Ramulus Cinnamomi Cassiae (*Gui Zhi*), 6g, mix-fried Radix Glycyrrhizae (*Gan Cao*), 6g, Semen Pruni Armeniacae (*Xing Ren*), 6g, Gypsum Fibrosum (*Shi Gao*), 20g, uncooked Rhizoma Zingiberis (*Sheng Jiang*), 3-6g, Fructus Zizyphi Jujubae (*Da Zao*), 2 pieces

Additions & subtractions: For mild aversion to wind and cold, subtract Cinnamon. For severe interior heat, increase Gypsum up to 30g and add Rhizoma Anemarrhenae Asphodeloidis (*Zhi Mu*), 9g.

8. Sore toxins

Symptoms: Aversion to cold, shivering in severe cases, fever, swelling, heat, and pain in the affected area, dark-colored urine, constipation, yellow tongue fur, and a bowstring, rapid or surging, rapid pulse

Therapeutic principles: Clear heat, drain fire, and resolve toxins

Acupuncture & moxibustion:

Shi Xuan (EX-UE-11) *Wei Zhong* (Bl 40)	Together, these points drain fire and resolve toxins when pricked to bleed.
Xue Hai (Sp 10) *Nei Ting* (St 44)	Together, these points clear heat in the blood when needled with draining method.

Additions & subtractions: For high fever, prick *Da Zhui* (GV 14) to bleed. For severe pain in the affected area, add *He Gu* (LI 4) and *Tai Chong* (Liv 3).

Chinese medicinal formula: Modified *Wu Wei Xiao Du Yin* (Five Flavors Disperse Toxins Drink)

Ingredients: Flos Lonicerae Japonicae (*Jin Yin Hua*), 15g, Flos Chrysanthemi Indici (*Ye Ju Hua*), 12g, Herba Taraxaci Mongolici Cum Radice (*Pu Gong Ying*), 9g, Herba Violae Yedoensitis Cum Radice (*Zi Hua Di Ding*), 9g, Radix Semiaquilegiae (*Tian Kui Zi*), 9g, Radix Ledebouriellae Divaricatae (*Fang Feng*), 9g, Fructus Forsythiae Suspensae (*Lian Qiao*), 9g, Herba Menthae Haplocalysis (*Bo He*), 3g, Radix Scutellariae Baicalensis (*Huang Qin*), 6g

9. Invasion of malaria evils (cold malaria)

Symptoms: Alternating aversion to wind cold and fever, severe aversion to wind and cold but no fever, or slight fever and sweating but no aversion to wind and cold, all of which recur at fixed intervals, lassitude of the spirit, fatigued limbs, chest and rib-side glomus, slimy, white tongue fur, and a bowstring, slow pulse

Therapeutic principles: Warm yang, scatter cold, and stop malaria

Acupuncture & moxibustion:

Da Zhui (GV 14) *Tao Dao* (GV 13)	Together, these points arouse yang to fight against the evils and scatter cold when needled with draining method and then moxaed on the heads of the needles.
Zu San Li (St 36) *Zhong Wan* (CV 12)	Together, these points support the righteous qi and dispel the evils when needled with supplementing method.
Jian Shi (Per 5)	An empirical point for malaria

Additions & subtractions: For headache, add *Tai Yang* (M-HN-5). For glomus and oppression in the stomach and abdomen, add *Pi Shu* (Bl 20). For vomiting of clear, thin water, abdominal distention, and no thirst, moxa *Shen Que* (CV 8) and needle *Gong Sun* (Sp 4) with supplementing method.

Chinese medicinal formula: Modified *Chai Hu Gui Zhi Gan Jiang Tang* (Bupleurum, Cinnamon & Dry Ginger Decoction)

Ingredients: Radix Bupleuri (*Chai Hu*), 9g, Ramulus Cinnamomi Cassiae (*Gui Zhi*), 9g, dry Rhizoma Zingiberis (*Gan Jiang*), 6g, Radix Trichosanthis Kirlowii (*Tian Hua Fen*), 12g, Radix Scutellariae Baicalensis (*Huang Qin*), 9g, uncooked Concha Ostreae (*Mu Li*), 20g, Radix Glycyrrhizae (*Gan Cao*), 3g, Radix Dichroae Febrifugae (*Chang Shan*), 9g, Fructus Amomi Tsao-ko (*Cao Guo*), 6g

Remarks: Because of increasing tourism to Africa, Asia, and South America, Western practitioners of Chinese medicine should not overlook the study of malaria.

2
Fear of Cold *(Wei Han)*

In Chinese medicine, fear of cold refers to a feeling of being chilled which *can* be improved by obtaining warmth.

Disease causes, disease mechanisms:

1. Yang vacuity

Yang vacuity usually develops from constitutional insufficiency, aging, enduring disease, overwork and taxation, or cold evils damaging yang. Yang is responsible for warming the body. Therefore, if yang becomes vacuous and insufficient, it may not be able to warm the body, thus leading to fear of cold. Therefore, it is said, "Yang vacuity causes external cold."

2. Cold striking the shao yin

This disease mechanism often develops from constitutional yang vacuity of the heart and kidneys coupled with external invasion of cold evils. In heat disease, external evils usually invade and enter the body from the exterior to the interior and from yang channels to yin. However, such evils can directly invade and enter the interior or the yin channels if the righteous qi is vacuous or when the evils are very strong. If cold evils take advantage of yang vacuity of the body and conquer yang, they may directly enter yin channels such as the shao yin. Cold is a yin evil which damages yang. The shao yin channel connects with the kidneys which are the water viscus. In addition, if there is a yang vacuity in the patient, all three mechanisms will lead to yin exuberance. "Yin exuberance causes cold." Therefore, fear of cold occurs.

3. Exuberant yang repelling yin

Exuberant yang repelling yin develops from heat evils depressed and deeply-lying in the interior which cannot flow freely to the exterior. Yin and yang are mutually rooted in each other, and should be in good balance. If either of them is too strong, they will not host each other, but rather repel each other. If yang is extremely exuberant in the interior, it will repel yin. In that case, yin cannot enter the interior to transform into yang. This then leads to a condition where yin stays in the outer while yang prevails in the inner. Yang is depressed in the inner and cannot stretch or flow freely to warm the outer, while yin stays in the outer giving rise to fear of cold.

4. Phlegm rheum collecting internally

Phlegm rheum collecting internally usually arises from dietary irregularities or vacuous yang which fails to transform dampness. Phlegm rheum is a kind of material evil which can easily cause obstruction. If phlegm rheum obstructs the flow of yang, fear of cold may occur since yang cannot flow freely to warm the body.

Treatment based on pattern discrimination:

1. Yang vacuity

Symptoms: Fear of cold, cold limbs, fatigue and lack of strength, reduced qi with disinclination to speak, a bland taste in the mouth, no thirst, clear urine, loose stools, a white facial complexion, a pale tongue, and a deep, slow, forceless pulse

Therapeutic principles: Warm yang and dispel cold

Acupuncture & moxibustion:

Guan Yuan (CV 4) *Shen Shu* (Bl 23)	Together, these points warm and supplement the original yang when moxaed.
Da Zhui (GV 14) *Bai Hui* (GV 20)	Together, these points arouse yang and dispel cold when moxaed.

Additions & subtractions: For predominant heart yang vacuity, add *Da Ling* (Per 7) and *Xi Men* (Per 3). For predominant spleen yang vacuity, add *Zu San Li* (St 36) and *Pi Shu* (Bl 20). For predominant kidney yang vacuity, moxa *Ming Men* (GV 4).

Chinese medicinal formulas: For predominant kidney yang vacuity: *You Gui Wan* (Restore the Right [Kidney] Pills)

Ingredients: Cooked Radix Rehmanniae (*Shu Di*), 12g, Radix Dioscoreae Oppositae (*Shan Yao*), 9g, Fructus Corni Officinalis (*Shan Zhu Yu*), 9g, Fructus Lycii Chinensis (*Gou Qi Zi*), 12g, Semen Cuscutae Chinensis (*Tu Si Zi*), 12g, Radix Angelicae Sinensis (*Dang Gui*), 6g, Gelatinum Cornu Cervi (*Lu Jiao Jiao*), 5g, Cortex Cinnamomi Cassiae (*Rou Gui*), 1g, salt stir-fried Cortex Eucommiae Ulmoidis (*Du Zhong*), 9g, and bland Radix Lateralis Praeparatus Aconiti Carmichaeli (*Fu Zi*), 6g

For predominant lung yang vacuity: Modified *Gan Cao Gan Jiang Tang* (Licorice & Dry Ginger Decoction)

Ingredients: Mix-fried Radix Glycyrrhizae (*Gan Cao*), 6g, dry Rhizoma Zingiberis (*Gan Jiang*), 6g, Herba Asari Cum Radice (*Xi Xin*), 3g, rice stir-fried Radix Codonopsitis Pilosulae (*Dang Shen*), 9g, Fructus Schisandrae Chinensis (*Wu Wei Zi*), 9g

For predominant spleen yang vacuity: *Fu Zi Li Zhong Tang* (Aconite Rectify the Center Decoction)

Ingredients: Blast-fried Radix Lateralis Praeparatus Aconiti Carmichaeli (*Fu Zi*), 6g, rice stir-fried Radix Codonopsitis Pilosulae (*Dang Shen*), 12g, dry Rhizoma Zingiberis (*Gan Jiang*), 9g, stir-fried Rhizoma Atractylodis Macrocephalae (*Bai Zhu*), 9g, honey mix-fried Radix Glycyrrhizae (*Gan Cao*), 6g

For predominant heart yang vacuity: Modified *Gui Zhi Gan Cao Tang* (Cinnamon & Licorice Decoction)

Ingredients: Stir-fried Ramulus Cinnamomi Cassiae (*Gui Zhi*), 9g, mix-fried Radix Glycyrrhizae (*Gan Cao*), 9g, Fructus Schisandrae Chinensis (*Wu Wei Zi*), 9g, bland Radix Lateralis Praeparatus Aconiti Carmichaeli (*Fu Zi*), 6g, Bulbus Allii (*Xie Bai*), 9g

Remarks: Patients with this pattern should avoid uncooked, chilled, excessively fluid-engendering foods, all which can damage kidney and spleen yang.

2. Cold striking the shao yin

Symptoms: Fear of cold, no fever, lassitude, cold limbs, listlessness, vomiting, diarrhea of clear grains, long voidings of clear urine, a pale tongue with white fur, and a deep, faint pulse

Therapeutic principles: Warm yang and scatter cold

Acupuncture & moxibustion:

Zhong Wan (CV 12) *Tian Shu* (St 25) *Guan Yuan* (CV 4)	The alarm points of the stomach, large intestine, and small intestines, respectively. Together, they warm yang and move the center to scatter cold when needled with simultaneous sparrow-pecking moxibustion.
Shen Que (CV 8)	Warms and supplements the original yang when moxaed with salt
Zu San Li (St 36)	Fortifies the spleen and harmonizes the center when needled with moxibustion on the needle heads

Additions & subtractions: For somnolence, moxa *Bai Hui* (GV 20). For vomiting immediately after eating, add *Nei Guan* (Per 6). For thirst, add *Fu Liu* (Ki 7).

Chinese medicinal formula: Modified *Si Ni Tang* (Four Counterflows Decoction)

Ingredients: Blast-fried Radix Lateralis Praeparatus Aconiti Carmichaeli (*Fu Zi*), 9g, dry Rhizoma Zingiberis (*Gan Jiang*), 9g, mix-fried Radix Glycyrrhizae (*Gan Cao*), 6g, stir-fried Rhizoma Atractylodis Macrocephalae (*Bai Zhu*), 9g

Additions & subtractions: For severe counterflow chilling of the limbs, severe fear of cold, a curled-up lying posture, and a faint pulse due to yang and qi desertion, add red Radix Panacis Ginseng (*Hong Shen*), 15g.

3. Exuberant yang repelling yin

Symptoms: Fear of cold, cold limbs, vexatious thirst with a liking for chilled drinks, vexatious heat in the chest, a burning hot abdomen when palpated by the palm, a dry throat, bad breath, dark-colored urine, dry stools, a red tongue with yellow fur, and a deep or deeply-lying pulse

Therapeutic principles: Clear and drain interior heat

Acupuncture & moxibustion:

Qu Chi (LI 11) *He Gu* (LI 4) *Nei Ting* (St 44)	Together, these points clear heat in the yang ming when needled with draining method.

Yong Quan (Ki 1)	Together, these points lead heat downward when
Yin Bai (Sp 1)	needled with draining method.

Qu Ze (Per 3)	Together, these points clear heat and nourish yin when
San Yin Jiao (Sp 6)	needled with even draining and even supplementing method.

Additions & subtractions: For constipation, add *Tian Shu* (St 25). For vexation, add *Nei Guan* (Per 6). For retching, add *Zhong Wan* (CV 12). For insomnia, add *Shen Men* (Ht 7).

Chinese medicinal formula: *Bai Hu Jia Ren Shen Tang* (White Tiger Plus Ginseng Decoction)

Ingredients: Uncooked Gypsum Fibrosum (*Shi Gao*), 30g, Rhizoma Anemarrhenae Asphodeloidis (*Zhi Mu*), 9g, Radix Glycyrrhizae (*Gan Cao*), 5g, Semen Oryzae Sativae (*Geng Mi*), 10g, Radix Panacis Ginseng (*Ren Shen*), 3g

Additions & subtractions: For constipation, abdominal distention, high fever, delirium, and heat not in the yang ming channel but in the yang ming bowels, replace *Bai Hu Jia Ren Shen Tang* with *Da Cheng Qi Tang* (Major Order the Qi Decoction): uncooked Radix Et Rhizoma Rhei (*Da Huang*), 12g, Mirabilitum (*Mang Xiao*), 6g, uncooked Fructus Immaturus Citri Aurantii (*Zhi Shi*), 12g, ginger mix-fried Cortex Magnoliae Officinalis (*Hou Po*), 12g.

4. Phlegm rheum collecting internally

Symptoms: Fear of cold, heavy limbs, chest and abdominal fullness and oppression, torpid intake, thirst with no desire to drink, a pale tongue with slimy fur, and a slippery pulse

Therapeutic principles: Free the flow of yang and transform rheum

Acupuncture & moxibustion:

Bai Hui (GV 20)	Together, these points warm and supplement yang
Guan Yuan (CV 4)	qi when needled with moxibustion. *Zu San Li* can
Zu San Li (St 36)	also move qi to help transform rheum.

Zhong Wan (CV 12)	Together, these points warm the center, fortify
Yin Ling Quan (Sp 9)	the spleen, and transform rheum when needled with moxibustion on the heads of the needles.

Additions & subtractions: For coughing with phlegm and panting, add *Fei Shu* (Bl 13). For pain in the rib-side which prevents one from turning over, add *Qi Men* (Liv 14). For rumbling in the intestines, add *Tian Shu* (St 25). For edema in the limbs, add *Shui Dao* (St 28).

Chinese medicinal formulas: For phlegm rheum in the chest and diaphragm with coughing of clear, thin phlegm and panting: Modified *Ling Gui Zhu Gan Tang* (Poria, Cinnamon, Atractylodes & Licorice Decoction)

Ingredients: Sclerotium Poriae Cocos (*Fu Ling*), 12g, stir-fried Ramulus Cinnamomi Cassiae (*Gui Zhi*), 9g, uncooked Rhizoma Atractylodis Macrocephalae (*Bai Zhu*), 6g, mix-fried Radix Glycyrrhizae (*Gan Cao*), 6g, dry Rhizoma Zingiberis (*Gan Jiang*), 3g, clear Rhizoma Pinelliae Ternatae (*Ban Xia*), 9g, uncooked Pericarpium Citri Reticulatae (*Chen Pi*), 6g

For phlegm rheum above the rib-side with rib-side pain worsening with cough: *Gan Sui Ban Xia Tang* (Euphorbia & Pinellia Decoction)

Ingredients: Radix Euphorbiae Kansui (*Gan Sui*), 0.5-1g (put the fine powder into capsules and take with the strained decoction), clear Rhizoma Pinelliae Ternatae (*Ban Xia*), 9g, Radix Albus Paeoniae Lactiflorae (*Bai Shao*), 9g, Fructus Zizyphi Jujubae (*Da Zao*) 10 pieces

Remarks: Euphorbia Kansui is very effective but very toxic. Beginners and laypersons should not prescribe this formula. The following modern instructions reduce this formula's toxicity but maintain its efficacy. Grind Euphorbia Kansui into fine powder. Put this fine powder into empty gelatin capsules. Take 0.5-1g before breakfast each day depending on the severity of the disease and the constitution of the patient. Swallow the capsules with a warm decoction made from 10 pieces of Fructus Zizyphi Jujubae (*Da Zao*). It is strictly forbidden to take Radix Glycyrrhizae (*Gan Cao*) with this formula, and it is dangerous to do so. Therefore, one cannot replace Red Dates with Licorice. Below 0.5g per dose, this formula's action is too weak, while at a dose of 1-1.5g, symptoms of toxicity can appear. During treatment, the doctor must keep a close eye on the patient. Stop this Chinese medicinal formula immediately if the urine and stools increase too much and as soon as chest and rib-side distention and pain begin to lessen. Two to three days is typically the maximum duration of administration of this formula.

For phlegm rheum in the stomach and intestines with borborygmus, a sloshing noise in the stomach or intestine, and mucous in the stools:

Modified *Ling Gui Zhu Gan Tang* (Poria, Cinnamon, Atractylodes & Licorice Decoction)

Ingredients: Sclerotium Poriae Cocos (*Fu Ling*), 12g, stir-fried Ramulus Cinnamomi Cassiae (*Gui Zhi*), 6g, uncooked Rhizoma Atractylodis Macrocephalae (*Bai Zhu*), 9g, mix-fried Radix Glycyrrhizae (*Gan Cao*), 6g, dry Rhizoma Zingiberis (*Gan Jiang*), 6g, clear Rhizoma Pinelliae Ternatae (*Ban Xia*), 9g, Fructus Amomi (*Sha Ren*), 6g

For phlegm rheum in the four limbs with heavy, painful, swollen limbs: Modified *Wu Pi San* (Five Peel Powder)

Ingredients: Pericarpium Arecae Catechu (*Da Fu Pi*), 9g, uncooked Pericarpium Citri Reticulatae (*Chen Pi*), 9g, Cortex Sclerotii Poriae Cocos (*Fu Ling Pi*), 9g, uncooked Cortex Zingiberis (*Sheng Jiang Pi*), 9g, uncooked Cortex Radicis Mori Albi (*Sang Bai Pi*), 9g, Rhizoma Alismatis (*Ze Xie*), 9g

Remarks: Fear of cold is a very common complaint in clinical practice. Many Westerners have a weak constitution and live in a overheated environment. Thus their defensive qi loses the habit of warming the skin-exterior. In such patients, fear of cold unaccompanied by other symptoms is not necessarily a symptom of yang vacuity.

In clinical practice, fear of cold may also be due to liver qi depression and stagnation or blood vacuity and cold. In the former case, yang is not insufficient but is depressed internally by qi stagnation. For this, one should use cool, moving medicinals to warm the body such as Modified *Si Ni San* (Four Counterflows Powder): Radix Bupleuri (*Chai Hu*), 6g, Radix Albus Paeoniae Lactiflorae (*Bai Shao*), 9g, Fructus Immaturus Citri Aurantii (*Zhi Shi*), 6g, Rhizoma Cyperi Rotundi (*Xiang Fu*), 6g, Herba Menthae Haplocalysis (*Bo He*), 3g, and mix-fried Radix Glycyrrhizae (*Gan Cao*), 6g.

In the latter case, blood vacuity allows the penetration of external cold into the vessels. In that case, fear of cold is combined with cold hands and feet, cyanosis of the tips of the fingers and toes, numbness in the four extremities, etc. The basic treatment is Modified *Dang Gui Si Ni Tang* (Dang Gui Four Counterflows Decoction): wine mix-fried Radix Angelicae Sinensis (*Dang Gui*), 12g, stir-fried Ramulus Cinnamomi Cassiae (*Gui Zhi*), 9g, wine mix-fried Radix Albus Paeoniae Lactiflorae (*Bai Shao*), 9g, Herba Asari Cum Radice (*Xi Xin*), 3g, Medulla Tetrapanacis Papyriferi

(*Tong Cao*), 3g, mix-fried Radix Glycyrrhizae (*Gan Cao*), 3g, Fructus Zizyphi Jujubae (*Da Zao*), 3 fruits, wine mix-fried Ramulus Mori Albi (*Sang Zhi*), 9g, and wine mix-fried Radix Ligustici Wallichii (*Chuan Xiong*), 9g.

3

Aversion to Cold with Shivering *(Wu Han Zhan Li)*

This refers to a subjective feeling of cold which is accompanied by uncontrollable shivering and which cannot be improved with warmth.

Disease causes, disease mechanisms:

1. Cold evils fettering the exterior

Cold is a yin evil which causes contracture and constriction. If cold evils invade the body, they will typically block and congest in the interstices and obstruct the defensive yang's free flow to the exterior. If defensive yang cannot warm the exterior, this typically leads to aversion to cold. Shivering, on the other hand, is due to the defensive qi's swift arising to fight against the invading evils. When the defensive qi is obstructed, the body will shiver in order to arouse the defensive qi to fight against and try to overcome the evils. Therefore, there is aversion to cold *with* shivering.

2. Shivering to sweat

In warm diseases, the righteous qi may become vacuous and weak if either evils overcome the righteous or the struggle between evil and righteous has been so strong that the righteous qi is damaged. The defensive qi is that part of the righteous qi whose job is to warm the body. Hence, if the righteous qi is vacuous, the defensive qi may be insufficient to warm the exterior and a feeling of cold may occur. However, even in such cases, the righteous qi may not give up the fight easily. Whenever there is a chance to overcome such evils, the body will shiver to arouse the righteous qi to counteract and overcome the invading evils. If the righteous qi wins, the invading evils will be expelled through sweating and the patient will be automatically cured. However, if this sweating damages the yang qi, one must return, *i.e,.* rescue, yang.

3. Sore toxins falling inward

If sore toxins become rampant, they may fall inward. The righteous qi is responsible for fighting against any evils in the body. If toxin evils are so strong that the righteous qi has difficulty counteracting them, the body will shiver to arouse the righteous qi. The violent fighting between the righteous qi and toxin evils in the interior will lead to weak defensive qi in the exterior thus resulting in aversion to cold. Therefore, there is a feeling of cold with shivering.

4. Heat accumulating & stagnating in the lungs

Heat in this case is often from warm or heat evils which invade the body externally and then shift inward to congest in the lungs. This heat may cook the fluids within the lungs into phlegm, leading to obstruction of the airways and thus impaired diffusing of the lungs. Because it is the diffusing of the lungs which promotes the circulation of the defensive qi in the exterior, there is a feeling of cold. If these heat evils bind with the phlegm, they may become even more exuberant. Because the heat evils are strong, the body will shiver to arouse the righteous qi to fight these evils. Therefore, there is aversion to cold with shivering.

5. Damp heat pouring downward

When damp heat is due to external contraction, it may invade the bladder, inhibiting the bladder's qi mechanism, and fight against the defensive qi. Because these evils obstruct the free flow of defensive yang, there is a feeling of being chilled. As described above, when heat is severe, the body will shiver to arouse the righteous qi to counteract the evils. Therefore, there is a feeling of being chilled with shivering.

6. Evils entering the shao yang

Malarial evils typically enter the shao yang. This means that external evils reside in both the exterior and interior. In the exterior, they obstruct the flow of the defensive yang, thus resulting in a cold feeling. In the interior, they engender heat. When the body tries to arouse the righteous qi to overcome these evils, shivering also occurs.

Treatment based on pattern discrimination:

I. Cold evils fettering the exterior

Symptoms: Aversion to cold with shivering, fever, no sweating, headache, body aches, thin, white fur, and a floating, tight pulse
Therapeutic principles: Resolve the exterior and scatter cold

Acupuncture & moxibustion:

Da Zhui (GV 14)   Together, these points arouse yang and scatter cold
Feng Men (Bl 12)   when moxaed.
Shen Zhu (GV 12)

Wai Guan (TB 5)   Together, these points resolve the exterior and
He Gu (LI 4)   scatter cold when needled with draining method.

Additions & subtractions: For coughing, add *Fei Shu* (Bl 13) or *Lie Que* (Lu 7). For nasal congestion, add *Ying Xiang* (LI 20).

Chinese medicinal formula: *Ma Huang Tang* (Ephedra Decoction)

Ingredients: Uncooked Herba Ephedrae (*Ma Huang*), 9g, uncooked Ramulus Cinnamomi Cassiae (*Gui Zhi*), 6g, Semen Pruni Armeniacae (*Xing Ren*), 12g, Radix Glycyrrhizae (*Gan Cao*), 3g

Additions & subtractions: For coughing and/or panting, subtract Cinnamon and add Fructus Perillae Frutescentis (*Su Zi*), 9g, and Cortex Radicis Mori Albi (*Sang Bai Pi*), 9g. For severe pain in the nape of the neck and upper back, add uncooked Radix Puerariae (*Ge Gen*), 9g. For slight condition with cough, phlegm, and fatigue, replace *Ma Huang Tang* with *Ren Shen Bai Du San* (Ginseng Vanquish Toxins Powder): Radix Codonopsitis Pilosulae (*Dang Shen*), 6g, Radix Bupleuri (*Chai Hu*), 9g, Radix Peucedani (*Qian Hu*), 9g, Radix Ligustici Wallichii (*Chuan Xiong*), 9g, Fructus Citri Aurantii (*Zhi Ke*), 6g, Radix Platycodi Grandiflori (*Jie Geng*), 9g, Radix Et Rhizoma Notopterygii (*Qiang Huo*), 9g, Sclerotium Poriae Cocos (*Fu Ling*), 9g, mix-fried Radix Glycyrrhizae (*Gan Cao*), 3g.

Remarks: In some rare cases when there is high fever, coughing and panting, and a floating, rapid pulse, one can see severe shivering in wind heat patterns. In that case, shivering is a defensive reaction to arouse the righteous qi to fight the evils, and one should use Modified *Ma Xing Shi Gan Tang* (Ephedra, Armeniaca, Gypsum & Licorice Decoction): uncooked Herba Ephedrae (*Ma Huang*), 9g, Semen Pruni Armeniacae (*Xing Ren*), 9g, uncooked Gypsum Fibrosum (*Shi Gao*), 30g, Radix Glycyrrhizae (*Gan Cao*), 6g, Flos Lonicerae Japonicae (*Jin Yin Hua*), 15g, Fructus Forsythiae Suspensae (*Lian Qiao*), 9g, Rhizoma Phragmitis Communis (*Lu Gen*), 12g, and Fructus Trichosanthis Kirlowii (*Gua Lou*), 12g.

2. Shivering to sweat

Symptoms: Seen in warm disease, there is sudden onset of aversion to cold with shivering, chilled limbs, a deep-lying pulse, and then cool sweating

Remarks: After sweating, no treatment is needed as long as there is no vacuity desertion. The symptoms of vacuity desertion are counterflow chilling in the limbs and a faint, dying pulse.

Therapeutic principles: If there is vacuity desertion, return yang and boost the qi

Acupuncture & moxibustion:

Shen Que (CV 8) *Guan Yuan* (CV 4) *Bai Hui* (GV 20)	Together, these points return yang when moxaed with sparrow-pecking method.
Qi Hai (CV 6) *Zu San Li* (St 36)	Together, these points boost the qi when needled with moxibustion on the heads of the needles.

Chinese medicinal formula: Modified *Fu Mai Tang* (Restore the Pulse Decoction)

Ingredients: Radix Panacis Ginseng (*Ren Shen*), 6g, stir-fried Ramulus Cinnamomi Cassiae (*Gui Zhi*), 6g, uncooked Radix Rehmanniae (*Sheng Di*), 9g, Tuber Ophiopogonis Japonici (*Mai Men Dong*), 9g, Gelatinum Corii Asini (*E Jiao*), 6g, Radix Lateralis Praeparatus Aconiti Carmichaeli (*Fu Zi*), 6g, mix-fried Radix Glycyrrhizae (*Gan Cao*), 9g, uncooked Rhizoma Zingiberis (*Sheng Jiang*), 6g, Fructus Zizyphi Jujubae (*Da Zao*), 2 pieces

3. Exterior cold & interior heat

Symptoms: Aversion to cold with shivering, counterflow chilling in the limbs, headache, body aches, no sweating, high fever, thirst, vexation and agitation, short voidings of dark-colored urine, a red tongue with yellow fur, and a surging, rapid pulse

Therapeutic principles: Resolve the exterior, dispel cold, and clear heat

Acupuncture & moxibustion:

Da Zhui (GV 14) *Wai Guan* (TB 5) *He Gu* (LI 4)	Together, these points course wind, scatter cold, and resolve the exterior when needled with draining method.
Chi Ze (Lu 5) *Qu Chi* (LI 11) *Fei Shu* (Bl 13)	Together, these points clear heat when needled with draining method.

Additions & subtractions: For nasal congestion, add *Ying Xiang* (LI 20). For constipation, moxa *Da Dun* (Liv 1).

Chinese medicinal formula: *Da Qing Long Tang* (Major Blue Dragon Decoction)

Ingredients: Uncooked Herba Ephedrae (*Ma Huang*), 9g, Ramulus Cinnamomi Cassiae (*Gui Zhi*), 6g, mix-fried Radix Glycyrrhizae (*Zhi Gan Cao*), 6g, Semen Pruni Armeniacae (*Xing Ren*), 6g, Gypsum Fibrosum (*Shi Gao*), 20g, uncooked Rhizoma Zingiberis (*Sheng Jiang*), 3g, Fructus Zizyphi Jujubae (*Da Zao*), 3 pieces

Additions & subtractions: For mild aversion to wind and cold, subtract Cinnamon. For severe interior heat, increase Gypsum up to 30g and add Rhizoma Anemarrhenae Asphodeloidis (*Zhi Mu*), 9g. For interior heat in the yang ming with dry stools, constipation, red urine, and red eyes, replace *Da Qing Long Tang* with *Fang Feng Tong Sheng San* (Ledebouriella Sagely Flow-freeing Powder): Radix Ledebouriellae Divaricatae (*Fang Feng*), 9g, Herba Schizonepetae Tenuifoliae (*Jing Jie*), 9g, Fructus Forsythiae Suspensae (*Lian Qiao*), 9g, uncooked Herba Ephedrae (*Ma Huang*), 6g, Herba Menthae Haplocalysis (*Bo He*), 6g, uncooked Radix Ligustici Wallichii (*Chuan Xiong*), 6g, Radix Angelicae Sinensis (*Dang Gui*), 3g, Radix Albus Paeoniae Lactiflorae (*Bai Shao*), 3g, bran stir-fried Rhizoma Atractylodis Macrocephalae (*Bai Zhu*), 3g, Radix Platycodi Grandiflori (*Jie Geng*), 6g, Fructus Gardeniae Jasminoidis (*Zhi Zi*), 9g, uncooked Radix Et Rhizoma Rhei (*Da Huang*), 9g, Mirabilitum (*Mang Xiao*), 6g, uncooked Gypsum Fibrosum (*Shi Gao*), 15g, Radix Scutellariae Baicalensis (*Huang Qin*), 12g, Talcum (*Hua Shi*), 15g, and Radix Glycyrrhizae (*Gan Cao*), 6g.

4. Sore toxins falling inward

Symptoms: Localized redness, swelling, heat, and pain, aversion to cold with shivering, fever, vexatious thirst, clouded spirit and delirium in severe cases, short voidings of dark-colored urine, constipation, a red tongue with yellow fur, and a surging, rapid pulse

Therapeutic principles: Clear heat, drain fire, and resolve toxins

Acupuncture & moxibustion:

Shi Xuan (EX-UE-11) Together, these points drain fire and resolve
Wei Zhong (Bl 40) toxins when pricked to bleed.

Xue Hai (Sp 10)	Together, these points clear heat in the blood
Nei Ting (St 44)	when needled with draining method.

Additions & subtractions: For delirium and clouded spirit, prick *Shui Gou* (GV 26) and use internally administered Chinese and/or Western medicinals.

Chinese medicinal formula: Modified *Wu Wei Xiao Du Yin* (Five Flavors Disperse Toxins Drink)

Ingredients: Flos Lonicerae Japonicae (*Jin Yin Hua*), 24g, Flos Chrysanthemi Indici (*Ye Ju Hua*), 18g, Herba Taraxaci Mongolici Cum Radice (*Pu Gong Ying*), 18g, Herba Violae Yedoensitis Cum Radice (*Zi Hua Di Ding*), 18g, Radix Semiaquilegiae (*Tian Kui Zi*), 18g, Fructus Forsythiae Suspensae (*Lian Qiao*), 9g, Radix Scutellariae Baicalensis (*Huang Qin*), 6g, Rhizoma Coptidis Chinensis (*Huang Lian*), 6g

5. Heat accumulating & stagnating in the lungs

Symptoms: Fever, shivering, chest pain, cough with yellow phlegm or pus and blood which has a fishy odor, a dry mouth and thirst with no desire to drink, possible vexation and fullness in the chest, a red tongue with yellow fur, and a slippery or slippery, rapid pulse

Note: This pattern is mainly seen in cases of pulmonary abscess. However, it may also be seen in severe bronchitis.

Therapeutic principles: Clear the lungs, resolve toxins, and expel pus

Acupuncture & moxibustion:

Chi Ze (Lu 5)	Together, these points clear the lungs, resolve
Fei Shu (Bl 13)	toxins, and help expel pus, when needled with
Gao Huang (Bl 43)	draining method. After needled, prick *Chi Ze* and
Da Zhui (GV 14)	*Da Zhui* to bleed.
He Gu (LI 4)	

Remarks: Acupuncture is only an adjunctive therapy for hacking up pus. Internally administered medicinal therapy should be used as the main treatment method for this condition.

Chinese medicinal formula: Modified *Wei Jing Tang* (Phragmites Decoction)

Ingredients: Rhizoma Phragmitis Communis (*Lu Gen*), 15g, Semen Coicis Lachryma-jobi (*Yi Yi Ren*), 15g, Semen Benincasae Hispidae (*Dong Gua*

Zi), 15g, Semen Pruni Persicae (*Tao Ren*), 6g, Herba Houttuyniae Cordatae Cum Radice (*Yu Xing Cao*), 30g, Herba Patriniae Heterophyllae Cum Radice (*Bai Jiang Cao*), 20g, Fructus Trichosanthis Kirlowii (*Gua Lou*), 9g, uncooked Radix Glycyrrhizae (*Gan Cao*), 6g, Flos Lonicerae Japonicae (*Jin Yin Hua*), 30g, Fructus Forsythiae Suspensae (*Lian Qiao*), 9g, Radix Platycodi Grandiflori (*Jie Geng*), 15g

Note: In case of pulmonary abscess, these large dosages must be respected.

Additions & subtractions: For profuse phlegm, add Bulbus Fritillariae Thunbergii (*Zhe Bei Mu*), 9g. For hemoptysis, add Rhizoma Bletillae Striatae (*Bai Ji*), 9g, and uncooked Rhizoma Imperatae Cylindricae (*Bai Mao Gen*), 9g. For heat damaging yin with vexatious heat in the five hearts, night sweats, and dry mouth and throat, add Tuber Ophiopogonis Japonici (*Mai Men Dong*), 9g, and Radix Adenophorae Strictae (*Nan Sha Shen*), 9g.

6. Damp heat pouring downward

Symptoms: High fever, shivering, short, yellow or reddish yellow urination, frequent, urgent, painful urination, possible urinary stoppage, pain or distention and pain in the lower abdomen, low back pain, a bitter taste in the mouth, dry throat, thirst with a desire for a little drink, constipation, a red tongue with yellow fur, and a slippery, rapid pulse

Therapeutic principles: Clear heat, eliminate dampness, and disinhibit urination

Acupuncture & moxibustion:

Zhong Ji (CV 3) *Pang Guang Shu* (Bl 28) *Nei Ting* (St 44)	Together, these points clear heat and disinhibit dampness when needled with draining method.
San Yin Jiao (Sp 6) *Yin Ling Quan* (Sp 9)	Together, these points clear and eliminate dampness and heat and disinhibit urination when needled with draining method.

Additions & subtractions: For high fever, prick *Wei Zhong* (Bl 40) to bleed. For low back pain, add *Wei Yang* (Bl 39). For hematuria, add *Ran Gu* (Ki 2).

Chinese medicinal formula: Modified *Ba Zheng San* (Eight Correcting [Ingredients] Powder)

Ingredients: Caulis Akebiae (*Mu Tong*), 5g, Herba Dianthi (*Qu Mai*), 9g, cooked Radix Et Rhizoma Rhei (*Da Huang*), 9g, Semen Plantaginis (*Che Qian Zi*), 9g, Talcum (*Hua Shi*), 12g, uncooked Fructus Gardeniae Jasminoidis (*Zhi Zi*), 9g, Herba Polygoni Avicularis (*Bian Xu*), 9g, Radix Tenuis Glycyrrhizae (*Gan Cao Shao*), 6g, Flos Lonicerae Japonicae (*Jin Yin Hua*), 15g, Fructus Forsythiae Suspensae (*Lian Qiao*), 12g

Additions & subtractions: For nausea and vomiting, subtract Akebia, replace uncooked with stir-fried Gardenia, and add uncooked Rhizoma Zingiberis (*Sheng Jiang*), 6g. For low back pain, add Radix Cyathulae (*Chuan Niu Xi*), 9g. For hematuria, add Herba Cephalanoploris Segeti (*Xiao Ji*), 9g, and Rhizoma Imperatae Cylindricae (*Bai Mao Gen*), 9g.

7. Invasion of malaria evils

Symptoms: Yawning and fatigue followed by aversion to cold with shivering, aching limbs, and then high fever, headache, a red facial complexion, thirst with a liking to drink, and, finally, sweating followed by abatement of fever, and a bowstring pulse

Note: This cycle of symptoms repeats itself regularly every one, two, or three days.

Therapeutic principles: Expel the evil and stop malaria

Acupuncture & moxibustion:

Da Zhui (GV 14) *Tao Dao* (GV 13)	Together, these points arouse yang to fight against evils and scatter cold when needled first with draining method and then with moxibustion on the heads of the needles.
Zu San Li (St 36) *Zhong Wan* (CV 12)	Together, these points support the righteous qi and dispel evils when needled with supplementing method.
Jian Shi (Per 5)	An empirical point for malaria

Additions & subtractions: For more heat than cold, add *Li Dui* (St 45). For more cold than heat, needle *Tai Xi* (Ki 3) with moxibustion on the heads of the needle. For enduring malaria, add *Pi Shu* (Bl 20) and *Wei Shu* (Bl 21). For glomus lump, add *Zhang Men* (Liv 13) and *Pi Gen* (M-BW-16).

Chinese medicinal formula: Modified *Xiao Chai Hu Tang* (Minor Bupleurum Decoction)

Ingredients: Uncooked Radix Bupleuri (*Chai Hu*), 9g, uncooked Radix Scutellariae Baicalensis (*Huang Qin*), 9g, lime-processed Rhizoma Pinelliae Ternatae (*Ban Xia*), 9g, uncooked Radix Codonopsitis Pilosulae (*Dang Shen*), 6g, Radix Glycyrrhizae (*Gan Cao*), 6g, uncooked Rhizoma Zingiberis (*Sheng Jiang*), 6g, Fructus Zizyphi Jujubae (*Da Zao*), 4 pieces, Radix Dichroae Febrifugae (*Chang Shan*), 9g, Fructus Amomi Tsao-ko (*Cao Guo*), 9g

4
Aversion to Cold with Fever *(Wu Han Fa Re)*

This refers to a subjective feeling of cold accompanied by fever. This pairing of symptoms is one of the main manifestations of exterior patterns. Since this disease category is made up of nothing other than aversion to cold plus fever, its disease causes and mechanisms are similar to those discussed above in terms of aversion to cold.

Disease causes, disease mechanisms:

1. Contraction of external evils

When evils enter the exterior of the body, they impede the free flow of the defensive yang. Thus the defensive yang is unable to warm the exterior properly and aversion to cold occurs. However, since the defensive yang is depressed in the exterior, it may transform into heat, thus giving rise to fever or, more literally, the emission of heat. However, the different varieties of external evils may each cause different severities of aversion to cold and fever. Cold and cool dryness are yin evils which damage yang and thus typically give rise to more pronounced aversion to cold and less fever. Dampness is also a yin evil. However, its nature is sticky and stagnant, and, therefore, it causes aversion to cold with generalized fever which is not easily emitted. Summerheat, wind, and heat are all yang evils. Therefore, they tend to cause more marked fever and less pronounced aversion to cold. Warm evils and epidemic toxins are even stronger yang evils and hence cause only a short duration of aversion to cold but a high fever.

2. Sore toxins

Sores usually develop from contraction of external heat toxins, fire toxins, or epidemic toxins or from internal heat which accumulates and congests in a local area. Within such sores, there is putrid flesh and vanquished blood which are recognized as evils by the body's righteous qi. In this case, the body will shiver (aversion to cold) in order to arouse the defensive qi to fight against the evils. This battle between the righteous and evils results in excessive movement of qi, *i.e.*, shivering, or congestion of qi, leading to fever.

Treatment based on pattern discrimination:

The signs and symptoms, treatment principles, and treatments of the first eight patterns of this condition are exactly the same as those listed under Chapter 1: "Aversion to Wind Cold" above. These are:

1. Wind evils assailing the exterior
2. Cold evils fettering the exterior
3. Summerheat & dampness damaging the defensive qi
4. Wind heat invading the lungs
5. Dry evils damaging the lungs
6. Cold dampness fettering the exterior
7. Exterior cold & interior heat
8. Sore toxins

9. Damp (warm) depressing the defensive qi

Symptoms: Aversion to cold with fever, generalized fever which is not easily emitted which is worse in the afternoon, heavy pain in the head and body, chest oppression, thirst but a distaste for drinking, no hunger, a pale yellow facial complexion, white, slimy tongue fur, and a soggy, moderate (*i.e.*, slightly slow) pulse

Therapeutic principles: Clear heat, transform dampness, and resolve the exterior

Acupuncture & moxibustion:

He Gu (LI 4) *Da Zhui* (GV 14) *Qu Chi* (LI 11)	Together, these points resolve the exterior and clear heat when needled with draining method.
Zhong Wan (CV 12) *Tai Chong* (Liv 3) *Qi Men* (Liv 14)	Together, these points move the qi, harmonize the center, and transform dampness when needled with draining method.

Additions & subtractions: For headache that feels as if the head had a tight band around it, add *Feng Chi* (GB 20). For stomach and abdominal fullness and distention, add *Zu San Li* (St 36). For loose stools, add *Gong Sun* (Sp 4).

Remarks: It is forbidden to strongly promote sweating to resolve the exterior in the treatment of damp warm patterns. The correct method is to transform dampness and free the flow of the defensive qi. This will result in slight sweating.

Chinese medicinal formula: *Huo Po Xia Ling Tang* (Agastaches, Magnolia, Pinellia & Poria Decoction)

Ingredients: Herba Agastachis Seu Pogostemi (*Huo Xiang*), 9g, clear Rhizoma Pinelliae Ternatae (*Ban Xia*), 6g, Sclerotium Rubrum Poriae Cocos (*Chi Fu Ling*), 12g, Semen Pruni Armeniacae (*Xing Ren*), 9g, Semen Coicis Lachryma-jobi (*Yi Yi Ren*), 18g, Fructus Cardamomi (*Bai Dou Kou*), 6g, Sclerotium Polypori Umbellati (*Zhu Ling*), 6g, warm Semen Praeparatus Sojae (*Dan Dou Chi*), 9g, Rhizoma Alismatis (*Ze Xie*), 6g, ginger mix-fried Cortex Magnoliae Officinalis (*Hou Po*), 6g

Additions & subtractions: For predominant heat, add uncooked Radix Scutellariae Baicalensis (*Huang Qin*), 9g, and Talcum (*Hua Shi*), 9g, and subtract Cardamon. For severe effusion of heat and aversion to cold, add Herba Eupatorei Fortunei (*Pei Lan*), 9g, and increase the dosages of Agastaches and prepared Soja.

10. Flooding of wind & water

Symptoms: Aversion to cold with fever, aching limbs, rapid onset of edema, inhibited urination, coughing and panting, thin, white tongue fur, and a floating, slippery or deep, tight pulse

Therapeutic principles: Course wind and resolve the exterior, diffuse the lungs and disinhibit water

Acupuncture & moxibustion:

Wai Guan (TB 5)	Together, these points course wind, resolve the
Feng Men (Bl 12)	exterior, and diffuse the lungs to disinhibit water
Fei Shu (Bl 13)	when needled with draining method.
Shui Dao (St 28)	Together, these points help free the waterways to
Shui Fen (CV 9)	disinhibit water when needled with draining method.

Additions & subtractions: For sore throat, prick *Shang Yang* (LI 1) to bleed. For vexatious thirst, fever, and scanty urine, add *Qu Chi* (LI 11) and *Chi Ze* (Lu 5). For body aches, add *Shen Zhu* (GV 12). For aversion to cold with sweating, add *Zu San Li* (St 36) and *He Gu* (LI 4).

Chinese medicinal formulas: For cold pattern: *Ma Huang Jia Zhu Tang* (Ephedra Plus Atractylodes Decoction)

Ingredients: Uncooked Herba Ephedrae (*Ma Huang*), 9g, uncooked Ramulus Cinnamomi Cassiae (*Gui Zhi*), 6g, Semen Pruni Armeniacae (*Xing Ren*), 9g, mix-fried Radix Glycyrrhizae (*Zhi Gan Cao*), 3g, uncooked Rhizoma Atractylodis Macrocephalae (*Bai Zhu*), 9g

For heat pattern: Modified *Yue Bi Jia Zhu Tang* (Maidservant from Yue Plus Atractylodes Decoction)

Ingredients: Honey stir-fried Herba Ephedrae (*Ma Huang*), 9g, uncooked Rhizoma Atractylodis Macrocephalae (*Bai Zhu*), 12g, uncooked Gypsum Fibrosum (*Shi Gao*), 25g, uncooked Rhizoma Zingiberis (*Sheng Jiang*), 6g, Fructus Zizyphi Jujubae (*Da Zao*), 4 fruits, Radix Glycyrrhizae (*Gan Cao*), 6g, Fructus Forsythiae Suspensae (*Lian Qiao*), 6g

11. Warm toxins invading the lung defensive

Symptoms: This pattern is often seen in the early stage of putrefying throat sand. Aversion to cold with fever is present. The throat is red, swollen, and sore, making swallowing difficult. As the disease develops, there are red, sand-like eruptions on the skin, mainly behind the ears and on the neck, chest, back and limbs. Other symptoms include a red tongue with thin, yellow fur, and a floating, rapid, forceful pulse

Therapeutic principles: Diffuse the lungs and clear heat, resolve toxins and disinhibit the throat

Acupuncture & moxibustion:

Shao Shang (Lu 11) *Chi Ze* (Lu 5) *Guan Chong* (TB 1)	Together, these points clear heat and resolve toxins when pricked to bleed. *Shao Shang* is a key point for throat problems.
He Gu (LI 4)	Resolves the exterior when needled with draining method
Xian Gu (St 43)	Drains heat from the yang ming when needled with draining method

Additions & subtractions: For headache, add *Feng Chi* (GB 20) and *Feng Fu* (GV 16). For convulsions, add *Tai Chong* (Liv 3) and *Bai Hui* (GV 20). For high fever, add *Da Zhui* (GV 14) and prick *Wei Zhong* (Bl 40) to bleed.

Remarks: Acupuncture is effective as an auxiliary therapy in this disease.

Chinese medicinal formula: *Pu Ji Xiao Du Yin* (*Universal Benefit* Disperse Toxins Drink)

Ingredients: Fructus Arctii Lappae (*Niu Bang Zi*), 9g, Fructificatio Lasiosphaerae (*Ma Bo*), 9g, Radix Isatidis Seu Baphicacanthi (*Ban Lan Gen*), 15g, Radix Scutellariae Baicalensis (*Huang Qin*), 9g, Rhizoma Coptidis Chinensis (*Huang Lian*), 6g, Fructus Forsythiae Suspensae (*Lian Qiao*), 15g, Herba Menthae Haplocalycis (*Bo He*), 3g, Radix Scrophulariae Ningpoensis (*Xuan Shen*), 9g, Bombyx Batryticatus (*Jiang Can*), 9g, Radix Platycodi Grandiflori (*Jie Geng*), 3g, Rhizoma Cimicifugae (*Sheng Ma*), 6g, Radix Bupleuri (*Chai Hu*), 6g, Pericarpium Citri Reticulatae (*Chen Pi*), 3g, Radix Glycyrrhizae (*Gan Cao*), 3g

Remarks: This is a contagious disease, and thus the patient should be quarantined.

12. Contraction of epidemic toxins

Symptoms: Aversion to cold with fever, headache, slight coughing, pain in the sides of the face below the earlobe which affects chewing followed by the occurrence of painful swelling in the cheeks with no clear margins, thin, white, slightly yellow tongue fur, and a floating, rapid pulse
Note: This pattern commonly corresponds to the early stage of mumps.

Therapeutic principles: Course wind and clear heat, scatter nodulation and disperse swelling

Acupuncture & moxibustion:

Jia Che (St 6)	Together, these local points dissipate the local
Yi Feng (TB 17)	congestion and stagnation of the qi and blood when needled with draining method.

Wai Guan (TB 5)	Together, these points course wind, clear heat, and
He Gu (LI 4)	resolve toxins when needled with draining method.

Additions & subtractions: For high fever, prick *Da Zhui* (GV 14) and *Shang Yang* (LI 1) to bleed.

Remarks: Juncibustion on *Jiao Sun* (TB 20) once per day for three days can help mumps. Pricking *Shao Shang* (Lu 11) to bleed 5-6 drops can also help mumps. Acupuncture is very effective for mumps when applied in the early stage within one day after its onset.

Chinese medicinal formula: Modified *Yin Qiao San* (Lonicera & Forsythia Powder)

Ingredients: Flos Lonicerae Japonicae (*Yin Hua*), 15g, Fructus Forsythiae Suspensae (*Lian Qiao*), 9g, Herba Menthae Haplocalycis (*Bo He*), 3g, Semen Praeparatus Sojae (*Dan Dou Chi*), 3g, Radix Platycodi Grandiflori (*Jie Geng*), 3g, Herba Schizonepetae Tenuifoliae (*Jing Jie*), 9g, Rhizoma Phragmitis Communis (*Lu Gen*), 9g, Folium Bambusae (*Zhu Ye*), 9g, Fructus Arctii Lappae (*Niu Bang Zi*), 15g, Radix Isatidis Seu Baphicacanthi (*Ban Lan Gen*), 21g, Bombyx Batryticatus (*Jiang Can*), 9g, Radix Glycyrrhizae (*Gan Cao*), 3g

Remarks: 1. Because mumps are contagious, patients with this condition should be quarantined. Because mumps can cause painful swelling of the testes and possible sterility, care should be taken in its treatment. Please see Volume Six of this series for a fuller exposition.

2. Aversion to cold with fever is a main symptom of exterior patterns, and these two symptoms can occur in many conditions in addition to those mentioned above. These include intestinal abscess, pulmonary abscess, and other such sores. Whenever these two symptoms manifest in an exterior pattern, their general therapeutic principles are to resolve the exterior and dispel evils. However, the disease evils involved in such exterior patterns may differ. For instance, wind, heat, summerheat, and warm toxins are yang, while cold, dampness, and cool dryness are yin. Therefore, specific therapeutic principles are needed for specific patterns in the treatment of real-life cases.

5

Fever without Cold *(Dan Re Bu Han)*

This refers to the sole occurrence of fever with no accompanying aversion to cold. This symptom may occur in both external and interior damage. In the early stage of externally contracted patterns, fever is typically accompanied by aversion to cold. However, if the invading evils enter the interior and transform into heat or fight violently with the righteous qi, fever may occur without chills. Therefore, fever without chills usually indicates that external evils have entered the interior in externally contracted conditions. All such cases are solely replete patterns. On the other hand, if there is internal damage due to qi, blood or yin vacuities, fever can also appear without aversion to cold or chills. Fever without chills is also present in tidal hectic fever which is discussed below. Nighttime fever due to blood stasis is included in tidal hectic fever.

Disease causes, disease mechanisms:

1. Heat evils brewing in the lungs

Heat evils brewing in the lungs usually develop from external contraction of heat evils or from cold which enters the interior and transforms into heat. Heat is a yang evil, and exuberant heat causes fever. Therefore, fever occurs without chills.

2. Heat flaming in the yang ming

This pattern usually develops from the tai yang pattern. In that case, invading cold evils shift into the yang ming. The yang ming has a lot of qi and a lot of blood. If invading cold evils shift into the yang ming, they usually transform into heat similar to the ruling or host qi. Heat is a yang evil and is hot by nature. If this heat burns in the channel, there will be exuberant heat in the qi division leading to fever without chills.

3. Intestinal heat binding

If heat evils are not cleared from the yang ming channel, they may shift into the yang ming bowel and bind in the intestinal tract. This will cause stoppage of the bowel qi and failure in its conveyance. In that case, the heat cannot find its way out but will steam internally, leading to fever without chills.

4. Damp heat depressing & steaming

Damp heat causing fever usually arises from external contraction of evils. Dampness is sticky and stagnant. Therefore, invading damp heat combined is difficult to dispel. If dampness and heat remain in the qi division or the middle burner and brew and steam there, there will be fever without chills.

5. Summerheat damaging the qi

Summerheat is a yang evil which easily damages the qi and exhausts liquids. Therefore, when it invades the body, it seldom presents a defensive division pattern. Rather, it typically presents a combined defensive and qi division pattern. The season of long summer corresponds to the earth phase. Therefore, summerheat easily enters the yang ming, since like attracts like. When invading summerheat enters the yang ming which has lots of qi and lots of blood, the heat will become even more exuberant. Therefore, there is fever without chills.

6. Heat entering the constructive & blood divisions

The constructive and blood divisions are the last two of the four divisions. Only strong heat evils can fight their way through to these final divisions. If strong heat enters these last two divisions, it will boil and burn the constructive and blood, the very yin fluids which are responsible for checking yang. In that case, exuberant heat will become even more effulgent, thus giving rise to fever without chills.

7. Exuberant heat toxins

Exuberant heat toxins usually result from invasion of toxic epidemic evils. Epidemic evils are typically very strong and can rapidly invade the body. The triple burner has a yang-fire nature. If heat toxins invade and bind in the triple burner, high fever may occur.

8. Qi vacuity

Qi vacuity may cause fever without chills by either of two mechanisms. First, if, for any reason, there is a severe qi vacuity, yin blood will not be adequately engendered and transformed. This results in a simultaneous qi and yin vacuity. Yin will thus fail to control yang which becomes hyperactive. Yang qi will thus move upward and outward in the body giving rise to low-grade fever. Because there is a simultaneous qi vacuity, there may be cold limbs, but there are no chills. Secondly, if, for any reason, the qi of the spleen and stomach is vacuous and weak, the central qi may fall downward and accumulate in the interior. Because it cannot upbear and ascend, it becomes depressed internally and may transform into heat, thus also giving rise to a low-grade fever but no particular chills.

9. Blood vacuity

Blood, which is yin by nature, participates in the balancing of yin and yang. Hence, if, for any reason, the blood becomes vacuous and insufficient, the harmony between yin and yang may be broken. Yin will not be able to control yang which then tends to spread towards the exterior, thus causing vacuity heat with low-grade fever and no chills but warm skin. As Wu Kun (1551-1620) said: "When the blood is full, the body is cool; when the blood is vacuous, the body is warm."

10. Yin vacuity

Yin vacuity usually develops from aging, constitutional yin vacuity, excessive thinking, enduring disease, febrile disease, excessive sexual activity, drug use, or from blood and/or liquid loss. Yin and yang promote and counterbalance each other. If yin becomes vacuous and insufficient, yang will become hyperactive and internal heat will be engendered. Therefore, there is low-grade fever with no chills.

Treatment based on pattern discrimination:

1. Heat evils brewing in the lungs

Symptoms: Fever without aversion to cold, coughing of thick phlegm, chest pain, flaring nostrils, hoarse breathing, thirst, sore throat, a red tongue with dry, yellow or slimy, yellow fur, and a slippery, rapid pulse

Therapeutic principles: Clear heat and drain the lungs

Acupuncture & moxibustion:

Chi Ze (Lu 5)	Together, these points clear and drain lung heat
Shao Shang (Lu 11)	when pricked to bleed and cupped.
Fei Shu (Bl 13)	

He Gu (LI 4)	Together, these points clear and drain the *yang*
Qu Chi (LI 11)	*ming* where there is plenty of qi and blood.
Li Dui (St 45)	

Additions & subtractions: For panting, add *Zhong Fu* (Lu 1). For chest and diaphragmatic glomus and fullness, add *Shang Wan* (CV 13). For vexation, add *Nei Guan* (Per 6). For constipation, add *Tian Shu* (St 25). For coughing of fishy, foul-smelling pus and phlegm, add *Yu Ji* (Lu 10).

Chinese medicinal formula: Modified *Ma Xing Shi Gan Tang* (Ephedra, Armeniaca, Gypsum & Licorice Decoction)

Ingredients: Uncooked Herba Ephedrae (*Ma Huang*), 9g, Semen Pruni Armeniacae (*Xing Ren*), 9g, uncooked Gypsum Fibrosum (*Shi Gao*), 24g, Radix Glycyrrhizae (*Gan Cao*), 6g, Herba Houttuyniae Cordatae Cum Radice (*Yu Xing Cao*), 15g, uncooked Radix Scutellariae Baicalensis (*Huang Qin*), 6g

Additions & subtractions: For severe lung heat, add honey stir-fried Cortex Radicis Mori Albi (*Sang Bai Pi*), 9g, and Lumbricus (*Di Long*), 6g. For profuse phlegm, add Radix Platycodi Grandiflori (*Jie Geng*), 9g, Bulbus Fritillariae Thunbergii (*Zhe Bei Mu*), 9g, Pericarpium Trichosanthis Kirlowii (*Gua Lou Pi*), 9g. For severe coughing, add honey stir-fried Cortex Radicis Mori Albi (*Sang Bai Pi*), 9g, and Folium Eriobotryae Japonicae (*Pi Pa Ye*), 9g. For coughing of blood, add Rhizoma Bletillae Striatae (*Bai Ji*), 9g, Herba Agrimoniae Pilosae (*Xian He Cao*), 9g, and Fructus Aristolochiae (*Ma Dou Ling*), 9g. For severe hasty panting, add Semen Lepidii Seu Descurainiae (*Ting Li Zi*), 9g, Rhizoma Belamcandae Chinensis (*She Gan*), 9g, and Bulbus Fritillariae Thunbergii (*Zhe Bei Mu*), 6g. For thirst, add Rhizoma Phragmitis Communis (*Lu Gen*), 9g, and Rhizoma Anemarrhenae Asphodeloidis (*Zhi Mu*), 9g. For constipation, add Radix Et Rhizoma Rhei (*Da Huang*), 9g.

2. Heat flaming in the yang ming

Symptoms: High fever with no chills but aversion to heat, a red facial complexion, profuse sweating, severe vexatious thirst, short voiding of dark-colored urine, a red tongue with yellow fur, and a surging, large pulse

Therapeutic principles: Clear heat and drain fire, boost the qi and engender liquids

Acupuncture & moxibustion:

He Gu (LI 4) *Qu Chi* (LI 11) *Nei Ting* (St 44)	Together, these points clear and drain the yang ming when needled with draining method.
Da Zhui (GV 14) *Shao Shang* (Lu 11)	Together, these points clear and drain heat evils when pricked to bleed.
Wei Shu (Bl 21)	It boosts the stomach and engenders liquid when needled with supplementing method.

Additions & subtractions: For thirst without profuse drinking and an aching, fatigued body, add *Yin Ling Quan* (Sp 9) to dry dampness. For hoarse breathing and panting, add *Fei Shu* (Bl 13) to drain lung heat. For counterflow chilling of the limbs, add *San Jiao Shu* (Bl 22) and prick *Shi Xuan* (EX-UE-1) to bleed.

Chinese medicinal formula: *Bai Hu Tang* (White Tiger Decoction)

Ingredients: Uncooked Gypsum Fibrosum (*Shi Gao*), 30g, uncooked Rhizoma Anemarrhenae Asphodeloidis (*Zhi Mu*), 12g, Radix Glycyrrhizae (*Gan Cao*), 6g, Semen Oryzae Sativae (*Geng Mi*), 15g

Additions & subtractions: For severe fever, increase the dosage of Gypsum to 30-60g. For great fever and great sweating damaging qi and yin, add white Radix Panacis Ginseng (*Bai Ren Shen*), 6g, or Radix Panacis Quinquifolii (*Xi Yang Shen*), 6g. For severe thirst, add Radix Trichosanthis Kirlowii (*Tian Hua Fen*), 9g, and Rhizoma Phragmitis Communis (*Lu Gen*), 9g.

3. Intestinal heat binding

Symptoms: High fever which gets worse in the afternoon, no chills, painful fullness in the abdomen which is hard and replete when touched, stoppage of defecation or heat bind with circumfluence, clouded spirit and delirium in severe cases, vexation and agitation, a red tongue with dry, yellow or scorched black fur, and a deep, replete, forceful pulse

Therapeutic principles: Free the flow of the bowels and drain heat, attack and precipitate dry binding

Acupuncture & moxibustion:

He Gu (LI 4)   Together, these points drain heat and attack heat
Shang Yang (LI 1)   binding when needled with draining method or pricked
Nei Ting (St 44)   to bleed for *Shang Yang* and *Li Dui*.
Li Dui (St 45)

Zhi Gou (TB 6)   Together, these points free the flow of the bowels and
Shang Ju Xu (St 37) precipitate binding when needled with draining method.

Additions & subtractions: For vexation, add *Nei Guan* (Per 6). For vomiting, add *Zhong Wan* (CV 12). For mania with desire to ascend to high places and sing, add *Jian Shi* (Per 5) and prick *Shui Gou* (GV 26) to bleed.

Chinese medicinal formula: *Da Cheng Qi Tang* (Major Order the Qi Decoction)

Ingredients: Uncooked Radix Et Rhizoma Rhei (*Da Huang*), 9g, Mirabilitum (*Mang Xiao*), 6g, uncooked Fructus Immaturus Citri Aurantii (*Zhi Shi*), 6g, ginger mix-fried Cortex Magnoliae Officinalis (*Hou Po*), 6g

Additions & subtractions: For fever, constipation accompanied with panting, chest oppression, profuse phlegm, and yellow, slimy tongue fur, replace *Da Cheng Qi Tang* with *Bai Cheng Qi Tang* (White Order the Qi Decoction): uncooked Gypsum Fibrosum (*Shi Gao*), 15g, uncooked Radix Et Rhizoma Rhei (*Da Huang*), 9g, Semen Pruni Armeniacae (*Xing Ren*), 6g, and Fructus Trichosanthis Kirlowii (*Gua Lou*), 9g. For a mild condition without dry stools, replace *Da Cheng Qi Tang* with *Xiao Cheng Qi Tang* (Minor Order the Qi Decoction): uncooked Radix Et Rhizoma Rhei (*Da Huang*), 9g, uncooked Fructus Immaturus Citri Aurantii (*Zhi Shi*), 6g, and ginger mix-fried Cortex Magnoliae Officinalis (*Hou Po*), 6g. For a mild condition without stomach and abdominal glomus and fullness, replace *Da Cheng Qi Tang* with *Tiao Wei Cheng Qi Tang* (Regulate the Stomach & Order the Qi Decoction): uncooked Radix Et Rhizoma Rhei (*Da Huang*), 9g, Mirabilitum (*Mang Xiao*), 9g, and mix-fried Radix Glycyrrhizae (*Gan Cao*), 6g. For a mild condition but heat damaging yin with thirst and very dry stools, replace *Da Cheng Qi Tang* with *Zeng Ye Cheng Qi Tang* (Increase Fluids & Order the Qi Decoction): Tuber Ophiopogonis Japonici (*Mai Men Dong*), 9g, uncooked Radix Rehmanniae (*Sheng Di*), 15g, Radix Scrophulariae Ningpoensis (*Xuan Shen*), 12g, Radix Et Rhizoma Rhei (*Da Huang*), 6-9g, and Mirabilitum (*Mang Xiao*), 3-6g.

4. Damp heat depressing & steaming

Symptoms: Fluctuating fever which gets worse in the afternoon and does not abate with sweating, no chills, thirst with not much desire to drink, chest oppression, stomach glomus, nausea, heavy or painful body, torpid intake, short voiding of red urine, loose stools which are, nonetheless difficult to defecate, a red tongue with slimy, yellow fur, and a bowstring, slippery, rapid pulse

Remarks: This is a generalized damp heat pattern. For specific damp heat patterns causing fever without aversion to cold, please see the additions & subtractions below.

Therapeutic principles: Diffuse qi and disinhibit dampness, clear heat and outthrust evils

Acupuncture & moxibustion:

Xia Xi (GB 43)	Together, these points clear heat and transform
Nei Ting (St 44)	dampness when needled with draining method.
Yang Ling Quan (GB 34)	
Zhong Wan (CV 12)	

Guan Chong (TB 1)	Together, these points diffuse the qi and outthrust
Zhi Gou (TB 6)	evils when needled with draining method.

Additions & subtractions: For jaundice, add *Zhi Yang* (GB 9). For constipation, add *Tian Shu* (St 25). For diarrhea with bloody, pussy stools, tenesmus, and abdominal pain, add *Cheng Shan* (Bl 57).

Chinese medicinal formula: *San Ren Tang* (Three Seeds Decoction)

Ingredients: Semen Pruni Armeniacae (*Xing Ren*), 9g, Fructus Cardamomi (*Bai Dou Kou*), 6g, Semen Coicis Lachryma-jobi (*Yi Yi Ren*), 15g, Talcum (*Hua Shi*), 18g, Medulla Tetrapanacis Papyriferi (*Tong Cao*), 6g, Folium Bambusae (*Zhu Ye*), 6g, ginger mix-fried Cortex Magnoliae Officinalis (*Hou Po*), 6g, ginger-processed Rhizoma Pinelliae Ternatae (*Ban Xia*), 6g

Additions & subtractions: For severe poor appetite, add Rhizoma Acori Graminei (*Shi Chang Pu*), 9g. For inhibited defecation of loose stools, add Fructus Immaturus Citri Aurantii (*Zhi Shi*), 12g. For severe damp heat, add Rhizoma Coptidis Chinensis (*Huang Lian*), 6g, and Herba Eupatorei

Fortunei (*Pei Lan*), 9g. For sliminess and a bland taste in the mouth, add Herba Agastachis Seu Pogostemi (*Huo Xiang*), 6g, and Herba Eupatorei Fortunei (*Pei Lan*), 9g. For nausea and vomiting, add ginger mix-fried Caulis Bambusae In Taeniis (*Zhu Ru*), 9g, and Herba Agastachis Seu Pogostemi (*Huo Xiang*), 9g. For fever, add Radix Scutellariae Baicalensis (*Huang Qin*), 6g, Rhizoma Coptidis Chinensis (*Huang Lian*), 6g, and Herba Agastachis Seu Pogostemi (*Huo Xiang*), 6g.

For damp heat in the liver channel with fever, damp, itchy scrotum, headache, red eyes, irascibility, vexation, a bitter taste in the mouth, and rib-side pain, replace *San Ren Tang* with *Long Dan Xie Gan Tang* (Gentiana Drain the Liver Decoction): Radix Gentianae Scabrae (*Long Dan Cao*), 6g, stir-fried Fructus Gardeniae Jasminoidis (*Zhi Zi*), 9g, wine stir-fried Radix Scutellariae Baicalensis (*Huang Qin*), 9g, uncooked Radix Bupleuri (*Chai Hu*), 6g, Caulis Akebiae (*Mu Tong*), 3g, Rhizoma Alismatis (*Ze Xie*), 9g, uncooked Radix Rehmanniae (*Sheng Di*), 9g, uncooked Radix Angelicae Sinensis (*Dang Gui*), 6g, Semen Plantaginis (*Che Qian Zi*), 9g, Radix Glycyrrhizae (*Gan Cao*), 6g. For damp heat in the liver channel with red, swollen, painful eyes, add Flos Chrysanthemi Morifolii (*Ju Hua*), 18g, and Spica Prunellae Vulgaris (*Xia Ku Cao*), 9g. For damp heat in the liver channel with yellow, thick, profuse pus from the ears, add Radix Istadis Seu Baphicacanthi (*Ban Lan Gen*), 15g, and Herba Cum Radice Taraxaci Mongolici (*Pu Gong Ying*), 15g.

For damp heat in the large intestine with fever, abdominal pain, tenesmus, profuse, foul-smelling diarrhea with pus and blood, and burning of the anus, replace *San Ren Tang* with Modified *Shao Yao Tang* (Peony Decoction): stir-fried till yellow Radix Albus Paeoniae Lactiflorae (*Bai Shao*), 15g, stir-fried Radix Angelicae Sinensis (*Dang Gui*), 6g, uncooked Rhizoma Coptidis Chinensis (*Huang Lian*), 6g, stir-fried till scorched Semen Arecae Catechu (*Bing Lang*), 9g, Radix Auklandiae Lappae (*Mu Xiang*), 9g, Radix Glycyrrhizae (*Gan Cao*), 6g, uncooked Radix Et Rhizoma Rhei (*Da Huang*), 6g, Radix Scutellariae Baicalensis (*Huang Qin*), 9g, and Radix Pulsatillae Chinensis (*Bai Tou Weng*), 12g.

For damp heat in the bladder with fever, short, yellow or reddish yellow urination, frequent, urgent, painful urination, possible urinary stoppage, and pain or distention and pain in the lower abdomen, replace *San Ren Tang* with *Ba Zheng San* (Eight Correcting [Ingredients] Powder): Caulis Akebiae (*Mu Tong*), 5g, Herba Dianthi (*Qu Mai*), 9g, cooked Radix Et Rhizoma Rhei (*Da Huang*), 9g, Semen Plantaginis (*Che Qian Zi*), 9g, Talcum (*Hua Shi*), 12g, uncooked Fructus Gardeniae Jasminoidis (*Zhi Zi*),

9g, Herba Polygoni Avicularis (*Bian Xu*), 9g, and Radix Tenuis Glycyrrhizae (*Gan Cao Shao*), 6g.

5. Summerheat damaging the qi

Symptoms: Fever with no aversion to cold, headache, a red facial complexion, hoarse breathing, chest oppression, vexation and agitation, thirst with a desire to drink, profuse sweating, fatigue, weakness, short voiding of red urine, a red tongue with dry, yellow fur, and a surging, rapid pulse

Therapeutic principles: Clear summerheat and drain heat, boost the qi and engender liquids

Acupuncture & moxibustion:

Er Jian (LI 2)	Together, these points clear summerheat and drain heat
Shang Yang (LI 1)	when needled with draining method or pricked to bleed
Shao Fu (Ht 8)	for *Shang Yang*.
Nei Ting (St 44)	

Zu San Li (St 36)	Together, these points boost the qi and engender
Wei Shu (Bl 21)	liquids when needled with supplementing method.

Additions & subtractions: For severe vexatious thirst, profuse sweating, and a vacuous, large, scallion-stalk pulse, add *Jian Shi* (Per 5) and *Qi Hai* (CV 6) to clear summerheat and boost the qi. For constipation, add *Tian Shu* (St 25). For high fever, headache, arched-back rigidity, panting and a scallion-stalk pulse, add *Bai Hui* (CV 20), *Yong Quan* (Ki 1) and *Guan Yuan* (CV 4) to supplement the original qi.

Chinese medicinal formula: *Qing Shu Yi Qi Tang* (Clear Summerheat & Boost Qi Decoction)

Ingredients: Herba Dendrobii (*Shi Hu*), 12g, Tuber Ophiopogonis Japonici (*Mai Men Dong*), 12g, Rhizoma Coptidis Chinensis (*Huang Lian*), 3g, Folium Bambusae (*Zhu Ye*), 6g, Folium Nelumbinis Nuciferae (*He Ye*), 9g, uncooked Rhizoma Anemarrhenae Asphodeloidis (*Zhi Mu*), 9g, Semen Oryzae Sativae (*Geng Mi*), 12g, Pericarpium Citrulli Vulgaris (*Xi Gua Pi*), 24g, Radix Glycyrrhizae (*Gan Cao*), 3g

Additions & subtractions: For severely damaged qi, add Radix Panacis Quinquefolii (*Xi Yang Shen*), 6g, and uncooked Fructus Schisandrae Chinensis

(*Wu Wei Zi*), 9g. For severely damaged fluids, add Radix Glehniae Littoralis (*Sha Shen*), 18g. For severe heat, add uncooked Gypsum Fibrosum (*Shi Gao*), 24g. For summerheat dampness with short, yellow or dark urination, nausea, vomiting, stomach and abdominal glomus and distention, slimy, yellow tongue fur, and a soggy pulse, replace *Qing Shu Yi Qi Tang* with *Lian Po Yin* (Coptis & Magnolia Drink): ginger mix-fried Cortex Magnoliae Officinalis (*Hou Po*), 6g, uncooked Rhizoma Coptidis Chinensis (*Huang Lian*), 3g, Rhizoma Acori Graminei (*Shi Chang Pu*), 3g, ginger stir-fried Rhizoma Pinelliae Ternatae (*Ban Xia*), 3g, clear Semen Praeparatus Sojae (*Dan Dou Chi*), 9g, Fructus Gardeniae Jasminoidis (*Zhi Zi*), 9g, and Rhizoma Phragmitis Communis (*Lu Gen*), 12g.

6. Heat entering the constructive & blood divisions

Symptoms: Fever which is worse at night, vexation and agitation, insomnia, dry mouth without desire to drink, mania, delirium, clouded spirit and eruption of macules and papules in severe cases, a red-purple tongue with scanty or peeled fur, and a fine, rapid pulse

Therapeutic principles: Clear the constructive and cool the blood, drain heat and resolve toxins

Acupuncture & moxibustion:

Shi Xuan (EX-UE-1) *Wei Zhong* (Bl 40)	Together, these points drain heat and resolve toxins when pricked to bleed.
Xue Hai (Sp 10) *San Yin Jiao* (Sp 6) *Qu Ze* (Per 3)	Together, these points clear the constructive and cool the blood when needled with draining method.

Additions & subtractions: For clouding collapse and loss of consciousness, add *Shui Gou* (GV 26). For convulsion, add *Feng Fu* (GV 16) and *Ya Men* (GV 15). For bloody urine, add *Zhong Ji* (CV 3). For bloody stool, moxa *Ge Shu* (Bl 17). For vomiting of blood, add *Liang Qiu* (St 34).

Chinese medicinal formula: Modified *Qing Ying Tang* (Clear the Constructive Decoction)

Ingredients: Cornu Bubali (*Shui Niu Jiao*), 25g, powdered, uncooked Radix Rehmanniae (*Sheng Di*), 15g, Radix Scrophulariae Ningpoensis (*Xuan Shen*), 12g, Folium Bambusae (*Zhu Ye*), 6g, Tuber Ophiopogonis Japonicae

(*Mai Dong*), 9g, uncooked Cortex Radicis Moutan (*Dan Pi*), 9g, uncooked Radix Salviae Miltiorrhizae (*Dan Shen*), 6g, uncooked Rhizoma Coptidis Chinensis (*Huang Lian*), 6g, Flos Lonicerae Japonicae (*Jin Yin Hua*), 15g, Fructus Forsythiae Suspensae (*Lian Qiao*), 10g

7. Exuberant heat toxins

Symptoms: Sudden high fever without aversion to cold, heart vexation, dry red lips, dry tongue fur, reddish urine, constipation, vomiting of blood or nose-bleeding in severe cases, delirium, a rapid and full or surging pulse

Therapeutic principles: Clear heat, drain fire, and resolve toxins

Acupuncture & moxibustion:

Shi Xuan (EX-UE-1) *Wei Zhong* (Bl 40) *Qu Ze* (Per 3)	Together, these points clear heat and resolve toxins when pricked to bleed.
Nei Ting (St 44) *He Gu* (LI 4)	Together, these points clear the heat and resolve toxins when needled with draining method.

Chinese medicinal formula: Modified *Huang Lian Jie Du Tang* (Coptis Resolve Toxins Decoction)

Ingredients: Uncooked Rhizoma Coptidis Chinensis (*Huang Lian*), 6g, uncooked Radix Scutellariae Baicalensis (*Huang Qin*), 6g, uncooked Cortex Phellodendri (*Huang Bai*), 6g, uncooked Fructus Gardeniae Jasminoidis (*Zhi Zi*), 9g, uncooked Radix Rehmanniae (*Sheng Di*), 9g, uncooked Radix Et Rhizoma Rhei (*Da Huang*), 9g, Radix Scrophulariae Ningpoensis (*Xuan Shen*), 9g, Folium Bambusae (*Zhu Ye*), 9g, Radix Glycyrrhizae (*Gan Cao*), 6g

Additions & subtractions: For thirst with dry mouth and lips, add Radix Trichosanthis Kirlowii (*Tian Hua Fen*), 9g, and Rhizoma Phragmitis Communis (*Lu Gen*), 9g. For heat entering the constructive and blood divisions with delirium, heart vexation, and insomnia, add *Qing Ying Tang* (Clear the Constructive Decoction) but subtract Water Buffalo Horn.

8. Qi vacuity

Symptoms: Fever, sometimes low, sometimes higher, fatigue, weakness, cold limbs, torpid intake, abdominal distention, loose stools, a sagging sensation in the lower abdomen, a pale tongue with thin, white fur, and a fine, weak pulse

Therapeutic principles: Fortify the spleen and boost the qi, eliminate fever with sweet and warm (medicinals)

Acupuncture & moxibustion:

He Gu (LI 4)
Qi Hai (CV 6)
Zu San Li (St 36)
Bai Hui (GV 20)

Together, these points supplement the center and boost the qi when needled with supplementing method.

Chinese medicinal formula: *Bu Zhong Yi Qi Tang* (Supplement the Center & Boost the Qi Decoction)

Ingredients: Honey mix-fried Radix Astragali Membranacei (*Huang Qi*), 18g, honey stir-fried Radix Codonopsis Pilosulae (*Dang Shen*), 12g, bran stir-fried Rhizoma Atractylodis Macrocephalae (*Bai Zhu*), 12g, honey mix-fried Radix Glycyrrhizae (*Zhi Gan Cao*), 6g, stir-fried Radix Angelicae Sinensis (*Dang Gui*), 6g, stir-fried Pericarpium Citri Reticulatae (*Chen Pi*), 6g, Radix Bupleuri (*Chai Hu*), 3g, Rhizoma Cimicifugae (*Sheng Ma*), 3g

Additions & subtractions: For cool body alternating with fever, spontaneous sweating, and aversion to wind, add stir-fried Ramulus Cinnamomi Cassiae (*Gui Zhi*), 9g, and Radix Albus Paeoniae Lactiflorae (*Bai Shao*), 9g. For spontaneous sweating, add Radix Ephedrae (*Ma Huang Gen*), 12g. For chest and abdominal oppression and distention, add Herba Agastachis Seu Pogostemi (*Huo Xiang*), 9g, Herba Eupatorei Fortunei (*Pei Lan*), 9g, and Rhizoma Acori Graminei (*Shi Chang Pu*), 6g.

9. Blood vacuity

Symptoms: Low-grade fever, warm skin when touched, red cheekbones but bright white face, thirst or dry mouth, dizziness, pale lips, nails, and tongue, weakness, torpid intake, heart palpitations, impaired memory, thin tongue with fine fur, and a fine, weak pulse

Therapeutic principles: Boost the qi and supplement the blood

Acupuncture & moxibustion:

Zu San Li (St 36)
Qi Hai (CV 6) Together, these points boost the qi to generate blood when needled with supplementing method.

San Yin Jiao (Sp 6)
Ge Shu (Bl 17) Together, these points supplement the blood to balance yin and yang when needled with supplementing method.

Chinese medicinal formulas: For a mild condition: *Dang Gui Bu Xue Tang* (Dang Gui Supplement the Blood Decoction)

Ingredients: Uncooked Radix Astragali Membranacei (*Huang Qi*), 30g, wine mix-fried Radix Angelicae Sinensis (*Dang Gui*), 10g

For heart blood vacuity and spleen qi vacuity: *Gui Pi Tang* (Return the Spleen Decoction)

Ingredients: Honey mix-fried Radix Astragali Membranacei (*Huang Qi*), 18g, stir-fried Radix Codonopsitis Pilosulae (*Dang Shen*), 12g, bran stir-fried Rhizoma Atractylodis Macrocephalae (*Bai Zhu*), 9g, stir-fried Radix Angelicae Sinensis (*Dang Gui*), 9g, Arillus Euphoriae Longanae (*Long Yan Rou*), 12g, licorice-processed Radix Polygalae Tenuifoliae (*Yuan Zhi*), 6g, stir-fried Semen Zizyphi Spinosae (*Suan Zao Ren*), 9g, Sclerotium Pararadicis Poriae Cocos (*Fu Shen*), 9g, mix-fried Radix Glycyrrhizae (*Gan Cao*), 3g, Radix Auklandiae Lappae (*Mu Xiang*), 3g

10. Yin vacuity

Symptoms: Low-grade fever, vexatious heat in the five hearts, night sweats, reddening of the cheekbones and lips, dizziness, tinnitus, dry throat, steaming bones, low back and knee soreness and weakness, lassitude of the spirit, vacuity vexation, insomnia, dry stools, a red tongue with scanty fur, and a fine, rapid pulse

Therapeutic principles: Enrich the yin and downbear fire

Acupuncture & moxibustion:

Yin Xi (Ht 6)
Nei Ting (St 44) Together, these points supplement yin and clear interior heat. (Supplement *Yin Xi,* while draining *Nei Ting.*)

He Gu (LI 4)
Fu Liu (Ki 7)
Together, these points balance yin and yang, supplement qi and yin, and stop sweating when needled with supplementing method.

Additions & subtractions: For vacuity heat damaging fluids, add *Wei Shu* (Bl 21) and *Pi Shu* (Bl 20). For vexation and agitation, add *Shen Men* (Ht 7). For low back pain, add *Shen Shu* (Bl 23).

Chinese medicinal formulas: For yin vacuity due to heat disease: *Qin Jiao Bie Jia San* (Gentiana Macrophylla & Carapax Amydae Powder)

Ingredients: Cortex Radicis Lycii Chinensis (*Di Gu Pi*), 12g, uncooked Radix Bupleuri (*Chai Hu*), 9g, Radix Gentianae Macrophyllae (*Qin Jiao*), 9g, uncooked Rhizoma Anemarrhenae Asphodeloidis (*Zhi Mu*), 9g, uncooked Radix Angelicae Sinensis (*Dang Gui*), 9g, Carapax Amydae Sinensis (*Bie Jia*), 15g, Fructus Pruni Mume (*Wu Mei*), 2 pieces, Herba Artemisiae Apiacae (*Qing Hao*), 6g

For kidney yin vacuity with fire effulgence: *Zhi Bai Di Huang Wan* (Anemarrhena & Phellodendron Rehmannia Pills)

Ingredients: Cooked Radix Rehmanniae (*Shu Di*), 18g, steamed Fructus Corni Officinalis (*Shan Zhu Yu*), 9g, stir-fried Radix Dioscoreae Oppositae (*Shan Yao*), 9g, Sclerotium Poriae Cocos (*Fu Ling*), 9g, Cortex Radicis Moutan (*Dan Pi*), 12g, salt mix-fried Rhizoma Alismatis (*Ze Xie*), 12g, salt mix-fried Rhizoma Anemarrhenae Asphodeloidis (*Zhi Mu*), 12g, salt mix-fried Cortex Phellodendri (*Huang Bai*), 12g

6

Tidal Hectic Fever *(Fa Re Ding Shi)*

This refers to fever that waxes and wanes at fixed times similar to the ocean's tides.

Disease causes, disease mechanisms:

1. Yin & blood vacuity

This vacuity usually develops from constitutional yin vacuity, excessive thinking, enduring disease, febrile disease, excessive sexual activity, aging, or from blood and/or liquid loss. Yin and yang promote and counterbalance each other. If one becomes vacuous, the other party will tend to become hyperactive. Blood belongs to yin. If, for any reason, yin and blood become vacuous and insufficient, yang will become hyperactive and internal heat will be engendered. Yang qi moves to the exterior during the daytime and enters the interior at night. This movement to the interior begins in the afternoon and is completed at night. Therefore, when yang qi enters the interior, vacuity heat due to yin vacuity will tend to get worse because yang is added to yang. Therefore, tidal hectic fever occurs.

2. Spleen-stomach qi vacuity

Spleen-stomach qi vacuity commonly arises due to internal damage from overwork taxation, dietary irregularities, or from enduring disease. The spleen qi is responsible for upbearing the clear. If the spleen becomes vacuous and weak, the central qi may fall downward and accumulate in the interior. Because it is depressed, it transforms into heat over time. Furthermore, because the yang qi cannot be upborne and ascend, it cannot move into the exterior as it should. This combination of mechanisms lead to tidal fever in the mornings.

3. Summerheat damaging the qi

In children, yin and yang are not fully developed, and thus they are susceptible to damage. In summer, summerheat is exuberant, and children especially cannot endure the fuming and steaming from this heat. This is because children have a pure yang constitution. As a result, qi and yin may be damaged. Qi is responsible for helping to engender and transform liquids. Therefore, if the qi is damaged, liquid formation may be affected. If liquids are not engendered, then damaged yin will become even worse. Yin's duty is to check yang. If yin is damaged and vacuous, yang will become hyperactive, thus leading to fever. Because summerheat causes qi and yin vacuity, when the qi vacuity predominates, tidal fever appears in the morning. When yin vacuity predominates, tidal fever appears in the evening.

4. Blood stasis depressed internally

Blood stasis usually forms from hits and falls, cold congealing, and qi stagnation or frenetic movement of the blood due to blood heat. If static blood becomes depressed internally, it will transform into heat over time, thus leading to the formation of internal heat. As stated above, yang enters the interior at night. When yang enters the interior, it will worsen this internal heat, hence giving rise to tidal hectic fever. Another explanation is that static blood prevents the engenderment of new blood. Therefore, blood stasis, step by step, leads to blood (and yin) vacuity. In this case, the balance between yin and yang is broken and yang becomes hyperactive, leading to internal vacuity heat. When yang qi enters the interior each afternoon and evening, vacuity heat becomes even more exuberant. Thus tidal fever occurs.

5. Intestinal heat binding

If heat evils are not cleared from the yang ming channel, they may shift into the yang ming bowel and bind in the intestinal tract. This will cause stoppage of the bowel qi and failure of conveyance. In that case, heat cannot find a way out but will steam internally, leading to fever. Because the yang ming channel has a lot of qi and a lot of blood, when yang starts to move into the interior in the afternoon, it will worsen the internal heat already in the yang ming channel, thus giving rise to tidal hectic fever.

6. Damp heat depressed & steaming

This damp heat usually arises from external contraction of evils. Dampness is sticky and stagnant. Thus heat combined with dampness may find it difficult to be expelled. In this case, dampness prevents heat from exiting through the skin. When the body's righteous yang retreats into the interior in the afternoon, heat added to heat results in tidal hectic fever.

7. Heat entering the constructive & blood divisions

This disease mechanism is mainly seen in the final stage of warm diseases when warm heat evils fall inward into the constructive and blood divisions. When heat enters these last two divisions, it will boil and burn the constructive and blood. These, being yin fluids, become damaged and consumed and yin is no longer able to restrain yang. In that case, the exuberant heat will become even more effulgent, giving rise to tidal hectic fever in the night when the body's righteous yang naturally accumulates internally.

Treatment based on pattern discrimination:

1. Yin & blood vacuity

Symptoms: Tidal fever in the afternoon or at night, heat in the palms and soles, bone steaming, vexation, insomnia, heart palpitations, night sweats, emaciation, a red tongue with scanty fur, and a fine, rapid pulse

Therapeutic principles: Enrich yin, nourish the blood, and downbear fire

Acupuncture & moxibustion:

Xin Shu (Bl 15)	Together, these points nourish the blood when needled
Pi Shu (Bl 20)	with supplementing method.
Gan Shu (Bl 18)	

Tai Xi (Ki 3)	Together, these points nourish yin and downbear fire
Yin Xi (Ht 6)	when needled with even draining and supplementing method.

Additions & subtractions: For dizziness and flowery vision, add *Feng Chi* (GB 20). For profuse dreams, add *Li Dui* (St 45). For seminal emission, add *San Yin Jiao* (Sp 6). For sore throat, add *Zhao Hai* (Ki 6). For coughing with no or scanty phlegm, add *Chi Ze* (Lu 5). For delayed menstruation, add *Xue Hai* (Sp 10).

Chinese medicinal formulas: For yin and blood vacuity due to warm disease: Modified *Qing Gu San* (Clear the Bones Powder)

Ingredients: Radix Stellariae Dichotomae (*Yin Chai Hu*), 12g, Rhizoma Picrorrhizae (*Hu Huang Lian*), 9g, Carapax Amydae Sinensis (*Bie Jia*), 9g, Herba Artemisiae Apiacae (*Qing Hao*), 9g, Radix Gentianae Macrophyllae

(*Qin Jiao*), 12g, Cortex Radicis Lycii Chinensis (*Di Gu Pi*), 9g, uncooked Rhizoma Anemarrhenae Asphodeloidis (*Zhi Mu*), 9g, Radix Glycyrrhizae (*Gan Cao*), 6g, uncooked Radix Angelicae Sinensis (*Dang Gui*), 9g

For yin vacuity due to kidney vacuity with effulgent heat: Modified *Zhi Bai Di Huang Wan* (Anemarrhena & Phellodendron Rehmannia Pills)

Ingredients: Cooked Radix Rehmanniae (*Shu Di*), 18g, steamed Fructus Corni Officinalis (*Shan Zhu Yu*), 9g, stir-fried Radix Dioscoreae Oppositae (*Shan Yao*), 9g, Sclerotium Poriae Cocos (*Fu Ling*), 9g, Cortex Radicis Moutan (*Dan Pi*), 12g, salt mix-fried Rhizoma Alismatis (*Ze Xie*), 12g, salt mix-fried Rhizoma Anemarrhenae Asphodeloidis (*Zhi Mu*), 12g, salt mix-fried Cortex Phellodendri (*Huang Bai*), 12g, Cortex Radicis Lycii Chinensis (*Di Gu Pi*), 9g

2. Spleen stomach qi vacuity

Symptoms: Tidal fever in the morning or low-grade fever which is worse in the morning or which worsens with overwork, reduced qi with laziness to speak, fatigued spirit and limbs, spontaneous perspiration, a bright white facial complexion, a pale, tender tongue, and a vacuous, fine, weak pulse

Therapeutic principles: Eliminate heat with sweet, warm (medicinals), supplement the center and boost the qi

Acupuncture & moxibustion:

Zhong Wan (CV 12) *Qi Hai* (CV 6) *Zu San Li* (St 36)	Together, these points supplement the center and boost the qi when needled with supplementing method.
Qu Chi (LI 11)	Clears heat when needled with draining method
Bai Hui (GV 20)	Upbears the central qi when moxaed

Additions & subtractions: For reduced food intake, add *Jian Li* (CV 11). For loose stools, add *Da Ju* (St 27). For headache and aversion to wind and cold, add *Lie Que* (Lu 7). For chest oppression and abdominal glomus, add *Feng Long* (St 40).

Chinese medicinal formula: *Bu Zhong Yi Qi Tang* (Supplement the Center & Boost the Qi Decoction)

Ingredients: Honey mix-fried Radix Astragali Membranacei (*Huang Qi*), 18g, honey stir-fried Radix Codonopsis Pilosulae (*Dang Shen*), 9g, bran stir-fried Rhizoma Atractylodis Macrocephalae (*Bai Zhu*), 12g, honey mix-fried Radix Glycyrrhizae (*Gan Cao*), 6g, stir-fried Radix Angelicae Sinensis (*Dang Gui*), 6g, stir-fried Pericarpium Citri Reticulatae (*Chen Pi*), 6g, Radix Bupleuri (*Chai Hu*), 6g, Rhizoma Cimicifugae (*Sheng Ma*), 3g

Additions & subtractions: For qi and blood vacuity with tidal hectic fever which is worse in the afternoon, frequent heart palpitations, spontaneous perspiration and night sweats, fatigue, weakness of the limbs, insomnia, shortage of qi, a pale tongue with scanty fur, and a fine, weak pulse, replace *Bu Zhong Yi Qi Tang* with Modified *Zhi Gan Cao Tang* (Licorice Decoction): mix-fried Radix Glycyrrhizae (*Gan Cao*), 12g, rice stir-fried Radix Codonopsitis Pilosulae (*Dang Shen*), 9g, uncooked Radix Rehmanniae (*Sheng Di*), 18g, Gelatinum Corii Asini (*E Jiao*), 9g, wine mix-fried Radix Angelicae Sinensis (*Dang Gui*), 9g, stir-fried Semen Zizyphi Spinosae (*Suan Zao Ren*), 9g, stir-fried Ramulus Cinnamomi Cassiae (*Gui Zhi*), 6g, Tuber Ophiopogonis Japonici (*Mai Men Dong*), 9g, and honey stir-fried Radix Astragali Membranacei (*Huang Qi*), 12g. For dual heart and spleen vacuity with tidal hectic fever which is worse at night, heart vexation, insomnia, impaired memory, night sweats, torpid intake, loose stools, a pale tongue, and a fine, weak pulse, replace *Bu Zhong Yi Qi Tang* with Modified *Gui Pi Tang* (Return the Spleen Decoction): honey mix-fried Radix Astragali Membranacei (*Huang Qi*), 15g, stir-fried Radix Codonopsitis Pilosulae (*Dang Shen*), 9g, bran stir-fried Rhizoma Atractylodis Macrocephalae (*Bai Zhu*), 15g, stir-fried Radix Angelicae Sinensis (*Dang Gui*), 9g, Arillus Euphoriae Longanae (*Long Yan Rou*), 15g, licorice-processed Radix Polygalae Tenuifoliae (*Yuan Zhi*), 3g, stir-fried Semen Zizyphi Spinosae (*Suan Zao Ren*), 15g, Sclerotium Poriae Cocos (*Fu Ling*), 12g, mix-fried Radix Glycyrrhizae (*Gan Cao*), 3g, Radix Auklandiae Lappae (*Mu Xiang*), 3g, stir-fried Radix Albus Paeoniae Lactiflorae (*Bai Shao*), 9g, and Cortex Phellodendri (*Huang Bai*), 6g.

3. Summerheat damaging the qi

Symptoms: Tidal fever in the morning or evening which is mainly seen in summertime diseases in children, profuse perspiration, thirst with a liking to drink, vexation and agitation, torpid intake, fatigued spirit, slimy tongue fur, and a soggy, rapid pulse

Therapeutic principles: Clear summerheat and boost the qi

Acupuncture & moxibustion:

He Gu (LI 4) *Nei Ting* (St 44)	Together, these points clear summerheat when needled with draining method.
Zhong Wan (CV 12) *Zu San Li* (St 36)	Together, these points boost the stomach and fortify the spleen to supplement the qi when needled with supplementing method.
San Yin Jiao (Sp 6) *Tai Xi* (Ki 3)	Together, these points nourish yin and clear heat when needled with supplementing method.

Chinese medicinal formula: Modified *Qing Shu Yi Qi Tang* (Clear Summerheat & Boost the Qi Decoction)

Ingredients: Radix Panacis Quinquefolii (*Xi Yang Shen*), 6g, Herba Dendrobii (*Shi Hu*), 12g, Tuber Ophiopogonis Japonici (*Mai Men Dong*), 12g, Rhizoma Coptidis Chinensis (*Huang Lian*), 3g, Folium Bambusae (*Zhu Ye*), 6g, Folium Nelumbinis Nuciferae (*He Ye*), 9g, uncooked Rhizoma Anemarrhenae Asphodeloidis (*Zhi Mu*), 9g, Semen Oryzae Sativae (*Geng Mi*), 12g, Pericarpium Citrulli Vulgaris (*Xi Gua Pi*), 24g, Radix Glycyrrhizae (*Gan Cao*), 3g

Additions & subtractions: For severe heat, add uncooked Gypsum Fibrosum (*Shi Gao*), 24g. For summerheat dampness with short, yellow or dark urination, nausea, vomiting, stomach and abdominal glomus and distention, slimy, yellow tongue fur, and a soggy pulse, replace *Qing Shu Yi Qi Tang* with *Lian Po Yin* (Coptis & Magnolia Drink): ginger mix-fried Cortex Magnoliae Officinalis (*Hou Po*), 6g, uncooked Rhizoma Coptidis Chinensis (*Huang Lian*), 6g, Rhizoma Acori Graminei (*Shi Chang Pu*), 3g, ginger stir-fried Rhizoma Pinelliae Ternatae (*Ban Xia*), 3g, clear Semen Praeparatus Sojae (*Dan Dou Chi*), 9g, Fructus Gardeniae Jasminoidis (*Zhi Zi*), 9g, and Rhizoma Phragmitis Communis (*Lu Gen*), 12g.

4. Blood stasis depressed internally

Symptoms: Tidal fever in the afternoon or at night, dry mouth and throat, rinsing the mouth with water but no desire to swallow it, lumps in the abdomen, possible local pain, dry, scaly skin in severe cases, dark rings around the eyes, possible fixed, stabbing pain in the head or chest, a greenish blue, purple tongue with static macules and spots, and a fine, choppy pulse

Therapeutic principles: Quicken the blood, transform stasis, and clear heat

Acupuncture & moxibustion:

He Gu (LI 4) *Qu Chi* (LI 11)	Together, these points clear heat when needled with draining method.
San Yin Jiao (Sp 6)	Quickens the blood and transforms stasis when combined with *He Gu*
Xue Hai (Sp 10)	Nourishes and quickens the blood when needled with supplementing method

Additions & subtractions: For local pain, add appropriate local and *a shi* points. For high fever, prick *Da Zhui* (GV 14) to bleed.

Chinese medicinal formula: *Xue Fu Zhu Yu Tang* (Blood Mansion Dispel Stasis Decoction)

Ingredients: Semen Pruni Persicae (*Tao Ren*), 12g, Flos Carthami Tinctorii (*Hong Hua*), 9g, wine mix-fried Radix Angelicae Sinensis (*Dang Gui*), 9g, wine mix-fried Radix Ligustici Wallichii (*Chuan Xiong*), 6g, wine mix-fried Radix Rubrus Paeoniae Lactiflorae (*Chi Shao*), 6g, Radix Bupleuri (*Chai Hu*), 6g, wine mix-fried Radix Cyathulae (*Chuan Niu Xi*), 9g, uncooked Radix Rehmanniae (*Sheng Di*), 9g, Fructus Citri Aurantii (*Zhi Ke*), 6g, mix-fried Radix Glycyrrhizae (*Gan Cao*), 3g

5. Intestinal heat binding

Symptoms: Tidal hectic fever in the afternoon, painful fullness in the abdomen which is hard and replete when touched, dry stools and constipation, clouded spirit and delirium in severe cases, vexation and agitation, a red tongue with dry, yellow or scorched black fur, and a deep, replete, forceful pulse

Therapeutic principles: Free the flow of the bowels and drain heat, attack and precipitate dry binding

Acupuncture & moxibustion:

He Gu (LI 4) *Nei Ting* (St 44)	Together, these points drain heat and attack heat binding when needled with draining method or

Shang Yang (LI 1) *Li Dui* (St 45)	pricked to bleed for *Shang Yang* and *Li Dui.*
Zhi Gou (TB 6) *Shang Ju Xu* (St 37)	Together, these points free the flow of the bowels and precipitate binding when needled with draining method.

Chinese medicinal formula: *Da Cheng Qi Tang* (Major Order the Qi Decoction)

Ingredients: Uncooked Radix Et Rhizoma Rhei (*Da Huang*), 9g, Mirabilitum (*Mang Xiao*), 6g, uncooked Fructus Immaturus Citri Aurantii (*Zhi Shi*), 6g, ginger mix-fried Cortex Magnoliae Officinalis (*Hou Po*), 6g

Additions & subtractions: For a mild condition without severe constipation, replace *Da Cheng Qi Tang* with *Xiao Cheng Qi Tang* (Minor Order the Qi Decoction): uncooked Radix Et Rhizoma Rhei (*Da Huang*), 9g, uncooked Fructus Immaturus Citri Aurantii (*Zhi Shi*), 6g, and ginger mix-fried Cortex Magnoliae Officinalis (*Hou Po*), 6g. For a mild condition without stomach and abdominal glomus and fullness, replace *Da Cheng Qi Tang* with *Tiao Wei Cheng Qi Tang* (Regulate the Stomach & Order the Qi Decoction): uncooked Radix Et Rhizoma Rhei (*Da Huang*), 9g, Mirabilitum (*Mang Xiao*), 9g, and mix-fried Radix Glycyrrhizae (*Gan Cao*), 6g. For a mild condition but heat damaging yin with thirst and very dry stools, replace *Da Cheng Qi Tang* with *Zeng Ye Cheng Qi Tang* (Increase Fluids & Order the Qi Decoction): Tuber Ophiopogonis Japonici (*Mai Men Dong*), 9g, uncooked Radix Rehmanniae (*Sheng Di*), 15g, Radix Scrophulariae Ningpoensis (*Xuan Shen*), 12g, Radix Et Rhizoma Rhei (*Da Huang*), 6-9g, and Mirabilitum (*Mang Xiao*), 3-6g.

6. Damp heat depressed & steaming

Symptoms: Tidal hectic fever in afternoon which does not abate with sweating, thirst but no great desire to drink, chest oppression, stomach glomus, nausea, heavy or painful body, torpid intake, short voidings of reddish urine, loose stools which are difficult to defecate, a red tongue with yellow, slimy fur, and a bowstring, slippery, rapid pulse

Therapeutic principles: Diffuse the qi and disinhibit dampness, clear heat and out-thrust evils

Acupuncture & moxibustion:

Yin Ling Quan (Sp 9)	Together, these points clear heat and transform
Yang Ling Quan (GB 34)	dampness when needled with draining method.
Nei Ting (St 44)	

Guan Chong (TB 1)	Together, these points diffuse the qi and out-
Zhi Gou (TB 6)	thrust evils when needled with draining method.

Chinese medicinal formula: *San Ren Tang* (Three Seeds Decoction)

Ingredients: Semen Pruni Armeniacae (*Xing Ren*), 9g, Fructus Cardamomi (*Bai Dou Kou*), 6g, Semen Coicis Lachryma-jobi (*Yi Yi Ren*), 15g, Talcum (*Hua Shi*), 18g, Medulla Tetrapanacis Papyriferi (*Tong Cao*), 6g, Folium Bambusae (*Zhu Ye*), 6g, ginger mix-fried Cortex Magnoliae Officinalis (*Hou Po*), 6g, ginger-processed Rhizoma Pinelliae Ternatae (*Ban Xia*), 9g

Additions & subtractions: For wind damp heat impediment causing tidal hectic fever in the afternoon, moving pain in the joints, red, hot, swollen joints, a red facial complexion, sweating, nausea, chest oppression, heart vexation, yellow, slimy tongue fur, and a slippery pulse, replace *San Ren Tang* with Modified *Jia Wei Er Miao San* (Added Flavors Two Marvels Powder): uncooked Cortex Phellodendri (*Huang Bai*), 12g, uncooked Rhizoma Atractylodis (*Cang Zhu*), 9g, wine mix-fried Radix Angelicae Sinensis (*Dang Gui*), 9g, Radix Achyranthis Bidentatae (*Niu Xi*), 9g, Radix Stephaniae Tetrandrae (*Han Fang Ji*), 9g, Rhizoma Dioscoreae Hypoglaucae (*Bei Xie*), 9g, Ramulus Mori Albi (*Sang Zhi*), 9g, Caulis Lonicerae Japonicae (*Ren Dong Teng*), 6g, and Radix Gentianae Macrophyllae (*Qin Jiao*), 9g. For severe poor appetite, add Rhizoma Acori Graminei (*Shi Chang Pu*), 9g. For inhibited defecation of loose stools, add Fructus Immaturus Citri Aurantii (*Zhi Shi*), 12g. For severe damp heat, add Rhizoma Coptidis Chinensis (*Huang Lian*), 6g, and Herba Eupatorei Fortunei (*Pei Lan*), 9g. For sliminess and a bland taste in the mouth, add Herba Agastachis Seu Pogostemi (*Huo Xiang*), 6g, and Herba Eupatorei Fortunei (*Pei Lan*), 9g. For nausea and vomiting, add ginger mix-fried Caulis Bambusae In Taeniis (*Zhu Ru*), 9g, and Herba Agastachis Seu Pogostemi (*Huo Xiang*), 9g. For fever, add Radix Scutellariae Baicalensis (*Huang Qin*), 6g, Rhizoma Coptidis Chinensis (*Huang Lian*), 6g, and Herba Agastachis Seu Pogostemi (*Huo Xiang*), 6g.

7. Heat entering the constructive & blood divisions

Symptoms: Fever which is worse at night, vexation and agitation, insomnia, a dry mouth with no desire to drink, delirium, clouded spirit and eruption of macules and papules in severe cases, a reddish purple tongue with scanty or peeled fur, and a fine, rapid pulse

Therapeutic principles: Clear the constructive and cool the blood

Acupuncture & moxibustion:

Shi Xuan (EX-UE-11) *Wei Zhong* (Bl 40)	Together, these points drain heat and resolve toxins when pricked to bleed.
Xue Hai (Sp 10) *San Yin Jiao* (Sp 6) *Qu Ze* (Per 3)	Together, these points clear the constructive and cool the blood when needled with draining method.

Chinese medicinal formula: Modified *Qing Ying Tang* (Clear the Constructive Decoction)

Ingredients: Cornu Bubali (*Shui Niu Jiao*), 25g, powdered, uncooked Radix Rehmanniae (*Sheng Di*), 15g, Radix Scrophulariae Ningpoensis (*Xuan Shen*), 9g, Folium Bambusae (*Zhu Ye*), 6g, Tuber Ophiopogonis Japonicae (*Mai Dong*), 9g, uncooked Cortex Radicis Moutan (*Dan Pi*), 9g, uncooked Radix Salviae Miltiorrhizae (*Dan Shen*), 6g, uncooked Rhizoma Coptidis Chinensis (*Huang Lian*), 6g, Flos Lonicerae Japonicae (*Jin Yin Hua*), 15g, Fructus Forsythiae Suspensae (*Lian Qiao*), 9g

7
Vexatious Heat in the Five Hearts *(Wu Xin Fan Re)*

This refers to a feeling of heat in the palms of the hands and soles of the feet accompanied by a feeling of vexatious heat in the heart and chest. In some cases, low-grade fever is also present.

Disease causes, disease mechanisms:

1. Yin vacuity

Yin vacuity can arise from constitutional yin vacuity, enduring disease, warm disease, aging, excessive sexual activity, and drug use. In addition, deep-lying evils due to the erroneous treatment of externally contracted disease may damage and consume yin blood, leading to yin vacuity. However, no matter what the reason, yin is responsible for controlling yang. If yin becomes vacuous, yang typically becomes hyperactive, thus giving rise to internal heat. The palms of the hands, soles of the feet, and the heart and chest all pertain to yin and the interior from the point of view of Chinese anatomy. Therefore, vexatious heat due to yin vacuity manifests in those areas described as anatomically yin.

2. Blood vacuity

Blood vacuity usually arises from constitutional vacuity of the spleen and stomach, enduring disease, excessive thinking, or excessive blood loss. Because the blood and essence on the one hand and the liver and kidneys on the other all share a common source, blood vacuity may also give rise to yang hyperactivity and the engenderment of internal heat. As mentioned above, the palms of the hands, soles of the feet, and the heart and chest are all categorized as relatively yin. Therefore, the internal heat due to yang hyperactivity as a result of blood vacuity often manifests as vexatious heat in the five hearts.

3. Fire heat depressed internally

Liver depression qi stagnation may be due to emotional disturbance, such as frustration, emotional depression, unfulfilled desires, or anger. When the liver becomes depressed, its qi becomes replete. Because qi is yang, when it accumulates, it may transform into heat. Because this heat is also depressed internally, it may have difficulty finding a way to the outside. As stated above, the palms of the hands, soles of the feet, and heart and chest all correspond to the yin interior of the body. Therefore, internal heat more easily manifests in these yin areas. Hence liver depression/depressive heat may also give rise to vexatious heat in the five hearts.

4. Stasis heat

Blood stasis may be due to a large number of causes. These include external injury severing the channels and vessels, heat in the blood causing the blood to move frenetically outside its pathways, qi stagnation failing to move the blood, qi vacuity failing to move the blood, yang vacuity resulting in vacuity cold which is constricting and contracting, or any other material depression, such as food, phlegm, or dampness, obstructing the free and uninhibited flow of qi and blood. Because the qi and blood move together, blood stasis typically results in the creation or worsening of qi stagnation. Because the qi is yang and, therefore, warm by nature, stagnant qi commonly transforms into depressive heat. Therefore, static blood is often complicated by depressive heat. This combination is then commonly referred to as stasis heat. Because this heat is depressed internally, it has trouble finding its way to the surface and frequently manifests externally in the yin portions of the body, such as the palms of the hands, soles of the feet, and heart and chest. Thus, blood stasis accompanied by depressive heat often results in vexatious heat in the five hearts.

Treatment based on pattern discrimination:

I. Yin vacuity

Symptoms: Vexatious heat in the five hearts which occurs or worsens in the afternoon, a desire to hold cold objects to relieve the feelings of heat, a tendency to sleep with one's hands and feet outside the covers, tidally red cheekbones, a dry mouth and throat, a red tongue with scanty fur, and a fine, rapid pulse

Therapeutic principles: Supplement the kidneys and enrich yin, clear heat and eliminate vexation

Acupuncture & moxibustion:

Fu Liu (Ki 7)   Together, these points nourish yin to clear heat

Tai Xi (Ki 3)
San Yin Jiao (Sp 6)   when needled with supplementing method.

Qu Chi (LI 11)   Together, these points clear heat in the blood
Xue Hai (Sp 10)   when needled with draining method.

Additions & subtractions: For vexation and agitation, reduced sleep, and thirst with no desire to drink, add *Gan Shu* (Bl 18) to nourish liver blood. For low back and knee aching and limpness, tinnitus, seminal emission, and night sweats, add *Shen Shu* (Bl 23) to enrich kidney yin. For coughing, night sweats, bone steaming, tidal fever, emaciation, spontaneous perspiration, and hoarse voice, add *Fei Shu* (Bl 13) to nourish lung yin. For toothache, add *Jia Che* (St 6). For constipation, add *Tian Shu* (St 25).

Chinese medicinal formulas: For heart yin vacuity with insomnia, vexation and agitation, impaired memory, heart palpitations, mental depression, and mouth sores: *Tian Wang Bu Xin Dan* (Heavenly Emperor Supplement the Heart Elixir)

Ingredients: Uncooked Radix Rehmanniae (*Sheng Di*), 12g, Radix Codonopsitis Pilosulae (*Dang Shen*), 9g, Tuber Asparagi Cochinensis (*Tian Men Dong*), 9g, Tuber Ophiopogonis Japonici (*Mai Men Dong*), 9g, Radix Scrophulariae Ningpoensis (*Xuan Shen*), 9g, Radix Salviae Miltiorrhizae (*Dan Shen*), 9g, Sclerotium Poriae Cocos (*Fu Ling*), 9g, Radix Polygalae Tenuifoliae (*Yuan Zhi*), 6g, Radix Angelicae Sinensis (*Dang Gui*), 9g, uncooked Fructus Schisandrae Chinensis (*Wu Wei Zi*), 9g, Semen Biotae Orientalis (*Bai Zi Ren*), 9g, stir-fried Semen Zizyphi Spinosae (*Suan Zao Ren*), 9g, and Radix Platycodi Grandiflori (*Jie Geng*), 3g

For non-interaction between the heart and kidneys with heart vexation, insomnia, heart palpitations, impaired memory, tinnitus, deafness, low back and knee aching and pain, and seminal emission: Modified *Huang Lian E Jiao Tang* (Coptis & Donkey Skin Glue Decoction)

Ingredients: Rhizoma Coptidis Chinensis (*Huang Lian*), 6g, Gelatinum Corii Asini (*E Jiao*), 6g, Radix Albus Paeoniae Lactiflorae (*Bai Shao*), 9g, Radix Scutellariae Baicalensis (*Huang Qin*), 6g, egg yolk, 1 piece, Cortex Radicis Lycii Chinensis (*Di Gu Pi*), 9g, Cortex Phellodendri (*Huang Bai*), 9g, Rhizoma Anemarrhenae Asphodeloidis (*Zhi Mu*), 9g, uncooked Radix Rehmanniae (*Sheng Di*), 15g

For lung yin vacuity with tuberculosis: Modified *Qin Jiao Bie Jia San* (Gentiana Macrophylla & Carapax Amydae Powder)

Ingredients: Cortex Radicis Lycii Chinensis (*Di Gu Pi*), 12g, uncooked Radix Bupleuri (*Chai Hu*), 9g, Radix Gentianae Macrophyllae (*Qin Jiao*), 9g, uncooked Rhizoma Anemarrhenae Asphodeloidis (*Zhi Mu*), 9g, uncooked Radix Angelicae Sinensis (*Dang Gui*), 9g, Carapax Amydae Sinensis (*Bie Jia*), 15g, Fructus Pruni Mume (*Wu Mei*), 2 pieces, Herba Artemisiae Apiacae (*Qing Hao*), 6g, Radix Stemonae (*Bai Bu*), 12g, Rhizoma Bletillae Striatae (*Bai Ji*), 12g

For lung yin vacuity with enduring cough: Modified *Bai He Gu Jin Tang* (Lily Secure Metal Decoction)

Ingredients: Bulbus Lilii (*Bai He*), 9g, uncooked Radix Rehmanniae (*Sheng Di*), 9g, Tuber Ophiopogonis Japonici (*Mai Dong*), 6g, cooked Radix Rehmanniae (*Shu Di*), 9g, Bulbus Fritillariae Cirrhosae (*Chuan Bei Mu*), 6g, Radix Scrophulariae Ningpoensis (*Xuan Shen*), 9g, uncooked Rhizoma Anemarrhenae Asphodeloidis (*Zhi Mu*), 9g, Radix Angelicae Sinensis (*Dang Gui*), 6g, Radix Albus Paeoniae Lactiflorae (*Bai Shao*), 6g, Radix Glycyrrhizae (*Gan Cao*), 6g

For liver yin vacuity with scanty menstruation, muscle spasms, blurred vision, dull rib-side pain, etc.: Modified *Yi Guan Jian* (One Link Decoction)

Ingredients: Radix Albus Paeoniae Lactiflorae (*Bai Shao*), 9g, processed Polygoni Multiflori (*He Shou Wu*), 9g, Radix Glehniae Littoralis (*Bei Sha Shen*), 9g, Tuber Ophiopogonis Japonici (*Mai Dong*), 9g, uncooked Radix Rehmanniae (*Sheng Di*), 9g, Fructus Lycii Chinensis (*Gou Qi Zi*), 9g, wine mix-fried Radix Angelicae Sinensis (*Dang Gui*), 9g, Fructus Meliae Toosendan (*Chuan Lian Zi*), 6g, uncooked Rhizoma Anemarrhenae Asphodeloidis (*Zhi Mu*), 9g, Cortex Radicis Lycii Chinensis (*Di Gu Pi*), 9g

For kidney yin vacuity with low back and knee aching and limpness, seminal emission, loose teeth, tinnitus, deafness, vertigo, and menopausal syndrome: Modified *Zhi Bai Di Huang Wan* (Anemarrhena & Phellodendron Rehmannia Pills)

Ingredients: Cooked Radix Rehmanniae (*Shu Di*), 18g, steamed Fructus Corni Officinalis (*Shan Zhu Yu*), 9g, stir-fried Radix Dioscoreae Oppositae (*Shan Yao*), 9g, Sclerotium Poriae Cocos (*Fu Ling*), 9g, Cortex Radicis Lycii

Chinensis (*Di Gu Pi*), 12g, salt mix-fried Rhizoma Alismatis (*Ze Xie*), 12g, salt mix-fried Rhizoma Anemarrhenae Asphodeloidis (*Zhi Mu*), 12g, salt mix-fried Cortex Phellodendri (*Huang Bai*), 12g, Radix Cynanchi Baiwai (*Bai Wai*), 9g

2. Blood vacuity

Symptoms: A subjective sensation of heat in the palms of the hands and soles of the feet in the afternoon which gets worse on slight overwork, fatigued spirit and lassitude, blurred vision, nightblindness, heart palpitations, dizziness and vertigo, pale nails and lips, a somber white or sallow yellow facial complexion, delayed menstruation, blocked menstruation, and/or scanty menstruation, a pale tongue, and a fine, weak or fine, weak, choppy pulse

Therapeutic principles: Supplement the liver and nourish the blood assisted by fortifying the spleen and boosting the qi

Acupuncture & moxibustion:

Pi Shu (Bl 20)	Together, these points supplement the liver and fortify
Gan Shu (Bl 18)	the spleen.
Ge Shu (Bl 17)	Together, these points nourish the blood and abate the
Gao Huang (Bl 43)	heat when needled with supplementing method.
Zu San Li (St 36)	Together, these points fortify the spleen to engender
Xue Hai (Sp 10)	the blood when needled with supplementing method

Additions & subtractions: For heart vexation, add *Xin Shu* (Bl 15).

Chinese medicinal formula: Modified *Bu Gan Tang* (Supplement the Liver Decoction)

Chinese medicinal formula: Wine mix-fried Radix Angelicae Sinensis (*Dang Gui*), 9g, wine mix-fried Radix Albus Paeoniae Lactiflorae (*Bai Shao*), 9g, prepared Radix Rehmanniae (*Shu Di*), 15g, wine mix-fried Radix Ligustici Wallichii (*Chuan Xiong*), 6g, bran stir-fried Rhizoma Atractylodis Macrocephalae (*Bai Zhu*), 9g, honey stir-fried Radix Astragali Membranacei (*Huang Qi*), 12g, Semen Zizyphi Spinosae (*Suan Zao Ren*), 9g, mix-fried Radix Glycyrrhizae (*Zhi Gan Cao*), 3g, Cortex Radicis Moutan (*Dan Pi*), 12g

3. Deep lying evils in the yin division

Symptoms: Heat in the palms of the hands and soles of the feet, heart vexation, reduced sleep, low-grade fever which gets worse in the evening, sometimes disappears in the morning, and abates without sweating, profuse food intake, emaciation, a red tongue with scanty fur, and a bowstring fine, slightly rapid pulse

Therapeutic principles: Enrich yin and nourish the blood, clear heat and out-thrust the evils

Acupuncture & moxibustion:

Zhong Zhu (TB 3) *Xian Gu* (St 43)	Together, these points clear heat and out-thrust evils when needled with draining method.
San Yin Jiao (Sp 6) *Fu Liu* (Ki 7)	Together, these points nourish yin to clear heat when needled with supplementing method.

Chinese medicinal formula: *Qing Hao Bie Jia Tang* (Artemisia Apiacea & Carapax Amydae Decoction)

Ingredients: Herba Artemisiae Apiacae (*Qing Hao*), 12g, Carapax Amydae Sinensis (*Bie Jia*), 9g, uncooked Radix Rehmanniae (*Sheng Di*), 9g, uncooked Rhizoma Anemarrhenae Asphodeloidis (*Zhi Mu*), 9g, Cortex Radicis Moutan (*Dan Pi*), 9g, Radix Scrophulariae Ningpoensis (*Xuan Shen*), 9g

Additions & subtractions: For a more severe condition, add Radix Stellariae Dichotomae (*Yin Chai Hu*), 9g, and Rhizoma Picrorrhizae (*Hu Huang Lian*), 9g, and replace Cortex Radicis Moutan (*Dan Pi*) with Cortex Radicis Lycii Chinensis (*Di Gu Pi*). For severe fluid damage with dry throat and mouth and severe thirst, add Tuber Ophiopogonis Japonici (*Mai Men Dong*), 9g, and uncooked Fructus Schisandrae Chinensis (*Wu Wei Zi*), 9g. For concomitant qi vacuity with shortness of breath, bodily weakness, and fatigue, add Radix Codonopsitis Pilosulae (*Dang Shen*), 12g, uncooked Fructus Schisandrae Chinensis (*Wu Wei Zi*), 9g, and honey stir-fried Radix Astragali Membranacei (*Huang Qi*), 12g. For heart vexation and insomnia, add stir-fried Semen Zizyphi Spinosae (*Suan Zao Ren*), 9g, and Semen Biotae Orientalis (*Bai Zi Ren*), 9g. For severe night sweats, subtract Artemisia Apiaca and add Cortex Radicis Lycii Chinensis (*Di Gu Pi*), 9g,

Semen Levis Tritici Aestivi (*Fu Xiao Mai*), 9g, and Radix Ephedrae (*Ma Huang Gen*), 9g.

4. Liver depression transforming heat

Symptoms: Vexatious heat in the five hearts, chest and rib-side fullness and oppression, emotional dysphoria, impatience, irascibility, head distention, a bitter taste in the mouth, dark-colored urine, menstrual irregularity in women, a red tongue with yellow fur, and a deep, rapid pulse

Therapeutic principles: Course the liver and rectify the qi, clear the liver and resolve depression

Acupuncture & moxibustion:

Shao Fu (Ht 8)	Together, these points drain fire when needled with
Xia Xi (GB 43)	draining method.
Zhong Zhu (TB 3)	Together, these points course the liver, resolve
Zhi Gou (TB 6)	depression, and clear heat when needled with
Xiang Jian (Liv 2)	draining method.

Additions & subtractions: For insomnia, add *Shen Men* (Ht 7). For bad breath, add *Lao Gong* (Per 8). For fever, pain in the rib-side, and a fine, rapid pulse, add *Qi Men* (Liv 14) and *San Yin Jiao* (Sp 6). For constipation, add *Shang Ju Xu* (St 37).

Chinese medicinal formula: Modified *Dan Zhi Xiao Yao San* (Moutan & Gardenia Rambling Powder)

Ingredients: Vinegar stir-fried Radix Bupleuri (*Chai Hu*), 9g, uncooked Radix Angelicae Sinensis (*Dang Gui*), 6g, Radix Albus Paeoniae Lactiflorae (*Bai Shao*), 6g, bran stir-fried Rhizoma Atractylodis Macrocephalae (*Bai Zhu*), 9g, Sclerotium Poriae Cocos (*Fu Ling*), 9g, mix-fried Radix Glycyrrhizae (*Gan Cao*), 6g, Herba Menthae Haplocalycis (*Bo He*), 3g, stir-fried till carbonized Cortex Radicis Moutan (*Dan Pi*), 9g, Fructus Gardeniae Jasminoidis (*Zhi Zi*), 12g, Rhizoma Cyperi Rotundi (*Xiang Fu*), 9g, stir-fried Fructus Meliae Toosendan (*Chuan Lian Zi*), 9g

Additions & subtractions: For liver depression without spleen qi vacuity, replace *Dan Zhi Xiao Yao San* with *Huo Yu Tang* (Fire Depression Decoction): Rhizoma Cimicifugae (*Sheng Ma*), 9g, Radix Bupleuri (*Chai Hu*), 9g,

Radix Puerariae (*Ge Gen*), 6g, uncooked Radix Albus Paeoniae Lactiflorae (*Bai Shao*), 6g, Radix Ledebouriellae Divaricatae (*Fang Feng*), 6g, Bulbus Allii Fistulosi (*Cong Bai*), 3g, and Radix Glycyrrhizae (*Gan Cao*), 6g. For menstrual irregularities with premenstrual head and breast pain and distention, add Rhizoma Cyperi Rotundi (*Xiang Fu*), 9g, and Pericarpium Citri Reticulatae Viride (*Qing Pi*), 9g. For severe internal heat with constipation, scanty urine, a dry mouth, and red eyes, subtract Atractylödes Macrocephala and add uncooked Radix Scutellariae Baicalensis (*Huang Qin*), 6g, and uncooked Rhizoma Anemarrhenae Asphodeloidis (*Zhi Mu*), 9g.

5. Stasis heat

Symptoms: Vexatious heat in the five hearts which worsens in the afternoon or at night, dry mouth and throat, rinsing the mouth with water but no desire to swallow it, dry, scaly skin in severe cases, dark rings around the eyes, possible fixed, stabbing pain in the head or chest, a greenish blue or purple tongue with static macules and spots, and a fine, choppy pulse

Therapeutic principles: Quicken the blood and transform stasis, clear heat and resolve depression

Acupuncture & moxibustion:

He Gu (LI 4)   Together, these points move the qi, quicken the blood,
San Yin Jiao (Sp 6) and transform stasis when needled with draining
        method.

Xue Hai (Sp 10) Together, these points nourish, quicken, and cool the
Ge Shu (Bl 17)   blood when needled with supplementing method.

Additions & subtractions: For local pain, add *a shi* points. For high fever, prick *Da Zhui* (GV 14) to bleed.

Chinese medicinal formula: Modified *Xue Fu Zhu Yu Tang* (Blood Mansion Dispel Stasis Decoction)

Ingredients: Semen Pruni Persicae (*Tao Ren*), 9g, Flos Carthami Tinctorii (*Hong Hua*), 9g, wine mix-fried Radix Angelicae Sinensis (*Dang Gui*), 9g, wine mix-fried Radix Ligustici Wallichii (*Chuan Xiong*), 9g, wine mix-fried Radix Rubrus Paeoniae Lactiflorae (*Chi Shao*), 9g, Radix Bupleuri

(*Chai Hu*), 9g, Fructus Citri Aurantii (*Zhi Ke*), 6g, Radix Cynanchi Baiwai (*Bai Wai*), 9g, wine mix-fried Radix Et Rhizoma Rhei (*Da Huang*), 6g

Additions & subtractions: For severe internal heat, add Cortex Radicis Moutan (*Dan Pi*), 9g, and Fructus Gardeniae Jasminoidis (*Zhi Zi*), 9g. For concomitant qi vacuity, add Radix Astragali Membranacei (*Huang Qi*), 15g, and rice stir-fried Radix Codonopsitis Pilosulae (*Dang Shen*), 9g.

8

Alternating Cold & Heat *(Han Re Wang Lai)*

This refers to alternating spells of fever and chills. This is different from fever and aversion to cold which occur simultaneously.

Disease causes, disease mechanisms:

1. Evils entering the shao yang

The shao yang is known as the pivot. In fact, a shao yang pattern describes a situation where evils are in two places in the body at the same time. Half the evils are located in the exterior and half are located in the interior. In other words, evils are neither entirely in the exterior nor entirely in the interior. This pattern is frequently seen in a number of febrile diseases. In the struggle between the righteous qi and evils, the battle may swing back and forth. When evils are relatively victorious, the defensive qi will be depressed and blocked. Hence the exterior is deprived of warming and chills occur. When the righteous qi is relatively victorious, heat will form leading to fever since yang added to yang engenders heat. As a result, alternating chills and fever are seen.

2. Heat entering the blood chamber

This disease mechanism is usually seen in women before, during, or after menstruation. Perimenstrually, the defensive qi is relatively weak and insecure. This is because the blood is the mother of the qi, and perimenstrually, the blood is accumulating in the uterus or, even worse, is being discharged from the body. Therefore, the defensive qi tends to be relatively vacuous and weak before, during, and after menstruation. In addition, the entire body opens during menstruation to allow the malign blood to be discharged. If external evils take advantage of this defensive qi vacuity and opening of the uterine gate to enter the body, attack the uterus, and bind with the blood, this will result in blood stasis. In addition, these evils may transform into heat whether they started as heat evils or not. As with the shao yang scenario presented above, when these evils overcome the righteous, there are chills. When the righteous overcomes these evils, there is fever since yang added to yang engenders heat.

Treatment based on pattern discrimination:

1. Evils entering the shao yang

Symptoms: Alternating fever and chills, chest and rib-side distention and pain, a bitter taste in the mouth, a dry throat, no desire to eat, heart vexation, frequent retching, nausea, possible deafness and vertigo, white or yellow tongue fur, and a bowstring pulse

Therapeutic principles: Harmonize the constructive and defensive and resolve the shao yang

Acupuncture & moxibustion:

Wai Guan (TB 5) *Qiu Xu* (GB 40) *Qi Men* (Liv 14)	Together, these points harmonize and resolve the shao yang when needled with even supplementing and draining method.
Jian Shi (Per 5) *He Gu* (LI 4)	Together, these points clear heat and eliminate vexation when needled with draining method.

Additions & subtractions: For deafness and vertigo, add *Jin Men* (GB 25) and *Ting Hui* (GB 2). For vexatious pain in the joints, add *Yang Fu* (GB 38) and *Da Shu* (Bl 11). For vomiting, add *Zhong Wan* (CV 12). For constipation, add *Zhi Gou* (TB 6) and *Shang Ju Xu* (St 37). For predominant fever, replace *Wai Guan* with *Zi Lin Qi* (GB 41).

Chinese medicinal formula: *Xiao Chai Hu Tang* (Minor Bupleurum Decoction)

Ingredients: Uncooked Radix Bupleuri (*Chai Hu*), 12g, uncooked Radix Scutellariae Baicalensis (*Huang Qin*), 9g, lime-processed Rhizoma Pinelliae Ternatae (*Ban Xia*), 9g, uncooked Radix Codonopsitis Pilosulae (*Dang Shen*), 6g, Radix Glycyrrhizae (*Gan Cao*), 6g, uncooked Rhizoma Zingiberis (*Sheng Jiang*), 3g, Fructus Zizyphi Jujubae (*Da Zao*), 4 pieces

Additions & subtractions: For severe chest and rib-side distention and pain, subtract Codonopsis and Licorice and add Fructus Citri Aurantii (*Zhi Ke*), 6g, Radix Platycodi Grandiflori (*Jie Geng*), 6g, and Pericarpium Citri Reticulatae Viride (*Qing Pi*), 6g. For frequent vomiting, fullness and pain in the stomach, constipation, and yellow tongue fur, subtract Codonopsis and Licorice and add uncooked Radix Et Rhizoma Rhei (*Da Huang*), 6g,

70

Fructus Immaturus Citri Aurantii (*Zhi Shi*), 9g, and uncooked Radix Albus Paeoniae Lactiflorae (*Bai Shao*), 9g. For damp heat with jaundice, add Herba Artemisiae Capillaris (*Yin Chen Hao*), 15g, and uncooked Fructus Gardeniae Jasminoidis (*Zhi Zi*), 9g. For severe thirst, subtract Pinellia and add Radix Trichosanthis Kirlowii (*Tian Hua Fen*), 15g. For abdominal pain, subtract Scutellaria and add Radix Albus Paeoniae Lactiflorae (*Bai Shao*), 9g.

2. External contraction of malaria evils

Symptoms: Alternating fever and chills which occur at fixed times, possibly once a day, every other day, or every third day. At the beginning, there are chills which cannot be relieved even with double quilts. Then there is high fever, vexatious thirst with a desire for lots of drinking, red lips and face, and, finally, sweating followed by a normal body temperature. The pulse is deep and bowstring during the shivering and surging, large, and rapid when there is fever. The pulse becomes normal again after sweating.[2]

Therapeutic principles: Dispel evils and eliminate malaria

Acupuncture & moxibustion:

Da Zhui (GV 14) *Hou Xi* (SI 3)	Together, these points arouse the yang and eliminate the evils when needled with draining method.
Zhong Zhu (TB 3) *Jian Shi* (Per 5)	Together, these points harmonize the constructive and defensive when needled with even supplementing and draining method.

Note: Treatment should be give 1-2 hours before the expected onset of the attack. Moxibustion after acupuncture improves its effectiveness. *Da Zhui*, *Hou Xi* and *Jian Shi* are traditional points for the treatment of malaria-like conditions.

Additions & subtractions: For splitting headache, add *Feng Chi* (GB 20) and *Tai Yang* (M-HN-5). For profuse sweating and thirst, add *Fu Liu* (Ki 7). For nausea and vomiting, add *Zhong Wan* (CV 12). For high fever, prick *Shi Xuan* (EX-UE-1) to bleed. For enduring malaria, add *Pi Shu* (Bl 21) and *Zu San Li* (St 36).

---

[2] The above are the signs and symptoms of what is called "normal malaria" in Chinese medicine. In Chinese medicine, there are a number of kinds of malaria. For more information on these, please see Nigel Wiseman & Feng Ye's *A Practical Dictionary of Chinese Medicine*, Paradigm Publications, Brookline, MA, 1998.

Chinese medicinal formula: *Zhi Nue Fang* (Treat Malaria Formula)

Ingredients: Radix Dichroae Febrifugae (*Chang Shan*), 9g, uncooked Radix Bupleuri (*Chai Hu*), 9g, Herba Artemisiae Apiacae (*Qing Hao*), 12g, Fructus Amomi Tsao-ko (*Cao Guo*), 9g, Rhizoma Anemarrhenae Asphodeloidis (*Zhi Mu*), 9g, Semen Arecae Catechu (*Bing Lang*), 6g, Radix Gentianae Macrophyllae (*Qin Jiao*), 6g, uncooked Radix Scutellariae Baicalensis (*Huang Qin*), 9g, Radix Auklandiae Lappae (*Mu Xiang*), 3g, Radix Glycyrrhizae (*Gan Cao*), 3g

Additions & subtractions: For profuse sweating and thirst, add Radix Panacis Ginseng (*Ren Shen*), 6g, Tuber Ophiopogonis Japonici (*Mai Men Dong*), 9g, and Radix Trichosanthis Kirlowii (*Tian Hua Fen*), 9g. For severe headache, add uncooked Radix Ligustici Wallichii (*Chuan Xiong*), 9g, and Radix Angelicae Dahuricae (*Bai Zhi*), 9g. For nausea and vomiting, add uncooked Pericarpium Citri Reticulatae (*Chen Pi*), 9g, ginger stir-fried Rhizoma Pinelliae Ternatae (*Ban Xia*), 9g, and Fructus Cardamomi (*Bai Dou Kou*), 6g. For crisis in summer, add Herba Elsholtziae Seu Moslae (*Xiang Ru*), 9g, and Rhizoma Coptidis Chinensis (*Huang Lian*), 6g. For crisis in winter, add Cortex Cinnamomi Cassiae (*Rou Gui*), 3g, and bland Radix Lateralis Praeparatus Aconiti Carmichaeli (*Fu Zi*), 6g. For heat malaria, add Gypsum Fibrosum (*Shi Gao*), 25g. For cold malaria, subtract Scutellaria and Anemarrhena and add Ramulus Cinnamomi Cassiae (*Gui Zhi*), 9g. For taxation malaria with qi vacuity, add Radix Astragali Membranacei (*Huang Qi*), 15g, and Radix Codonopsitis Pilosulae (*Dang Shen*), 9g. In case of blood vacuity, add Radix Angelicae Sinensis (*Dang Gui*), 9g, and Radix Albus Paeoniae Lactiflorae (*Bai Shao*), 9g.

3. Deep lying summerheat & dampness invading the shao yang

Symptoms: Alternating fever and chills, sweating does not abate the fever, thirst but drinking just a little, heart vexation, possible headache, possible sour vomiting, chest and stomach glomus and oppression, possible rib-side and abdominal distention, short voidings of dark-colored urine, red tongue edges with slimy, white fur, and a bowstring pulse

Therapeutic principles: Clear heat, transform dampness, and disinhibit the qi mechanism

Acupuncture & moxibustion:

Da Zhui (GV 14)   Together, these points clear heat when needled with
Tao Dao (GV 13)   draining method.

Qu Chi (LI 11) *Hou Xi* (SI 3)	Together, these points clear heat and prevent contrary shifting of evils to the pericardium when needled with draining method.
Zhi Gou (TB 6) *Zhong Wan* (CV 12)	Together, these points transform dampness and dis-inhibit the qi mechanism when needled with draining method.

Additions & subtractions: For nausea and vomiting, add *Nei Guan* (Per 6). For inhibited defecation, add *Tian Shu* (St 25). For loose stools, add *Gong Sun* (Sp 4).

Chinese medicinal formula: *Hao Qin Qing Dan Tang* (Artemesia Apiacea & Scutellaria Clear the Gallbladder Decoction)

Ingredients: Herba Artemisiae Apiacae (*Qing Hao*), 6g, ginger stir-fried Caulis Bambusae In Taeniis (*Zhu Ru*), 9g, ginger stir-fried Rhizoma Pinelliae Ternatae (*Ban Xia*), 6g, Sclerotium Rubrum Poriae Cocos (*Chi Fu Ling*), 9g, Radix Scutellariae Baicalensis (*Huang Qin*), 6g, Fructus Citri Aurantii (*Zhi Ke*), 6g, uncooked Pericarpium Citri Reticulatae (*Chen Pi*), 6g, Talcum (*Hua Shi*), 3g, Radix Glycyrrhizae (*Gan Cao*), 3g, Pulvis Indigonis (*Qing Dai*), 3g (Pulvis means powdered.)

Additions & subtractions: For severe vomiting, add uncooked Rhizoma Zingiberis (*Sheng Jiang*), 6g, and Flos Inulae Racemosae (*Xuan Fu Hua*), 9g. For vertigo, add uncooked Concha Haliotidis (*Shi Jue Ming*), 15g, and uncooked Radix Albus Paeoniae Lactiflorae (*Bai Shao*), 9g. For jaundice, add Tuber Curcumae (*Yu Jin*), 9g, Herba Artemisiae Capillaris (*Yin Chen Hao*), 15g, and Fructus Gardeniae Jasminoidis (*Zhi Zi*), 9g. For tinnitus or deafness, add Rhizoma Acori Graminei (*Shi Chang Pu*), 9g, and Radix Bupleuri (*Chai Hu*), 6g. For short, dark-colored urination or astringent, painful urination, add Semen Plantaginis (*Che Qian Zi*), 9g, Fructus Gardeniae Jasminoidis (*Zhi Zi*), 9g, and Rhizoma Alismatis (*Ze Xie*), 9g. For severe heat, replace with Modified *Huang Lian Wen Dan Tang* (Coptis Warm the Gallbladder Decoction): Caulis Bambusae In Taeniis (*Zhu Ru*), 9g, clear Rhizoma Pinelliae Ternatae (*Ban Xia*), 6g, Fructus Immaturus Citri Aurantii (*Zhi Shi*), 6g, Sclerotium Poriae Cocos (*Fu Ling*), 9g, Pericarpium Citri Reticulatae (*Chen Pi*), 6g, Rhizoma Coptidis Chinensis (*Huang Lian*), 6g, Radix Glycyrrhizae (*Gan Cao*), 3g, bile-processed Rhizoma Arisaematis (*Dan Nan Xing*), 6g, Radix Scutellariae Baicalensis (*Huang Qin*), 6g, and Herba Artemisiae Apiacae (*Qing Hao*), 6g.

4. Heat entering the blood chamber

Symptoms: Alternating fever and chills, hard fullness in the lower abdomen or below the chest and rib-side, clear mind during the day but delirium at night, heart vexation, headache, dizziness, dry mouth and throat, thin, yellow or dry, yellow tongue fur, and a deep and rapid, deep and replete, bowstring and rapid, or forceful pulse

Therapeutic principles: Clear the constructive and drain heat, quicken the blood and transform stasis

Acupuncture & moxibustion:

Da Dun (Liv 1) *Yin Bai* (Sp 1)	Together, these points clear the constructive and drain heat when pricked to bleed.
Zhong Ji (CV 3) *He Gu* (LI 4) *San Yin Jiao* (Sp 6)	Together, these points quicken the blood and transform stasis when needled with draining method.

Additions & subtractions: For high fever, prick *Wei Zhong* (Bl 40) and *Da Zhui* (GV 14) to bleed. For a bitter taste in the mouth, add *Yang Ling Quan* (GB 34). For vomiting, add *Nei Guan* (Per 6) and *Xia Xi* (GB 43). For profuse sweating, add *Xia Xi* (GB 43). For delirium, prick *Bai Hui* (GV 20) to bleed.

Chinese medicinal formula: Modified *Xiao Chai Hu Tang* (Minor Bupleurum Decoction)

Ingredients: Uncooked Radix Bupleuri (*Chai Hu*), 9g, uncooked Radix Scutellariae Baicalensis (*Huang Qin*), 9g, lime-processed Rhizoma Pinelliae Ternatae (*Ban Xia*), 6g, uncooked Radix Codonopsitis Pilosulae (*Dang Shen*), 6g, Radix Glycyrrhizae (*Gan Cao*), 6g, uncooked Rhizoma Zingiberis (*Sheng Jiang*), 3g, Fructus Zizyphi Jujubae (*Da Zao*), 3 pieces, Radix Salviae Miltiorrhizae (*Dan Shen*), 9g, uncooked Radix Rubrus Paeoniae Lactiflorae (*Chi Shao*), 9g, Herba Lycopi Lucidi (*Ze Lan*), 9g.

Additions & subtractions: For severe heat, subtract Codonopsis and add Fructus Gardeniae Jasminoidis (*Zhi Zi*), 9g. For severe dryness, subtract Codonopsis and add uncooked Radix Rehmanniae (*Sheng Di*), 15g

9

Absence of Sweating *(Wu Han)*

This refers to absence of sweating when external evils invade the exterior and negatively affect the normal opening and closing of the pores.

Disease causes, disease mechanisms:

If external cold evils enter the body and fetter the exterior, they will typically result in absence of sweating. Commonly, external cold combines with either wind or dampness. In either case, cold is a yin evil which causes contracture and constriction. When wind cold or cold damp evils invade the body, as long as cold is predominant, they typically first fetter the exterior. This is because cold contracts and constricts the interstices. If the exterior is fettered, the defensive qi will become depressed and will not be able to perform its functions. One of its functions is to open and close the pores. With cold constricting the interstices and the defensive dysfunctional, there is absence of sweating.

Treatment based on pattern discrimination:

1. Wind cold invasion with exterior repletion

Symptoms: Absence of sweating, aversion to cold, fever, headache, body aches, nasal congestion, heaviness of the body, sneezing, nasal discharge, itchy throat, thin, white tongue fur, and a floating, tight pulse

Therapeutic principles: Resolve the exterior and promote sweating

Acupuncture & moxibustion:

Feng Men (Bl 12)	Together, these points arouse yang and course
Da Zhui (GV 14)	and resolve the evils in the exterior when needled
Feng Chi (GB 20)	with draining method.

He Gu (LI 4)	Together, these points promote sweating when draining
Fu Liu (Ki 7)	*He Gu* and supplementing *Fu Liu*.

Additions & subtractions: For coughing, add *Fei Shu* (Bl 13). If fever does not abate, add *Qu Chi* (LI 11) and *Zhi Gou* (TB 6). For severe headache, add *Feng Chi* (GB 20).

Chinese medicinal formula: *Ma Huang Tang* (Ephedra Decoction)

Ingredients: Uncooked Herba Ephedrae (*Ma Huang*), 9g, uncooked Ramulus Cinnamomi Cassiae (*Gui Zhi*), 6g, Semen Pruni Armeniacae (*Xing Ren*), 12g, Radix Glycyrrhizae (*Gan Cao*), 3g

Remarks: *Ma Huang Tang*'s diaphoretic action is enhanced when followed by fresh ginger and rice congee. Then the patient should go to bed and cover themselves with blankets to induce sweating.

2. Exterior cold & interior heat

Symptoms: Absence of sweating, fever and aversion to cold, vexatious pain in the limbs, nasal congestion, a husky voice, vexatious thirst, coughing of yellow phlegm, dark-colored urine, white or thin, yellow tongue fur, and a floating, rapid pulse

Therapeutic principles: Course wind, dispel cold, and clear heat

Acupuncture & moxibustion:

Feng Men (Bl 12)	Together, these points course wind, scatter cold,
Wai Guan (TB 5)	and promote sweating when needled with
He Gu (LI 4)	draining method.
Jian Shi (Per 5)	Together, these points clear heat when needled
Nei Ting (St 44)	with draining method.

Additions & subtractions: For sore throat, prick *Shao Shang* (Lu 11) to bleed. For constipation, add *Shang Ju Xu* (St 37) and *Zhi Gou* (TB 6). For headache, add *Feng Chi* (GB 20). For body aches, add *Shen Zhu* (GV 12).

Chinese medicinal formula: *Da Qing Long Tang* (Major Blue Dragon Decoction)

Ingredients: Uncooked Herba Ephedrae (*Ma Huang*), 9g, Ramulus Cinnamomi Cassiae (*Gui Zhi*), 6g, mix-fried Radix Glycyrrhizae (*Zhi Gan Cao*), 6g, Semen Pruni Armeniacae (*Xing Ren*), 6g, Gypsum Fibrosum (*Shi Gao*),

20g, uncooked Rhizoma Zingiberis (*Sheng Jiang*), 3g, Fructus Zizyphi Jujubae (*Da Zao*), 2 pieces

3. Cold dampness fettering the exterior

Symptoms: Absence of sweating, head distention as if the head were wrapped by a band, encumbered, heavy limbs, vexatious pain in the joints, fear of cold, slight fever which gets worse in the afternoon, white, slimy tongue fur, and a floating, tight or slow pulse

Therapeutic principles: Scatter cold and eliminate dampness

Acupuncture & moxibustion:

Feng Chi (GB 20) *Wai Guan* (TB 5) *He Gu* (LI 4)	Together, these points scatter cold, promote sweating, and resolve the exterior when needled with draining method.
Zu San Li (St 36) *Yin Ling Quan* (Sp 9)	Together, these points harmonize the center and transform dampness when needled with draining method.

Additions & subtractions: For loose stools, add *Tian Shu* (St 25). For stomachache, add *Zhong Wan* (CV 12). For abdominal distention, add *Gong Sun* (Sp 4).

Chinese medicinal formula: *Qiang Huo Sheng Shi Tang* (Notopterygium Overcome Dampness Decoction)

Ingredients: Radix Et Rhizoma Notopterygii (*Qiang Huo*), 9g, Radix Angelicae Pubescentis (*Du Huo*), 9g, Radix Et Rhizoma Ligustici Chinensis (*Gao Ben*), 6g, Radix Ledebouriellae Divaricatae (*Fang Feng*), 6g, Radix Ligustici Wallichii (*Chuan Xiong*), 6g, Fructus Viticis (*Man Jing Zi*), 6g, Radix Glycyrrhizae (*Gan Cao*), 3g

10
Shivering & Sweating *(Zhan Han)*

This refers to sweating immediately after shivering in an externally contracted febrile disease.

Disease causes, disease mechanisms:

Shivering and sweating is usually seen in externally contracted febrile disease where the invading evils (commonly cold and epidemic pestilential qi) fight with the righteous qi in the exterior or qi levels. In response to the presence of evils in the exterior, the defensive qi rushes to the exterior to combat these evils. This means that the defensive qi, which already is described as being violent or rash in nature, rushes even more forcefully into battle. One of the functions of qi is to move and stir. Therefore, rushing defensive qi results in shivering. If the righteous qi wins this battle, the defensive qi then opens the pores and expels the evils along with sweat. This is because qi moves body fluids. As the defensive qi out-thrusts the evils, it also moves some of the body's fluids outside the body. Therefore, shivering and then sweating occur.

Treatment based on pattern discrimination:

1. Tai yang pattern yet to be resolved

Symptoms: Fever, aversion to cold, aching limbs, thin, white tongue fur, and a floating, rapid, forceless pulse are followed by shivering. Uninhibited sweating after the shivering will dispel the evils and result in a cure, but inhibited sweating will fail to dispel the evils and thus requires further treatment.

Therapeutic principles: Harmonize the constructive and defensive, resolve the flesh and diffuse the exterior

Acupuncture & moxibustion:

Wai Guan (TB 5)
He Gu (LI 4)
Together, these points resolve the flesh and diffuse the exterior when needled with draining method.

Feng Men (Bl 12) *Zu San Li* (St 36)	Together, these points arouse yang, help the righteous qi, and harmonize the constructive and defensive qi when needled with even draining and supplementing method.

Additions & subtractions: For headache, add *Tai Yang* (M-HN-5). For fever not yet abated, add *Da Zhui* (GV 14). For sore throat, prick *Shao Shang* (Lü 11) to bleed.

Chinese medicinal formula: *Gui Zhi Tang* (Cinnamon Twig Decoction)

Ingredients: Uncooked Ramulus Cinnamomi Cassiae (*Gui Zhi*), 9g, uncooked Radix Albus Paeoniae Lactiflorae (*Bai Shao*), 9g, mix-fried Radix Glycyrrhizae (*Zhi Gan Cao*), 6g, uncooked Rhizoma Zingiberis (*Sheng Jiang*), 9g, Fructus Zizyphi Jujubae (*Da Zao*), 3 pieces

Note: As with *Ma Huang Tang* above, the diaphoretic action of *Gui Zhi Tang* is much better when followed by fresh ginger and rice congee, etc.

2. Epidemic pestilential evils remaining in the qi division yet to be resolved

Symptoms: High fever, aversion to heat, vexatious thirst with possible desire to drink, yellow tongue fur, and a surging, large pulse followed by shivering. If the shivering leads to a calm pulse and cool body, it means that the evils have been dispelled. If there is still fever after shivering and sweating, it means that the evils remain in the channels and further treatment is needed.

Therapeutic principles: Resolve the exterior and clear heat

Acupuncture & moxibustion:

Da Zhui (GV 14) *He Gu* (LI 4) *Wai Guan* (TB 5) *Qu Chi* (LI 11)	Together, these points resolve the exterior and clear heat when needled with draining method.
Zu San Li (St 36) *San Yin Jiao* (Sp 6)	Together, these points boost the qi and support the righteous when needled with supplementing method.

Additions & subtractions: For coughing, add *Chi Ze* (Lu 5). For constipation, add *Tian Shu* (St 25). For sore throat, prick *Shang Yang* (LI 1) to bleed.

Chinese medicinal formula: *Chai Hu Qing Zao Tang* (Bupleurum Clear Dryness Decoction)

Ingredients: Uncooked Radix Bupleuri (*Chai Hu*), 9g, uncooked Radix Scutellariae Baicalensis (*Huang Qin*), 9g, uncooked Rhizoma Anemarrhenae Asphodeloidis (*Zhi Mu*), 9g, Radix Trichosanthis Kirlowii (*Tian Hua Fen*), 12g, Pericarpium Citri Reticulatae (*Chen Pi*), 3g, Radix Glycyrrhizae (*Gan Cao*), 3g, uncooked Rhizoma Zingiberis (*Sheng Jiang*), 6g, Fructus Zizyphi Jujubae (*Da Zao*), 3 pieces

11
Spontaneous Perspiration *(Zi Han)*

This refers to spontaneous sweating not due to either exertion, hot surroundings, heavy clothing, or administration of diaphoretic medicinals. Spontaneous perspiration during menopause is not included here. For that, please refer to "Hot Flashes in the Head & Face" in Volume 1 and "Night Sweats" in the present volume.

Disease causes, disease mechanisms:

1. Disharmony between the constructive & defensive qi

Disharmony between the constructive and defensive is usually due to external contraction of wind evils. Wind is a yang evil which is opening and discharging by nature. The defensive qi is responsible for securing the interstices. When wind evils invade the exterior of the body, the defensive qi becomes depressed and cannot flow to the exterior. One of the functions of the defensive qi is the opening and closing of the pores. If the defensive qi cannot reach the exterior, it will not be able to open or close the pores properly and secure the exterior. Hence the interstices become loose, the pores open, and spontaneous perspiration occurs.

2. Summerheat damage

This pattern is often seen in summer when summerheat is predominant. Summerheat is a yang evil which is hot by nature. Heat causes relaxation of the skin, and this relaxation of the skin gives rise to loose interstices. In addition, heat can force the fluids to move outside the body. Therefore, contraction of summerheat often leads to spontaneous perspiration.

3. Flaming heat in the yang ming

Flaming heat in the yang ming usually develops from contraction of external evils which are not resolved but rather shift into the interior where they transform into heat. On one hand, exuberant yang causes frenetic movement leading to the opening of the pores. On the other hand, flaming heat forces body fluids outside the body. Therefore, there will be spontaneous perspiration.

4. Damp heat depressed & steaming

Damp heat usually arises from external contraction of damp heat evils, external contraction of cold dampness which transforms into heat over time, or from excessive consumption of fried, greasy, sweet foods or alcohol which ferment dampness and engender heat. Dampness is a yin evil which is sticky and stagnant by nature. Therefore, it obstructs the flow of the defensive yang to the exterior, thus causing the exterior to be insecure and the interstices loose. On the other hand, heat is a yang evil which is hot and diffusing by nature and forces the fluids outside the body. Therefore, the combination of these two mechanisms can easily lead to spontaneous perspiration.

5. Qi vacuity

Qi vacuity may be due to enduring disease, overwork taxation, excessive thinking, or aging. One of the five functions of the qi is to secure and constrain. Therefore, if, for any reason, the qi becomes vacuous and weak, it may fail to constrain the interstices and secure the exterior, and spontaneous perspiration may occur.

6. Yang vacuity

Yang vacuity usually develops from enduring disease, overwork taxation, constitutional insufficiency, or aging. Yang is nothing other than a lot of qi. In other words, yang vacuity always includes qi vacuity. As we have explained above, if qi becomes vacuous, it may not secure the exterior and close the pores. Hence, spontaneous perspiration may also be seen in yang vacuity patterns.

7. Water rheum

Water rheum usually results from vacuity of the spleen, lungs, and/or kidneys. If the spleen becomes vacuous, it cannot move and transform water dampness. If the lungs become vacuous, they cannot distribute fluids. And if the kidneys become vacuous, they cannot warm and transform water dampness. Any of these may lead to internal accumulation of water rheum. The heart is located in the clear and spacious cavity above. When water rheum accumulates in this cavity, it may trap heart yang leading to inhibited qi and blood flow. This results in insufficient nourishment to the heart. When the heart is vacuous, it cannot restrain its humor, *i.e.*, sweat, and spontaneous perspiration occurs.

Treatment based on pattern discrimination:

I. Disharmony between the constructive & defensive qi

Symptoms: A small amount of sweating, aversion to wind, slight fever, body aches, headache, nasal congestion, nasal discharge, thin, white tongue fur, and a floating, moderate (*i.e.*, slightly slow) pulse

Therapeutic principles: Harmonize the constructive and defensive qi

Acupuncture & moxibustion:

Da Zhui (GV 14) *Feng Men* (Bl 12)	Together, these points arouse yang, course wind, and scatter cold when needled with draining method.
Wai Guan (TB 5) *He Gu* (LI 4) *Jian Shi* (Per 5)	Together, these points resolve the exterior and harmonize the constructive and defensive when needled with draining method.

Additions & subtractions: For dry retching, add *Zhong Wan* (CV 12). For headache, add *Feng Chi* (GB 20).

Chinese medicinal formula: *Gui Zhi Tang* (Cinnamon Twig Decoction)

Ingredients: Uncooked Ramulus Cinnamomi Cassiae (*Gui Zhi*), 9g, uncooked Radix Albus Paeoniae Lactiflorae (*Bai Shao*), 9g, mix-fried Radix Glycyrrhizae (*Gan Cao*), 6g, uncooked Rhizoma Zingiberis (*Sheng Jiang*), 3g, Fructus Zizyphi Jujubae (*Da Zao*), 3 pieces

Additions & subtractions: For coughing and/or panting, add ginger mix-fried Cortex Magnoliae Officinalis (*Hou Po*), 9g, and Semen Pruni Armeniacae (*Xing Ren*), 9g. For severe body aches, add uncooked Radix Puerariae (*Ge Gen*), 9g. For incessant sweating, add Radix Lateralis Praeparatus Aconiti Carmichaeli (*Fu Zi*), 6g.

2. Externally invading wind heat

Symptoms: Inhibited sweating, slight aversion to wind and cold, persistent fever that is not abated by sweating, headache, a red, painful, possibly swollen throat, a dry mouth with slight thirst, coughing, a red tongue tip with thin, yellow fur, and a floating, rapid pulse

Therapeutic principles: Course wind and clear heat

Acupuncture & moxibustion:

Da Zhui (GV 14) *He Gu* (LI 4) *Wai Guan* (TB 5)	Together, these points course wind, clear heat, and resolve the exterior when needled with draining method.
Chi Ze (Lu 5)	Clears lung heat and stops coughing when needled with draining method

Additions & subtractions: For high fever, add *Qu Chi* (LI 11). For thirst, add *Fu Liu* (Ki 7). For sore throat, prick *Shao Shang* (Lu 11) to bleed. For symptoms due to heat toxins, prick *Shi Xuan* (EX-UE-1). For coughing with profuse phlegm, add *Fei Shu* (Bl 13).

Chinese medicinal formula: Modified *Sang Ju Yin* (Morus & Chrysanthemum Drink)

Ingredients: Uncooked Folium Mori Albi (*Sang Ye*), 9g, uncooked Flos Chrysanthemi Morifolii (*Ju Hua*), 9g, Herba Menthae Haplocalycis (*Bo He*), 3g, Semen Pruni Armeniacae (*Xing Ren*), 9g, uncooked Fructus Forsythiae Suspensae (*Lian Qiao*), 9g, uncooked Radix Platycodi Grandiflori (*Jie Geng*), 6g, Rhizoma Phragmitis Communis (*Lu Gen*), 6g, Radix Glycyrrhizae (*Gan Cao*), 6g, Herba Schizonepetae Tenuifoliae (*Jing Jie*), 9g

Additions & subtractions: For sore throat, add Fructus Arctii Lappae (*Niu Bang Zi*), 9g, and Radix Isatidis Seu Baphicacanthi (*Ban Lan Gen*), 9g. For coughing, add Folium Eriobotryae Japonicae (*Pi Pa Ye*), 9g, and Radix Peucedani (*Qian Hu*), 9g. For severe thirst with a red tongue and scanty fur, add uncooked Rhizoma Polygonati Odorati (*Yu Zhu*), 9g, and Radix Trichosanthis Kirlowii (*Tian Hua Fen*), 9g. For headache, add Fructus Viticis (*Man Jing Zi*), 9g. For severe aversion to wind and cold, add Radix Ledebouriellae Divaricatae (*Fang Feng*), 9g. For high fever, add uncooked Rhizoma Anemarrhenae Asphodeloidis (*Zhi Mu*), 15g, and uncooked Radix Scutellariae Baicalensis (*Huang Qin*), 6g.

3. Wind dampness damaging the exterior

Symptoms: Off and on sweating which is not profuse but is more severe on the palms and forehead, aversion to wind and cold, heavy, numb limbs, thirst with no thought of drinking, dizziness, tinnitus, scanty urination, thin, white tongue fur, and a floating, moderate (*i.e.*, slightly slow) pulse

Therapeutic principles: Dispel wind and overcome dampness

Acupuncture & moxibustion:

Feng Men (Bl 12)	Together, these points course wind and resolve
Wai Guan (TB 5)	the exterior when needled with draining method.
He Gu (LI 4)	Together, these points boost the qi, transform
Zu San Li (St 36)	dampness, and secure the exterior when needled
	with supplementing method.

Additions & subtractions: For headache which feels as if the head were swathed or tied with a band, add *Feng Chi* (GB 20). For chest oppression, add *Dan Zhong* (CV 17) and *Yin Ling Quan* (Sp 9).

Chinese medicinal formula: *Fang Ji Huang Qi Tang* (Stephania & Astragalus Decoction)

Ingredients: Radix Stephaniae Tetrandrae (*Han Fang Ji*), 12g, uncooked Radix Astragali Membranacei (*Huang Qi*), 15g, uncooked Rhizoma Atractylodis Macrocephalae (*Bai Zhu*), 9g, uncooked Rhizoma Zingiberis (*Sheng Jiang*), 3g, Fructus Zizyphi Jujubae (*Da Zao*), 3 pieces

Additions & subtractions: For severe heaviness and numbness of the limbs, add Rhizoma Atractylodis (*Cang Zhu*), 9g, and Radix Et Rhizoma Notopterygii (*Qiang Huo*), 9g. For severe aversion to wind, add Radix Ledebouriellae Divaricatae (*Fang Feng*), 9g, and Radix Et Rhizoma Notopterygii (*Qiang Huo*), 9g. For edema in the limbs, add stir-fried Ramulus Cinnamomi Cassiae (*Gui Zhi*), 9g, and Sclerotium Poriae Cocos (*Fu Ling*), 12g. For inhibited urination, add Sclerotium Poriae Cocos (*Fu Ling*), 9g, and Rhizoma Alismatis (*Ze Xie*), 9g.

4. Summerheat damage

Symptoms: Profuse, incessant sweating, great thirst with a liking for profuse drinking, fever, chest and diaphragmatic glomus and oppression, heart vexation, shortness of breath, fatigue, a red tongue with dry, yellow fur, and a floating, large, forceless pulse

Therapeutic principles: Clear summerheat and drain heat, boost the qi and engender liquids

Acupuncture & moxibustion:

Da Zhui (GV 14) *Qu Chi* (LI 11) *Nei Ting* (St 44)	Together, these points clear summerheat and drain heat when needled with draining method.
He Gu (LI 4) *Fu Liu* (Ki 7)	Together, these points boost the qi and engender liquids when needled with supplementing method.

Additions & subtractions: For heart vexation, add *Nei Guan* (Per 6). For nausea and stomach glomus, add *Zhong Wan* (CV 12). For heavy-headedness and distention and pain in the head, add *Feng Chi* (GB 20) and *Bai Hui* (GV 20).

Chinese medicinal formula: Modified *Qing Shu Yi Qi Tang* (Clear Summerheat & Boost the Qi Decoction)

Ingredients: Radix Panacis Quinquefolii (*Xi Yang Shen*), 6g, Herba Dendrobii (*Shi Hu*), 12g, Tuber Ophiopogonis Japonici (*Mai Men Dong*), 9g, Rhizoma Coptidis Chinensis (*Huang Lian*), 3g, Folium Bambusae (*Zhu Ye*), 6g, Folium Nelumbinis Nuciferae (*He Ye*), 9g, uncooked Rhizoma Anemarrhenae Asphodeloidis (*Zhi Mu*), 9g, Semen Oryzae Sativae (*Geng Mi*), 12g, Pericarpium Citrulli Vulgaris (*Xi Gua Pi*), 24g, Radix Glycyrrhizae (*Gan Cao*), 3g

Additions & subtractions: For a slight summerheat pattern, subtract Coptis and Anemarrhena. For severe heat, add uncooked Gypsum Fibrosum (*Shi Gao*), 24g. For severely damaged qi, add uncooked Fructus Schisandrae Chinensis (*Wu Wei Zi*), 9g. For severely damaged fluids, add Radix Glehniae Littoralis (*Sha Shen*), 15g, and uncooked Radix Rehmanniae (*Sheng Di*), 15g. For fatigue, reduced food intake, loose stools, and abdominal fullness, subtract Ophiopogon, Anemarrhena, Coptis, and Citrullus and add uncooked Radix Astragali Membranacei (*Huang Qi*), 12g, bran stir-fried Rhizoma Atractylodis Macrocephalae (*Bai Zhu*), 9g, and stir-fried Pericarpium Citri Reticulatae (*Chen Pi*), 9g.

5. Flaming heat in the yang ming

Symptoms: Extremely profuse perspiration, high fever, aversion to heat, a red facial complexion, vexatious thirst with a liking for profuse drinking, a red or crimson tongue with dry, yellow fur, and a surging, large, forceful pulse

Therapeutic principles: Clear heat and drain fire

Acupuncture & moxibustion:

Da Zhui (GV 14) Together, these points clear heat and drain fire
Qu Chi (LI 11) when needled with draining method.
Nei Ting (St 44)
Jie Xi (St 41)

Additions & subtractions: For severe pain in the forehead, add *Yin Tang* (M-HN-3) and *Tou Wei* (St 8). For enduring high fever, prick *Wei Zhong* (Bl 40) to bleed. For constipation, add *Zhi Gou* (TB 6) and *Shang Ju Xu* (St 37).

Chinese medicinal formula: *Bai Hu Tang* (White Tiger Decoction)

Ingredients: Uncooked Gypsum Fibrosum (*Shi Gao*), 30g, uncooked Rhizoma Anemarrhenae Asphodeloidis (*Zhi Mu*), 12g, Radix Glycyrrhizae (*Gan Cao*), 6g, Semen Oryzae Sativae (*Geng Mi*), 15g

Additions & subtractions: For high fever, increase the dosage of Gypsum to 30-60g. For great fever and great sweating damaging the qi and yin, add white Radix Panacis Ginseng (*Ren Shen*), 6g, or Radix Panacis Quinguifolii (*Xi Yang Shen*), 6g, and Tuber Ophiopogonis Japonici (*Mai Men Dong*), 9g, and uncooked Fructus Schisandrae Chinensis (*Wu Wei Zi*), 9g. For severe thirst, add Radix Trichosanthis Kirlowii (*Tian Hua Fen*), 9g, and Rhizoma Phragmitis Communis (*Lu Gen*), 9g.

6. Damp heat depressed & steaming

Symptoms: Slight sweating, inhibited, sticky perspiration, tidal hectic fever in the afternoon which does not abate with sweating, thirst with no desire for drinking, chest oppression, stomach glomus, nausea, heavy or painful body, possible heavy, painful joints, possible edema, torpid intake, short voidings of red urine, loose stools which are difficult to defecate, slimy, white tongue fur, and a bowstring, slippery, rapid pulse

Therapeutic principles: Clear and disinhibit dampness and heat

Acupuncture & moxibustion:

Yin Ling Quan (Sp 9)
San Yin Jiao (Sp 6)
Yang Ling Quan (GB 34)
Nei Ting (St 44)
Zhong Wan (CV 12)

Together, these points clear heat and transform dampness when needled with draining method.

Chinese medicinal formula: *San Ren Tang* (Three Seeds Decoction)

Ingredients: Semen Pruni Armeniacae (*Xing Ren*), 9g, Fructus Cardamomi (*Bai Dou Kou*), 6g, Semen Coicis Lachryma-jobi (*Yi Yi Ren*), 18g, Talcum (*Hua Shi*), 18g, Medulla Tetrapanacis Papyriferi (*Tong Cao*), 6g, Folium Bambusae (*Zhu Ye*), 6g, ginger mix-fried Cortex Magnoliae Officinalis (*Hou Po*), 6g, ginger-processed Rhizoma Pinelliae Ternatae (*Ban Xia*), 9g

Additions & subtractions: For severe damp heat, add Rhizoma Coptidis Chinensis (*Huang Lian*), 6g, Radix Scutellariae Baicalensis (*Huang Qin*), 6g, and Fructus Gardeniae Jasminoidis (*Zhi Zi*), 6g. For fever with aversion to cold and headache, add Herba Agastachis Seu Pogostemi (*Huo Xiang*), 9g, Herba Eupatorei Fortunei (*Pei Lan*), 9g, and warm Semen Praeparatus Sojae (*Dan Dou Chi*), 9g. For reduced appetite, add Rhizoma Acori Graminei (*Shi Chang Pu*), 9g. For inhibited defecation of loose stools, add Fructus Immaturus Citri Aurantii (*Zhi Shi*), 12g. For inhibited urination, add Rhizoma Alismatis (*Ze Xie*), 9g, Semen Plantaginis (*Che Qian Zi*), 9g, and Cortex Sclerotii Poriae Cocos (*Fu Ling Pi*), 9g. For sliminess and a bland taste in the mouth, add Herba Agastachis Seu Pogostemi (*Huo Xiang*), 6g, and Herba Eupatorei Fortunei (*Pei Lan*), 9g. For nausea and vomiting, add ginger mix-fried Caulis Bambusae In Taeniis (*Zhu Ru*), 9g, and Herba Agastachis Seu Pogostemi (*Huo Xiang*), 9g.

7. Qi vacuity

Symptoms: Frequent spontaneous perspiration which gets worse on exertion, fear of cold, fatigue, shortage of qi with laziness to speak, possible low-grade fever, thirst with a liking for warm beverages, a bright white facial complexion, susceptibility to invasion by wind cold, a pale tongue with thin, white fur, and a moderate (*i.e.*, slightly slow), forceless pulse

Therapeutic principles: Boost the qi and secure the exterior

Acupuncture & moxibustion:

Qi Hai (CV 6)
Dan Zhong (CV 17)
Zu San Li (St 36)
He Gu (LI 4)

Together, these points boost the qi and secure the exterior when needled with supplementing method.

Additions & subtractions: For heart palpitations and shortage of qi, add *Xin Shu* (Bl 15). For fatigued limbs and lack of strength, fullness in the abdomen, and loose stools, add *Pi Shu* (Bl 20). For coughing with clear, thin phlegm, add *Fei Shu* (Bl 13).

Chinese medicinal formula: *Bu Zhong Yi Qi Tang* (Supplement the Center & Boost the Qi Decoction)

Ingredients: Uncooked mix-fried Radix Astragali Membranacei (*Huang Qi*), 18g, honey stir-fried Radix Codonopsis Pilosulae (*Dang Shen*), 12g, bran stir-fried Rhizoma Atractylodis Macrocephalae (*Bai Zhu*), 12g, honey mix-fried Radix Glycyrrhizae (*Gan Cao*), 6g, stir-fried Radix Angelicae Sinensis (*Dang Gui*), 6g, stir-fried Pericarpium Citri Reticulatae (*Chen Pi*), 6g, Radix Bupleuri (*Chai Hu*), 3g, Rhizoma Cimicifugae (*Sheng Ma*), 3g

Additions & subtractions: For severe sweating, subtract Bupleurum and Cimicifuga and add Radix Ephedrae (*Ma Huang Gen*), 9g, Fructus Levis Tritici Aestivi (*Fu Xiao Mai*), 9g, and Fructus Schisandrae Chinensis (*Wu Wei Zi*), 9g. For reduced food intake, eructation, and stomach fullness after eating, add stir-fried Fructus Germinatus Hordei Vulgaris (*Mai Ya*), 6g, stir-fried Massa Medica Fermentata (*Shen Qu*), 6g, and stir-fried Fructus Crataegi (*Shan Zha*), 6g. For severe qi vacuity, replace Codonopsis with Radix Panacis Ginseng (*Ren Shen*), 6g. For constitutional insufficiency with susceptibility to invasion by wind cold, add *Yu Ping Feng San* (Jade Windscreen Powder), *i.e.*, uncooked Radix Astragali Membranacei (*Huang Qi*), 24g, Rhizoma Atractylodis Macrocephalae (*Bai Zhu*), 15g, and Radix Ledebouriellae Divaricatae (*Fang Feng*), 9g. For concomitant blood vacuity with heart palpitations, a white, lusterless facial complexion, pale lips and fingers and a fine pulse, replace *Bu Zhong Yi Qi Tang* with Modified *Ba Zhen Tang* (Eight Pearls Decoction): cooked Radix Rehmanniae (*Shu Di*), 18g, Radix Albus Paeoniae Lactiflorae (*Bai Shao*),

9g, wine mix-fried Radix Angelicae Sinensis (*Dang Gui*), 9g, wine mix-fried Radix Ligustici Wallichii (*Chuan Xiong*), 6g, Radix Codonopsitis Pilosulae (*Dang Shen*), 9g, bran stir-fried Rhizoma Atractylodis

Macrocephalae (*Bai Zhu*), 9g, Sclerotium Poriae Cocos (*Fu Ling*), 9g, mix-fried Radix Glycyrrhizae (*Gan Cao*), 6g, and uncooked Radix Astragali Membranacei (*Huang Qi*), 15g. For concomitant heart blood vacuity with insomnia, easy fright, mental depression, and profuse dreams, replace *Bu Zhong Yi Qi Tang* with *Ren Shen Yang Rong Tang* (Ginseng Nourish the Constructive Decoction): Radix Codonopsitis Pilosulae (*Dang Shen*), 9g, uncooked Radix Astragali Membranacei (*Huang Qi*), 18g, uncooked Radix Albus Paeoniae Lactiflorae (*Bai Shao*), 15g, Radix Angelicae Sinensis (*Dang Gui*), 9g, stir-fried Pericarpium Citri Reticulatae (*Chen Pi*), 6g, Cortex Cinnamomi Cassiae (*Rou Gui*), 3g, stir-fried Rhizoma Atractylodis Macrocephalae (*Bai Zhu*), 15g, cooked Radix Rehmanniae (*Shu Di*), 9g, Fructus Schisandrae Chinensis (*Wu Wei Zi*), 9g, licorice-processed Radix Polygalae Tenuifoliae (*Yuan Zhi*), 6g, Sclerotium Pararadicis Poriae Cocos (*Fu Shen*), 9g, and mix-fried Radix Glycyrrhizae (*Gan Cao*), 6g.

8. Yang vacuity

Symptoms: Spontaneous perspiration which gets worse on exertion, cold body and limbs, reduced food intake, abdominal distention, a liking for hot drinks, loose stools, a bright white facial complexion, a pale tongue with white fur, and a vacuous, weak pulse

Therapeutic principles: Warm yang and constrain yin

Acupuncture & moxibustion:

He Gu (LI 4)	Together, these points warm yang and constrain
Zu San Li (St 36)	yin when moxaed.
Guan Yuan (CV 4)	Together, these points warm yang and constrain
Qi Hai (CV 6)	yin when moxaed.

Additions & subtractions: For cold sweating, heart palpitations, and chilled limbs, add *Ju Que* (CV 14) and *Nei Guan* (Per 6). For panting, add *Tian Tu* (CV 22). For chest pain, add *Jiu Wei* (CV 15). For daybreak diarrhea, moxa *Ming Men* (GV 4). For pain in the lower abdomen, moxa *Zhong Ji* (CV 3).

Chinese medicinal formulas: For spleen yang vacuity: Modified *Zheng Yuan Tang* (Correct the Origin Decoction)

Ingredients: Mix-fried Radix Astragali Membranacei (*Huang Qi*), 18g, honey stir-fried Radix Codonopsis Pilosulae (*Dang Shen*), 12g, bran stir-fried

Rhizoma Atractylodis Macrocephalae (*Bai Zhu*), 12g, stir-fried Pericarpium Citri Reticulatae (*Chen Pi*), 6g, stir-fried Radix Dioscoreae Oppositae (*Shan Yao*), 9g, Cortex Cinnamomi Cassiae (*Rou Gui*), 3g, bland Radix Lateralis Praeparatus Aconiti Carmichaeli (*Fu Zi*), 6g, dry Rhizoma Zingiberis (*Gan Jiang*), 6g, honey mix-fried Radix Glycyrrhizae (*Gan Cao*), 6g

For kidney yang vacuity: Modified *You Gui Wan* (Restore the Right [Kidney] Pills)

Ingredients: Cooked Radix Rehmanniae (*Shu Di*), 9g, stir-fried Radix Dioscoreae Oppositae (*Shan Yao*), 9g, steamed Fructus Corni Officinalis (*Shan Zhu Yu*), 12g, stir-fried Semen Cuscutae Chinensis (*Tu Si Zi*), 9g, salt stir-fried Cortex Eucommiae Ulmoidis (*Du Zhong*), 9g, Radix Lateralis Praeparatus Aconiti Carmichaeli (*Fu Zi*), 6g, Cortex Cinnamomi Cassiae (*Rou Gui*), 3g, Gelatinum Cornu Cervi (*Lu Jiao Jiao*), 6g, wine-steamed Fructus Schisandrae Chinensis (*Wu Wei Zi*), 15g

Additions & subtractions: For low back pain, add salt stir-fried Cortex Eucommiae Ulmoidis (*Du Zhong*), 9g. For enduring yang vacuity with enduring spontaneous perspiration leading to yin vacuity, replace *You Gui Wan* with Modified *Zuo Gui Wan* (Restore the Left [Kidney] Pills): cooked Radix Rehmanniae (*Shu Di*), 18g, stir-fried Radix Dioscoreae Oppositae (*Shan Yao*), 12g, steamed Fructus Corni Officinalis (*Shan Zhu Yu*), 15g, Fructus Lycii Chinensis (*Gou Qi*), 9g, Radix Achyranthis Bidentatae (*Niu Xi*), 9g, Semen Cuscutae Chinensis (*Tu Si Zi*), 9g, Gelatinum Cornu Cervi (*Lu Jiao Jiao*), 6g, Gelatinum Plastri Testudinis (*Gui Ban Jiao*), 6g, salt mix-fried Cortex Phellodendri (*Huang Bai*), 9g, and salt mix-fried Rhizoma Anemarrhenae Asphodeloidis (*Zhi Mu*), 9g.

9. Water rheum

Symptoms: Spontaneous perspiration, usually in small amounts, heart palpitations, dizziness, nausea, chest and epigastric fullness and glomus, shortness of breath, sometimes cold body and limbs, lassitude of the spirit, loose stools, reduced food intake, a pale tongue with a white, slimy fur, and a bowstring, slippery pulse

Note: This pattern is often seen in those with cardiovascular disease accompanied by high blood pressure and heart palpitations.

Therapeutic principles: Transform phlegm and quiet the heart

Acupuncture & moxibustion:

Feng Long (St 40) *Yin Ling Quan* (Sp 9) *Zu San Li* (St 36)	Together, these points dry dampness and transform phlegm.
Nei Guan (Per 6)	Quiets the heart and harmonizes the center
Xin Shu (Bl 15)	Supplements the heart and quiets the spirit

Additions & subtractions: For lung vacuity, add *Fei Shu* (Bl 13). For kidney vacuity, add *Shen Shu* (Ki 23). For abdominal pain, borborygmus, and diarrhea, moxa *Ming Men* (GV 4). For frequent heart palpitations, add *Ju Que* (CV 14). For severe dizziness, add *Qu Chi* (LI 11). When *Qu Chi* is combined with *Zu San Li*, it is a special combination for treating high blood pressure.

Chinese medicinal formula: *Shi Wei Wen Dan Tang* (Ten Flavors Warm the Gallbladder Decoction)

Ingredients: Lime-processed Rhizoma Pinelliae Ternatae (*Ban Xia*), 9g, Fructus Immaturus Aurantii (*Zhi Shi*), 6g, Sclerotium Poriae Cocos (*Fu Ling*), 9g, uncooked Pericarpium Citri Reticulatae (*Chen Pi*), 9g, stir-fried Semen Zizyphi Spinosae (*Suan Zao Ren*), 6g, processed Radix Polygalae Tenuifoliae (*Yuan Zhi*), 6g, uncooked Fructus Schizandrae Chinensis (*Wu Wei Zi*), 6g, cooked Radix Rehmanniae (*Shu Di*), 3g, rice stir-fried Radix Codonopsis Pilosulae (*Dang Shen*), 6g, mix-fried Radix Glycyrrhizae (*Gan Cao*), 3g

Additions & subtractions: For dizziness and vertigo, add Rhizoma Gastrodiae Elatae (*Tian Ma*), 9g, and bran stir-fried Rhizoma Atractylodis Macrocephalae (*Bai Zhu*), 9g, and increase the dosage of Pinellia up to 9g. For severe heart palpitations, increase the dosage of Polygala, Schizandra, and Ziziphus Spinosa up to 9g. For severe qi vacuity, add honey stir-fried Radix Astragali Membranacei (*Huang Qi*), 12g, and increase the dosage of Codonopsis and Licorice up to 9g. For heart blood vacuity, add wine mix-fried Radix Angelicae Sinensis (*Dang Gui*), 9g. For abdominal pain, borborygmus, cold limbs, and diarrhea, add dry Rhizoma Zingiberis (*Gan Jiang*), 6g. For chest fullness and glomus, replace Immature Aurantium with Fructus Citri Aurantii (*Zhi Ke*), 6g, and add Radix Platycodi Grandiflori (*Jie Geng*), 6g. For coughing, add Flos Inulae Racemosae (*Xuan Fu Hua*), 9g, and Semen Pruni Armeniacae (*Xing Ren*), 6g.

12
Night Sweats *(Dao Han)*

This refers to sweating while sleeping which then stops when one wakes. After this sweating, there is no aversion to cold but sometimes there is vexatious heat.

Disease causes, disease mechanisms:

1. Yin vacuity with internal heat

Yin vacuity arises from the loss of blood and/or essence, enduring disease such as enduring coughing due to pulmonary tuberculosis, excessive sexual activity, or aging. "Yin vacuity causes internal heat, and overstrong yang causes failure to constrain." If internal heat is strong enough to cause non-constrainment of the interstices and forces fluids out, sweating may occur. Yang flows outward when awake and inward when sleeping. Therefore, yin vacuity with internal heat may cause night sweats because any internal heat will become even stronger when yang flows inward at night. Because "sweat is the liquid of the heart," "the lungs are connected with the skin and body hair," and "the kidneys store the original yin," sweating from yin vacuity with internal heat mainly involves three viscera: the heart, lungs and kidneys.

2. Heart blood vacuity

Heart blood vacuity usually develops from overwork taxation, over-thinking, enduring disease, enduring bleeding, or spleen vacuity failing to engender and transform the blood. During sleep, the blood returns to and is treasured in the liver. If the blood is already insufficient, when what blood there is returns to the liver, this may cause a temporary yin vacuity. If yin fails to control yang, yang will become hyperactive and counterflow upward and outward. Because fluids are moved and dispersed by yang qi, sweat may follow the yang qi upward and outward during sleep at night, thus resulting in night sweats.

3. Spleen vacuity & damp obstruction

Here, dampness is mainly due to dietary irregularity, *i.e.*, excessive consumption of alcohol, sweet foods, uncooked and/or chilled foods, or dairy products. In this case, the damaged spleen fails to move and transform water dampness. If dampness accumulates and obstructs the center, the clear cannot be upborne, while the turbid will fail to be downborne. Because the qi is not upborne, the defensive qi may fail to constrain fluids which flow out. Because the qi moves to the interior during sleep, the circulation of fluids in the exterior is even more sluggish at night than in the day. That means that at night, there is even more dampness to flow outward if the interstices are not secured by the qi. Hence night sweats may occur.

4. Damp heat depressed & steaming

Damp heat usually arises from external contraction of evils, from external contraction of cold dampness which transforms into heat over time, or from excessive consumption of fried, greasy, sweet foods or alcohol which ferment dampness and engender heat. Dampness is a yin evil which is sticky and stagnant by nature. During the daytime, dampness can prevent the effusion of heat. In that case, heat may accumulate in the interior during the day. At night, when the yang qi returns inward to circulate in the interior, yang added to yang makes this evil heat even worse. This heat must find a way to exit the body. Therefore, it moves upward and outward. Since heat is nothing other than yang qi, this yang qi moves fluids upward and outward along with it. Therefore, if damp heat fumes and steams from the interior outward to the skin, this may lead to night sweats.

5. Evils obstructing the shao yang

If evil qi has not been eliminated but the righteous qi has become vacuous, evils and the righteous qi will fight, half in the exterior and half in the interior. Evils in the interior typically engender heat. Because the yang qi retreats inward with the setting sun, it A) is less capable of securing the interstices and closing the pores, and B) will add yang to yang. This means, the retreating yang qi will make any internal heat all the worse. This heat will naturally move upward and outward. Thus evils located half in the exterior and half in the interior may also provoke night sweats.

Treatment based on pattern discrimination:

1. Heart yin vacuity

Symptoms: Night sweats, heart palpitations, heart vexation, profuse dreams, insomnia, impaired memory, a hot sensation in the palms of the hands and soles of the feet, a red tongue with scanty liquids, and a fine, rapid pulse

Therapeutic principles: Nourish the heart, enrich the yin, and constrain sweat

Acupuncture & moxibustion:

Yin Xi (Ht 6) *Hou Xi* (SI 3)	Together, these points nourish heart yin and constrain sweat when needled with supplementing method.
Xin Shu (Bl 15) *Shen Shu* (Bl 23) *San Yin Jiao* (Sp 6)	Together, these points supplement the blood and nourish yin when needled with supplementing method.

Additions & subtractions: For fatigued spirit and shortage of qi, add *Dan Zhong* (CV 17). For a sallow yellow facial complexion, add *Zu San Li* (St 36). For severe yin vacuity, add *Fu Liu* (Ki 7).

Chinese medicinal formula: *Tian Wang Bu Xin Dan* (Heavenly Emperor Supplement the Heart Elixir)

Ingredients: Uncooked Radix Rehmanniae (*Sheng Di*), 12g, Radix Codonopsitis Pilosulae (*Dang Shen*), 6g, Tuber Asparagi Cochinensis (*Tian Men Dong*), 9g, Tuber Ophiopogonis Japonici (*Mai Men Dong*), 9g, Radix Scrophulariae Ningpoensis (*Xuan Shen*), 9g, Radix Salviae Miltiorrhizae (*Dan Shen*), 9g, Sclerotium Pararadicis Poriae Cocos (*Fu Shen*), 9g, Radix Polygalae Tenuifoliae (*Yuan Zhi*), 6g, Radix Angelicae Sinensis (*Dang Gui*), 6g, uncooked Fructus Schisandrae Chinensis (*Wu Wei Zi*), 9g, Semen Biotae Orientalis (*Bai Zi Ren*), 9g, stir-fried Semen Zizyphi Spinosae (*Suan Zao Ren*), 9g, Radix Platycodi Grandiflori (*Jie Geng*), 3g

2. Lung yin vacuity

Symptoms: Night sweats, coughing, shortness of breath, scanty, sticky phlegm, vexatious heat in the five hearts, afternoon tidal fever, red cheekbones, thirst, a red tongue with scanty fur, and a fine, rapid pulse

Therapeutic principles: Enrich yin, moisten the lungs, and constrain sweat

Acupuncture & moxibustion:

Fei Shu (Bl 13) *Chi Ze* (Lu 5) *Gao Huang* (Bl 43)	Together, these points enrich yin, moisten the lungs, and constrain sweat when needled with supplementing method.
Fu Liu (Ki 7)	Supplements the son so as to help the mother when needled with supplementing method

Additions & subtractions: For fatigue, lack of strength, and torpid intake, add *Pi Shu* (Bl 20). For coughing of blood, add *Kong Zui* (Lu 6). For seminal emission, add *Zhi Shi* (Bl 52). For vexation and insomnia, add *Shen Men* (Ht 7).

Chinese medicinal formula: Modified *Bai He Gu Jin Tang* (Lily Secure Metal Decoction)

Ingredients: Bulbus Lilii (*Bai He*), 9g, uncooked Radix Rehmanniae (*Sheng Di*), 9g, Tuber Ophiopogonis Japonici (*Mai Dong*), 9g, cooked Radix Rehmanniae (*Shu Di*), 9g, Bulbus Fritillariae Cirrhosae (*Chuan Bei Mu*), 6g, Radix Scrophulariae Ningpoensis (*Xuan Shen*), 9g, Radix Angelicae Sinensis (*Dang Gui*), 6g, Radix Platycodi Grandiflori (*Jie Geng*), 6g, uncooked Radix Albus Paeoniae Lactiflorae (*Bai Shao*), 9g, Radix Glycyrrhizae (*Gan Cao*), 6g, uncooked Fructus Schisandrae Chinensis (*Wu Wei Zi*), 9g

3. Kidney yin vacuity

Symptoms: Night sweats, low back and knee aching and limpness, possible seminal emission, emaciation, vexatious heat in the five hearts, sore throat, a red tongue with scanty fur, and a fine, rapid pulse

Therapeutic principles: Supplement the kidneys, enrich yin, and constrain sweat

Acupuncture & moxibustion:

Shen Shu (Bl 23) *Fu Liu* (Ki 7) *San Yin Jiao* (Sp 6)	Together, these points supplement and enrich kidney yin and constrain sweat when needled with supplementing method.

Yong Quan (Ki 1)   Downbears effulgent fire when needled with draining method.

Additions & subtractions: For dizziness and vertigo, add *Guan Yuan* (CV 4). For insomnia and profuse dreams, add *Shen Men* (Ht 7). For easy erection, add *Zhong Ji* (CV 3). For seminal emission, add *Zhi Shi* (Bl 52). For scanty menstruation, add *Gui Lai* (St 29) and *Xue Hai* (Sp 10). For sore throat, add *Zhao Hai* (Ki 6).

Chinese medicinal formula: Modified *Zhi Bai Di Huang Wan* (Anemarrhena & Phellodendron Rehmannia Pills)

Ingredients: Cooked Radix Rehmanniae (*Shu Di*), 18g, steamed Fructus Corni Officinalis (*Shan Zhu Yu*), 12g, stir-fried Radix Dioscoreae Oppositae (*Shan Yao*), 12g, Sclerotium Poriae Cocos (*Fu Ling*), 9g, Cortex Radicis Moutan (*Dan Pi*), 6g, salt mix-fried Rhizoma Alismatis (*Ze Xie*), 9g, salt mix-fried Rhizoma Anemarrhenae Asphodeloidis (*Zhi Mu*), 9g, salt mix-fried Cortex Phellodendri (*Huang Bai*), 9g, uncooked Fructus Schisandrae Chinensis (*Wu Wei Zi*), 9g, Fructus Levis Tritici Aestivi (*Fu Xiao Mai*), 12g

Additions & subtractions: For severe night sweats, replace Schisandra and Wheat with calcined Os Draconis (*Long Gu*), 30g, and calcined Concha Ostreae (*Mu Li*), 30g. For effulgent fire due to yin vacuity with fever, mouth and lip dryness, a red facial complexion, and constipation, temporally replace *Zhi Bai Di Huang Wan* with *Dang Gui Liu Huang Tang* (Dang Gui Six Yellows Decoction): uncooked Radix Angelicae Sinensis (*Dang Gui*), 9g, uncooked Radix Rehmanniae (*Sheng Di*), 9g, cooked Radix Rehmanniae (*Shu Di*), 9g, Radix Scutellariae Baicalensis (*Huang Qin*), 9g, Rhizoma Coptidis Chinensis (*Huang Lian*), 6g, Cortex Phellodendri (*Huang Bai*), 9g, uncooked Radix Astragali Membranacei (*Huang Qi*), 18g, and Fructus Levis Tritici Aestivi (*Fu Xiao Mai*), 15g. For febrile disease damaging yin fluids with bone steaming, emaciation, and red lips, replace *Zhi Bai Di Huang Wan* with *Qin Jiao Bie Jia San* (Gentiana Macrophylla & Carapax Amydae Powder): Cortex Radicis Lycii Chinensis (*Di Gu Pi*), 15g, uncooked Radix Bupleuri (*Chai Hu*), 9g, Radix Gentianae Macrophyllae (*Qin Jiao*), 9g, uncooked Rhizoma Anemarrhenae Asphodeloidis (*Zhi Mu*), 9g, uncooked Radix Angelicae Sinensis (*Dang Gui*), 9g, Carapax Amydae Sinensis (*Bie Jia*), 15g, Fructus Pruni Mume (*Wu Mei*), 2 pieces, and Herba Artemisiae Apiaceae (*Qing Hao*), 6g.

4. Heart blood vacuity

Symptoms: Night sweats, heart palpitations, insomnia, pale lips and nails, a pale, lusterless facial complexion, shortness of breath, fatigue, a pale thin tongue, and a fine, forceless pulse

Therapeutic principles: Supplement the blood and nourish the heart, fortify the spleen and boost the qi

Acupuncture & moxibustion:

Xin Shu (Bl 15)	Together, these points supplement the heart, liver, and
Ge Shu (Bl 17)	spleen to nourish the blood when needled with
Gan Shu (Bl 18)	supplementing method.
Pi Shu (Bl 20)	
Yin Xi (Ht 6)	Nourishes heart fluids and constrains sweat when needled with supplementing method.

Chinese medicinal formula: Modified *Gui Pi Tang* (Return the Spleen Decoction)

Ingredients: Radix Codonopsitis Pilosulae (*Dang Shen*), 9g, uncooked Radix Astragali Membranacei (*Huang Qi*), 15g, bran stir-fried Rhizoma Atractylodis Macrocephalae (*Bai Zhu*), 15g, stir-fried Radix Angelicae Sinensis (*Dang Gui*), 9g, Arillus Euphoriae Longanae (*Long Yan Rou*), 9g, Sclerotium Pararadicis Poriae Cocos (*Fu Shen*), 9g, Radix Auklandiae Lappae (*Mu Xiang*), 3g, stir-fried Semen Zizyphi Spinosae (*Suan Zao Ren*), 15g, Semen Biotae Orientalis (*Bai Zi Ren*), 9g, uncooked Fructus Schisandrae Chinensis (*Wu Wei Zi*), 9g, mix-fried Radix Glycyrrhizae (*Gan Cao*), 3g

5. Spleen vacuity & damp obstruction

Symptoms: Night sweats, heavy-headedness, headache with a sensation of something tight bound around the head, encumbered, heavy limbs, fatigue, stomach oppression, abdominal distention, torpid intake, nausea, sliminess in the mouth, loose stools, inhibited urination, a slimy, white tongue fur, and a slippery or soggy, moderate (*i.e.*, slightly slow) pulse

Therapeutic principles: Transform dampness, harmonize the center, and fortify the spleen

Acupuncture & moxibustion:

San Yin Jiao (Sp 6)	Together, these points transform dampness and
Yin Ling Quan (Sp 9)	harmonize the center when needled with even
Zhong Wan (CV 12)	supplementing draining methods.

Pi Shu (Bl 20)	Together, these points fortify the spleen and dry
Tai Bai (Sp 3)	dampness when needled with supplementing method.

Additions & subtractions: For loose stools, add *Xia Ju Xu* (St 39). For severe heavy-headedness, add *Feng Long* (St 40). For fatigued spirit and fear of cold, moxa *Guan Yuan* (CV 4). For somnolence, add *San Jian* (LI 3).

Chinese medicinal formula: Modified *Huo Po Xia Ling Tang* (Agastaches, Magnolia, Pinellia & Poria Decoction)

Ingredients: Herba Agastachis Seu Pogostemi (*Huo Xiang*), 9g, clear Rhizoma Pinelliae Ternatae (*Ban Xia*), 6g, Sclerotium Rubrum Poriae Cocos (*Chi Fu Ling*), 12g, Semen Coicis Lachryma-jobi (*Yi Yi Ren*), 18g, Fructus Cardamomi (*Bai Dou Kou*), 6g, Sclerotium Polypori Umbellati (*Zhu Ling*), 6g, ginger mix-fried Cortex Magnoliae Officinalis (*Hou Po*), 6g, Radix Ephedrae (*Ma Huang Gen*), 15g

Additions & subtractions: For severe damp accumulation, add Rhizoma Atractylodis (*Cang Zhu*), 9g, and uncooked Pericarpium Citri Reticulatae (*Chen Pi*), 9g. For severe qi vacuity, add bran stir-fried Rhizoma Atractylodis Macrocephalae (*Bai Zhu*), 9g, and uncooked Radix Astragali Membranacei (*Huang Qi*), 15g.

6. Damp heat depressed & steaming

Symptoms: Night sweats, tidal hectic fever, encumbered limbs, stomach oppression, torpid intake, heavy-headedness, dryness and stickiness in the mouth with a bitter taste, dark-colored urine, a red tongue with slimy, yellow fur, and a soggy, rapid or slippery, rapid pulse

Therapeutic principles: Clear heat and transform dampness

Acupuncture & moxibustion:

Yin Ling Quan (Sp 9)	Together, these points clear heat and transform
Yang Ling Quan (GB 34)	dampness when needled with draining method.
Zhi Gou (TB 6)	
Nei Ting (St 44)	

Chinese medicinal formula: Modified *Lian Po Yin* (Coptis & Magnolia Drink)

Ingredients: Fructus Gardeniae Jasminoidis (*Zhi Zi*), 9g, clear Semen Praeparatus Sojae (*Dan Dou Chi*), 9g, uncooked Rhizoma Coptidis Chinensis (*Huang Lian*), 6g, ginger mix-fried Cortex Magnoliae Officinalis (*Hou Po*), 6g, Rhizoma Acori Graminei (*Shi Chang Pu*), 6g, ginger stir-fried Rhizoma Pinelliae Ternatae (*Ban Xia*), 6g, Sclerotium Poriae Cocos (*Fu Ling*), 9g

Additions & subtractions: For severe heat, add Radix Scutellariae Baicalensis (*Huang Qin*), 9g. For severe dampness, add Rhizoma Alismatis (*Ze Xie*), 9g, and Sclerotium Polypori Umbellati (*Zhu Ling*), 9g. For concomitant spleen vacuity, add bran stir-fried Rhizoma Atractylodis Macrocephalae (*Bai Zhu*), 9g, and stir-fried Radix Dioscoreae Oppositae (*Shan Yao*), 9g. For torpid intake, add stir-fried Massa Medica Fermentata (*Shen Qu*), 9g.

7. Evils obstructing the shao yang

Symptoms: Sweating during sleep, alternating fever and chills, chest and rib-side pain and fullness, a bitter taste in the mouth, a dry throat, no desire to eat, heart vexation, frequent retching, nausea, possible deafness and vertigo, white or yellow tongue fur, and a bowstring pulse

Therapeutic principles: Harmonize and resolve the shao yang

Acupuncture & moxibustion:

Wai Guan (TB 5) *Qiu Xu* (GB 40) *Qi Men* (Liv 14)	Together, these points harmonize and resolve the *shao yang* when needled with even supplementing and draining method.
Yin Xi (Ht 6) *He Gu* (LI 4)	Together, these points clear heat, expel evils, and stop the sweating when needled with draining method.

Additions & subtractions: For deafness and vertigo, add *Jin Men* (GB 25) and *Ting Hui* (GB 2). For vomiting, add *Zhong Wan* (CV 12). For constipation, add *Zhi Gou* (TB 6) and *Shang Ju Xu* (St 37).

Chinese medicinal formula: *Xiao Chai Hu Tang* (Minor Bupleurum Decoction)

Ingredients: Uncooked Radix Bupleuri (*Chai Hu*), 12g, uncooked Radix Scutellariae Baicalensis (*Huang Qin*), 9g, lime-processed Rhizoma

Pinelliae Ternatae (*Ban Xia*), 9g, uncooked Radix Codonopsitis Pilosulae (*Dang Shen*), 6g, Radix Glycyrrhizae (*Gan Cao*), 6g, uncooked Rhizoma Zingiberis (*Sheng Jiang*), 3g, Fructus Zizyphi Jujubae (*Da Zao*), 4 pieces, Radix Glycyrrhizae (*Gan Cao*), 3g

Additions & subtractions: For severe heat, subtract Codonopsis and add Rhizoma Coptidis Chinensis (*Huang Lian*), 6g. For severe night sweats, add calcined Os Draconis (*Long Gu*), 18g, and Concha Ostreae (*Mu Li*), 18g. For severe pain and fullness in the chest and rib-side, subtract Codonopsis and Licorice and add Fructus Citri Aurantii (*Zhi Ke*), 6g, Radix Platycodi Grandiflori (*Jie Geng*), 6g, and Pericarpium Citri Reticulatae Viride (*Qing Pi*), 6g. For fullness and pain in the stomach, constipation, and yellow tongue fur, subtract Codonopsis and Licorice and add uncooked Radix Et Rhizoma Rhei (*Da Huang*), 6g, Fructus Immaturus Citri Aurantii (*Zhi Shi*), 9g, and uncooked Radix Albus Paeoniae Lactiflorae (*Bai Shao*), 9g. For severe thirst, subtract Pinellia and add Radix Trichosanthis Kirlowii (*Tian Hua Fen*), 15g.

13
Hemilateral Sweating *(Ban Shen Han Chu)*

Hemilateral sweating refers to perspiration on one side of the body only.

Disease causes, disease mechanisms:

1. Qi & blood vacuity

Qi and blood vacuity usually develops from overwork taxation, enduring disease, and great loss of the blood. Qi is responsible for securing the exterior of the body, while the blood is responsible for nourishing the body. In addition, qi is the commander of the blood, while the blood is the mother of qi. Thus qi and blood are mutually dependent and work together to secure and defend the body. If one becomes greatly vacuous, so typically will the other. If they become vacuous and insufficient, they may fail to circulate all around the body. In that case, one or more parts of the body may not receive sufficient nourishment and securing. Thus insecurity of the interstices may occur in that part of the body. If this happens on only one side of the body, hemilateral sweating may be seen.

2. Cold dampness impeding & obstructing

Cold dampness resulting in hemilateral sweating usually arises from external contraction of these evils. Cold is a yin evil which causes contracture and constriction. Dampness is also a yin evil which is sticky and fixed in nature. Therefore, both cold and dampness can easily cause obstruction. If these evils invade the body and impede and obstruct the channels and network vessels on one side of the body only, the qi on that side of the body may be insufficient to secure the exterior. Instead, the pores fall open and fluids exit, thus resulting in hemilateral sweating.

3. Disharmony between the constructive & defensive qi

Disharmony, literally "non-union," between the constructive and defensive may be due to either external contraction of wind evils or overwork taxation. The constructive qi flows inside the vessels, while the defensive qi moves outside the vessels. However, these two are united and do accompany one another on their rounds. The exterior defensive or the interstices are only secured when both the constructive and defensive flow freely and work in harmony. If this relationship becomes disharmonious, then the defensive qi cannot secure the exterior efficiently, thus leading to loosely packed interstices and open pores. If such disharmony occurs on only one side of the body, then hemilateral sweating may occur.

4. Yin vacuity with fire effulgence

Yin vacuity with fire effulgence usually develops from aging, congenital insufficiency, enduring disease, febrile disease, or excessive sexual activity. Because yin is supposed to control yang, if yin becomes vacuous and insufficient, yang may become exuberant and hyperactive. Because yang's nature is warm or hot, such yin vacuity may lead to effulgent fire. If such effulgent fire is strong enough to cause non-constrainment of the interstices and forces the fluids outside the body, sweating may occur. If such yin vacuity affects only a single side of the body, hemilateral sweating may occur.

Treatment based on pattern discrimination:

1. Qi & blood vacuity

Symptoms: Hemilateral sweating, reduced qi with laziness to speak, fatigue, lack of strength, a somber, lusterless facial complexion, dizziness and vertigo, tingling in the hands and feet, a pale tongue with white fur, and a fine, weak pulse

Therapeutic principles: Supplement both the qi and blood

Acupuncture & moxibustion:

He Gu (LI 4) *Zu San Li* (St 36)	Together, these points boost the qi and constrain sweat when needled with supplementing method.
Xue Hai (Sp 10) *Pi Shu* (Bl 20) *Wei Shu* (Bl 21) *San Yin Jiao* (Sp 6)	Together, these points nourish the blood when needled with supplementing method.

Additions & subtractions: For heart palpitations, add *Nei Guan* (Per 6). For insomnia, add *Shen Men* (Ht 7) or *Xin Shu* (Bl 15). For incessant uterine bleeding, add *Guan Yuan* (CV 4). For reduced food intake, add *Jian Li* (CV 11).

Chinese medicinal formula: *Ren Shen Yang Rong Tang* (Ginseng Nourish the Constructive Decoction)

Ingredients: Radix Codonopsitis Pilosulae (*Dang Shen*), 9g, uncooked Radix Astragali Membranacei (*Huang Qi*), 18g, stir-fried Rhizoma Atractylodis Macrocephalae (*Bai Zhu*), 15g, uncooked Radix Albus Paeoniae Lactiflorae (*Bai Shao*), 18g, cooked Radix Rehmanniae (*Shu Di*), 9g, Radix Angelicae Sinensis (*Dang Gui*), 9g, stir-fried Pericarpium Citri Reticulatae (*Chen Pi*), 6g, Cortex Cinnamomi Cassiae (*Rou Gui*), 3g, uncooked Fructus Schisandrae Chinensis (*Wu Wei Zi*), 12g, licorice-processed Radix Polygalae Tenuifoliae (*Yuan Zhi*), 6g, Sclerotium Poriae Cocos (*Fu Ling*), 9g, mix-fried Radix Glycyrrhizae (*Gan Cao*), 6g

Additions & subtractions: For profuse sweating, add Fructus Levis Tritici Aestivi (*Fu Xiao Mai*), 12g, and Radix Ephedrae (*Ma Huang Gen*), 15g.

2. Cold dampness impeding & obstructing

Symptoms: Hemilateral sweating, painful hypertonicity of the sinews, inhibited bending and stretching of the hands and feet, heavy limbs, difficulty turning over in severe cases, slimy, white tongue fur, and a soggy or slow pulse

Therapeutic principles: Warm and scatter cold and dampness, quicken the blood and free the flow of the network vessels

Acupuncture & moxibustion:

Bi Nao (LI 14)	Together, these points quicken the blood and free
Shou San Li (LI 10)	the flow of the network vessels when needled with
Zu San Li (St 36)	draining method.

He Gu (LI 4)	Together, these points warm and scatter cold
Qi Hai (CV 6)	dampness when needled with moxibustion on the
	heads of the needles.

Note: This treatment is only applied to the affected side.

Additions & subtractions: For encumbered, heavy head and body, add *Zhi Gou*

(TB 6) and *Yin Ling Quan* (Sp 9). For fatigued spirit and fear of cold, moxa *Ming Men* (GV 4). For stomachache, add *Zhong Wan* (CV 12). For clear, thin vaginal discharge, add *San Yin Jiao* (Sp 6).

Chinese medicinal formula: Modified *Juan Bi Tang* (Alleviate Impediment Decoction)

Ingredients: Uncooked Radix Astragali Membranacei (*Huang Qi*), 15g, wine mix-fried Radix Angelicae Sinensis (*Dang Gui*), 9g, wine mix-fried Radix Rubrus Paeoniae Lactiflorae (*Chi Shao*), 9g, Radix Et Rhizoma Notopterygii (*Qiang Huo*), 9g, Rhizoma Curcumae Longae (*Jiang Huang*), 9g, Radix Albus Paeoniae Lactiflorae (*Bai Shao*), 12g, Radix Ledbouriellae Divaricatae (*Fang Feng*), 9g, uncooked Rhizoma Zingiberis (*Sheng Jiang*), 3g, Caulis Piperis Futokadsurae (*Hai Feng Teng*), 9g, wine mix-fried Radix Ligustici Wallichii (*Chuan Xiong*), 6g, processed Radix Aconiti Carmichaeli (*Chuan Wu Tou*), 3g, mix-fried Radix Glycyrrhizae (*Gan Cao*), 6g

Additions & subtractions: For stubborn impediment, replace *Juan Bi Tang* with *Xiao Huo Luo Dan* (Minor Quicken the Network Vessels Elixir): processed Radix Aconiti Kusnezofii (*Cao Wu Tou*) and processed Radix Aconiti Carmichaeli (*Chuan Wu Tou*), 60g each (decocted at least 30 minutes before adding the other medicinals), processed Rhizoma Arsiaematis (*Tian Nan Xing*), 60g, Resina Myrrhae (*Mo Yao*), 20g, and Resina Olibani (*Ru Xiang*), 20g. Grind into powder and mix the medicinals. Boil six grams of this powder in 250cc of water for 15 minutes. Take the resulting preparation (*i.e.*, water and powder) in two divided doses. The Aconite used must be processed.

3. Disharmony between the constructive & defensive qi

Symptoms: Hemilateral sweating, fever, aversion to wind, headache, moist, white tongue fur, and a moderate (*i.e.*, slightly slow), weak pulse

Therapeutic principles: Regulate and harmonize the constructive and defensive qi

Acupuncture & moxibustion:

Wai Guan (TB 5)   Together, these points course wind and resolve the
Feng Men (Bl 12)   exterior when needled with draining method.

He Gu (LI 4)
Zu San Li (St 36)
Yin Xi (Ht 6)

Together, these points regulate and harmonize the constructive-blood and stop sweating when needled with supplementing method.

Additions & subtractions: For body aches, add *Shen Zhu* (GV 12). For rigidity of the nape of the neck, add *Feng Chi* (GB 20).

Chinese medicinal formula: *Gui Zhi Tang* (Cinnamon Twig Decoction)

Ingredients: Uncooked Ramulus Cinnamomi Cassiae (*Gui Zhi*), 9g, uncooked Radix Albus Paeoniae Lactiflorae (*Bai Shao*), 9g, mix-fried Radix Glycyrrhizae (*Gan Cao*), 6g, uncooked Rhizoma Zingiberis (*Sheng Jiang*), 9g, Fructus Zizyphi Jujubae (*Da Zao*), 3 pieces

Additions & subtractions: For coughing and/or panting, add ginger mix-fried Cortex Magnoliae Officinalis (*Hou Po*), 9g, and Semen Pruni Armeniacae (*Xing Ren*), 9g. For severe body aches, add uncooked Radix Puerariae (*Ge Gen*), 9g. For incessant sweating, add Radix Lateralis Praeparatus Aconiti Carmichaeli (*Fu Zi*), 6g.

Remarks: This pattern can also be seen in patients without fever or an acute disorder. In that case, it is usually seen in those with a weak constitution accompanied by fatigue and susceptibility to contraction of wind cold evils. For such cases, one can add the following medicinals to the above formula: rice stir-fried Radix Codonopsitis Pilosulae (*Dang Shen*), 9g, Tuber Ophiopogonis Japonici (*Mai Men Dong*), 9g, and uncooked Fructus Schisandrae Chinensis (*Wu Wei Zi*), 9g, *i.e., Sheng Mai Yin* (Engender the Pulse Drink).

4. Yin vacuity with fire effulgence

Symptoms: Hemilateral sweating especially in the afternoon or at night, low-grade fever, vexatious heat in the five hearts, red cheekbones and lips, dizziness, tinnitus, a dry throat, steaming bones, low back and knee soreness and weakness, lassitude of the spirit, vacuity vexation, insomnia, seminal emission, scanty, dark-colored urine, dry stools, a red tongue with scanty fur, and a fine, rapid pulse

Therapeutic principles: Nourish yin and downbear fire

Acupuncture & moxibustion:

Yin Xi (Ht 6) *Shen Shu* (Bl 23) *San Yin Jiao* (Sp 6) *Gan Shu* (Bl 18)	Together, these points nourish yin and downbear fire, supplement and nourish the liver and kidneys when needled with supplementing method.
He Gu (LI 4) *Fu Liu* (Ki 7)	Together, these points balance yin and yang, supplement the qi and yin, and stop sweating.

Additions & subtractions: For heart palpitations, add *Nei Guan* (Per 6). For dry, sore throat, add *Zhao Hai* (Ki 6). For insomnia, add *Shen Men* (Ht 7). For vacuity heat damaging fluids, add *Wei Shu* (Bl 21) and *Pi Shu* (Bl 20).

Chinese medicinal formula: Modified *Zhi Bai Di Huang Wan* (Anemarrhena & Phellodendron Rehmannia Pills)

Ingredients: Cooked Radix Rehmanniae (*Shu Di*), 18g, steamed Fructus Corni Officinalis (*Shan Zhu Yu*), 12g, stir-fried Radix Dioscoreae Oppositae (*Shan Yao*), 12g, Sclerotium Poriae Cocos (*Fu Ling*), 9g, Cortex Radicis Moutan (*Dan Pi*), 6g, salt mix-fried Rhizoma Alismatis (*Ze Xie*), 9g, salt mix-fried Rhizoma Anemarrhenae Asphodeloidis (*Zhi Mu*), 9g, salt mix-fried Cortex Phellodendri (*Huang Bai*), 9g, uncooked Fructus Schisandrae Chinensis (*Wu Wei Zi*), 9g, Fructus Levis Tritici Aestivi (*Fu Xiao Mai*), 12g

Additions & subtractions: For severe hemilateral sweating, replace Moutan with Cortex Radicis Lycii Chinensis (*Di Gu Pi*) and add calcined Concha Ostreae (*Mu Li*), 18g. For severe heart vexation or insomnia, add stir-fried Semen Zizyphi Spinosae (*Suan Zao Ren*), 12g, and Semen Biotae Orientalis (*Bai Zi Ren*), 9g. For low-grade or tidal hectic fever, add Cortex Radicis Lycii Chinensis (*Di Gu Pi*), 9g, and Radix Cynanchi Baiwai (*Bai Wai*), 9g.

Remarks: When hemilateral sweating occurs in those over 50 years of age, it suggests the possibility of wind stroke. Therefore, one should be careful to treat the patient's condition speedily and comprehensively. In addition, prevention of contracting wind evils or overworking is strongly advised in such patients.

14

Yellow Sweat *(Huang Han)*

Yellow sweat refers to perspiration of yellow-colored sweat which often even stains the patient's clothes.

Disease causes, disease mechanisms:

1. Congestion & obstruction of the constructive & defensive

Congestion and obstruction of the constructive and defensive causing yellow sweating usually develop from a combination of two factors. The first is a preexisting internal heat condition. This heat moves upward and outward, forcing the body fluids to follow, thus leading to sweating. The second is a subsequent exposure to external damp evils, such as being caught in the rain or from showering in cold water while still sweating. This causes sudden closure of the pores and thus depression of the constructive and defensive qi. Since the fluids in the body are moved by and with the qi, if the constructive and defensive qi become depressed, so do body fluids. If the preexisting internal heat and the subsequently accumulating water dampness mutually struggle and bind in the flesh, the tissue corresponding to the earth phase, heat may turn the sweat yellow, *i.e.*, the color of earth.

2. Damp heat brewing & accumulating

Damp heat causing yellow sweat may develop from either external contraction of evils or from enduring accumulation of internal dampness which transforms into heat. Dampness is yin, while heat is yang. Thus these two evils mutually struggle with each other. Heat stews the juices and makes dampness even thicker and more obstructing, while dampness blocks heat's scattering and dissipation. Thus heat becomes even more intense. Because the fluids moving through the flesh, the body tissue which corresponds to the earth phase, is fumed and steamed by this damp heat, it becomes the color of earth, *i.e.*, yellow.

Treatment based on pattern discrimination:

1. Congestion & obstruction of the constructive & defensive

Symptoms: Sweat as yellow as the juice of Cortex Phellodendri (*Huang Bai*) after having been caught in rain or after taking a cold shower while sweating, fever, thirst, an encumbered, heavy body with edema, formication, thirst, inhibited urination, white tongue fur, and a deep pulse

Therapeutic principles: Diffuse and free the flow of the depressed and harmonize the constructive and defensive

Acupuncture & moxibustion:

San Jiao Shu (Bl 22) *Zhi Gou* (TB 6)	Together, these points diffuse and free depression and stagnation when needled with draining method.
He Gu (LI 4) *Wai Guan* (TB 5) *Qu Chi* (LI 11)	Together, these points harmonize the constructive and defensive when needled with even draining and supplementing method.

Additions & subtractions: For body aches, add *Shen Zhu* (GV 12). For headache, add *Feng Chi* (GB 20). For high fever, add *Da Zhui* (GV 14).

Chinese medicinal formula: *Huang Qi Shao Yao Gui Zhi Ku Jiu Tang* (Astragalus, Peony, Cinnamon & Bitter Wine Decoction)

Ingredients: Uncooked Radix Astragali Membranacei (*Huang Qi*), 18g, Radix Albus Paeoniae Lactiflorae (*Bai Shao*), 6g, uncooked Ramulus Cinnamomi Cassiae (*Gui Zhi*), 6g, rice vinegar, 20ml

2. Damp heat brewing & accumulating

Symptoms: Yellow sweat, fever, slight edema, rib-side pain, torpid intake, a bitter taste in the mouth, dark-colored urine, slimy, yellow tongue fur, and a bowstring, slippery pulse

Remarks: There may be absence of fever if yellow sweating is a chronic, enduring condition. In addition to the generalized symptoms listed above, there may also be strong odor, sticky, hot, bad-smelling underarm perspiration, and stickiness and sliminess in the mouth.

Therapeutic principles: Clear heat and disinhibit dampness

Acupuncture & moxibustion:

He Gu (LI 4) *Qu Chi* (LI 11)	Together, these points clear heat when needled with draining method.
Zu San Li (St 36) *Pi Shu* (Bl 20) *Yin Ling Quan* (Sp 9)	Together, these points fortify the spleen and disinhibit dampness when needled with supplementing method.
San Jiao Shu (Bl 22)	Frees the flow of qi of the three burners to help clear heat and disinhibit dampness when needled with draining method.

Additions & subtractions: For heart vexation, add *Nei Guan* (Per 6). For abdominal oppression and distention, add *Zhong Wan* (CV 12). For constipation, add *Nei Ting* (St 44).

Chinese medicinal formula: Modified *Yin Chen Wu Ling Tang* (Artemisia Capillaris Five [Ingredients] Poria Decoction)

Ingredients: Herba Artemisiae Capillaris (*Yin Chen Hao*), 18g, Rhizoma Alismatis (*Ze Xie*), 9g, Sclerotium Poriae Cocos (*Fu Ling*), 9g, Sclerotium Polypori Umbellati (*Zhu Ling*), 9g, uncooked Rhizoma Atractylodis Macrocephalae (*Bai Zhu*), 6g, uncooked Radix Scutellariae Baicalensis (*Huang Qin*), 6g, Fructus Gardeniae Jasminoidis (*Zhi Zi*), 9g

15
Incessant Sweating *(Han Chu Bu Shi)*

This refers to profuse, persistent sweating with oily, pear-shaped droplets of sweat. Incessant sweating is usually seen in critical cases. It is also known as "leaking sweating," "expiry sweating," or "desertion sweating."

Disease causes, disease mechanisms:

1. Yin desertion

Yin desertion usually develops from high fever with profuse sweating, great vomiting and/or diarrhea, great loss of blood, or from enduring disease, any of which may greatly consume yin. Yin desertion is not due to heat, but it certainly will engender heat which then forces fluids outside the body, leading to sweating. Secondarily, yang desertion may follow yin desertion, since yin and yang are mutually rooted and interdependent. In that case, incessant sweating is due to yang qi failing to secure the exterior and close the pores.

2. Yang desertion

Yang desertion is due to either severe enduring disease which exhausts yang or from yin desertion as described above. Yang is supposed to constrain yin and, only when yang is sound, can the exterior be secured. If yang deserts, yin and yang will separate. Thus, yang fails to constrain yin but rather floats outward and disperses. Because qi moves fluids, fluids may follow the yang qi exiting from the body. Therefore, incessant sweating occurs.

Remarks: Because yin and yang are mutually rooted, it is rare for one of these to desert without the other also deserting. Therefore, the above two mechanisms often occur in a single patient. In that case, one plays the primary and the other plays a secondary role.

Treatment based on pattern discrimination:

1. Yin desertion

Symptoms: Great persistent sweating which is hot and sticky or oily, possible fever, warm limbs, thirst with a liking for cold drinks, rough breathing, fatigued spirit and lassitude, red, dry lips and tongue, and a vacuous, rapid or fine, rapid, forceless pulse

Therapeutic principles: Foster yin and engender liquids, boost the qi and stem desertion

Acupuncture & moxibustion:

Shui Gou (GV 26) *Guan Yuan* (CV 4) *Zu San Li* (St 36)	Together, these points regulate yin and yang, boost the qi, and stem desertion when needled with supplementing method.
Yong Quan (Ki 1) *Tai Xi* (Ki 3)	Together, these points foster yin and engender liquids when needled with supplementing method.

Additions & subtractions: For heart vexation, add *Nei Guan* (Per 6). For shortness of breath, add *Dan Zhong* (CV 17). For coma, add *Bai Hui* (GV 20).

Chinese medicinal formula: Modified *Sheng Mai Yin* (Engender the Pulse Drink)

Ingredients: Radix Panacis Ginseng (*Ren Shen*), 10g, uncooked Fructus Schisandrae Chinensis (*Wu Wei Zi*), 10g, Tuber Ophiopogonis Japonici (*Mai Dong*), 15g, uncooked Fructus Corni Officinalis (*Shan Zhu Yu*), 10g

Additions & subtractions: For severe qi vacuity, add uncooked Radix Astragali Membranacei (*Huang Qi*), 20g. For severe sweating, add Fructus Levis Tritici Aestivi (*Fu Xiao Mai*), 12g, and Radix Ephedrae (*Ma Huang Gen*), 12g. For heart palpitations, add calcined Dens Draconis (*Long Chi*), 15g, uncooked Concha Ostreae (*Mu Li*), 15g, and Magnetitum (*Ci Shi*), 12g.

2. Yang desertion

Symptoms: Great incessant sweating which is bead-like in shape, clear, thin, and cold, fear of cold, a curled-up lying posture, counterflow chilling in the limbs, listlessness of the essence spirit, a somber white facial complexion, faint breathing, thirst with a liking for hot drinks, a moist tongue, and a faint pulse verging on expiry or a floating, rapid, scallion-stalk pulse

116

Therapeutic principles: Supplement yang and stem desertion, return yang and stem counterflow

Acupuncture & moxibustion:

Su Liao (GV 25) *Guan Yuan* (CV 4)	Together, these points regulate yin and yang and stem desertion when needled with even supplementing and draining method.
Shen Que (CV 8) *Qi Hai* (CV 6)	Together, these points supplement yang, return yang, and stem counterflow when strongly moxaed.

Additions & subtractions: For coma, strongly moxa *Bai Hui* (GV 20).

Chinese medicinal formula: *Jia Wei Shen Fu Tang* (Added Flavors Ginseng & Aconite Decoction)

Ingredients: Radix Panacis Ginseng (*Ren Shen*), 12g, blast-fried Radix Lateralis Praeparatus Aconiti Carmichaeli (*Fu Zi*), 9g, calcined Os Draconis (*Long Gu*), 30g, calcined Concha Ostreae (*Mu Li*), 30g

Additions & subtractions: For severe chilled limbs and cold body, add dry Rhizoma Zingiberis (*Gan Jiang*), 9g. For severe sweating, add uncooked Radix Astragali Membranacei (*Huang Qi*), 20g.

16

Hemilateral Numbness *(Ban Shen Ma Mu)*

This refers to numbness of the skin on one side of the body only.

Disease causes, disease mechanisms:

1. Central qi vacuity

Central qi vacuity arises from overwork taxation, dietary irregularity, enduring disease, or from enduring administration of bitter, cold medicinals. Central qi refers to the qi of the spleen and stomach. If, for any reason, the central qi becomes vacuous and weak, the engenderment and transformation of qi and blood will be reduced and qi and blood vacuity will occur. If the qi and blood become vacuous, they will fail to fill the vessels in the skin. If the skin fails to obtain sufficient blood, it cannot perform its functions, one of which is tactile sensation. Thus qi and especially blood vacuity may lead to numbness. Because the spleen lives on the right side, spleen vacuity often causes hemilateral numbness on the right side of the body.

2. Blood vacuity

Blood vacuity usually develops from excessive loss of blood, including meno- and metrorrhagia, excessive sexual activity, multiple births, or febrile disease, all of which greatly consume blood and yin. The blood is responsible for nourishing the skin. If the blood becomes vacuous, the skin will obtain sufficient nourishment and, therefore, will hypofunction. One of the skin's functions is tactile sensation. Hence blood vacuity may result in numbness of the skin. The liver stores the blood and lives on the left. Therefore, liver blood vacuity often causes hemilateral numbness on the left side of the body.

3. Wind cold assailing externally

External evils usually assail the body through the skin. Wind is the chief of the hundreds of diseases, and cold is a yin evil which causes contraction and tension by its very nature. When these two evils enter the network vessels through the skin and hair, they cause obstruction therein.

Consequently, the skin may not receive sufficient nourishment, thus giving rise to numbness as described above. Because the channels and network vessels on the two sides of the body are semi-independent, evils may attack only one side of the body and not affect the other. Therefore, hemilateral numbness may occur only on the affected side.

4. Liver wind stirring internally

The liver wind usually arises from yin vacuity of the liver-kidneys, extreme vacuity of liver blood, or from extremely exuberant heat. If liver wind stirs internally and scurries into the network vessels, it may create obstruction in the vessels. Hence the skin may be deprived of sufficient nourishment and numbness may occur. Because wind is a yang evil and the liver is a yin viscus, internally engendered wind typically shifts into the liver's paired yang channel, the shao yang gallbladder channel. The shao yang rules the sides of the body and is often associated with one-sided pathologies. This is why liver wind causing obstruction in the channels and network vessels commonly only affects one or the other side of the body.

5. Dampness & phlegm obstructing the network vessels

Dietary irregularities, such as addiction to sweet, fatty, chilled, and/or uncooked food or alcohol, can damage the spleen. This may lead to the spleen's failure to control movement and transformation. Failure of movement and transformation then results in collection and accumulation of dampness. If dampness endures, it will tend to congeal into phlegm. Because phlegm is a turbid yin evil, once it is formed, it tends to obstruct the free flow of the qi and blood. Thus, the qi and blood cannot fill the vessels in the skin, leading to hemilateral numbness when phlegm obstruction occurs on only one side of the body.

Treatment based on pattern discrimination:

I. Central qi vacuity

Symptoms: Hemilateral numbness, limp, forceless limbs, heart palpitations, shortness of breath, aversion to wind, spontaneous perspiration, a pale tongue with thin, white fur, and a weak pulse

Therapeutic principles: Supplement the qi and free the flow of the network vessels

Acupuncture & moxibustion:

Zu San Li (St 36)   Together, these points supplement the center, boost the
San Yin Jiao (Sp 6) qi, and free the flow of the channels and network
He Gu (LI 4)   vessels when needled with supplementing method.
Shou San Li (LI 10)

Qi Hai (CV 6)   Together, these points supplement the qi and lift the
Bai Hui (GV 20)   fallen when needled with supplementing method.

Additions & subtractions: For reduced food intake, add *Jian Li* (CV 11). For abdominal distention, add *Fu Tong Gu* (Ki 20). For loose stools, add *Gong Sun* (Sp 4).

Chinese medicinal formula: Modified *Shen Xiao Huang Qi Tang* (Miraculous Effect Astragalus Decoction)

Ingredients: Uncooked Radix Astragali Membranacei (*Huang Qi*), 24g, Radix Panacis Ginseng (*Ren Shen*), 6g, mix-fried Radix Glycyrrhizae (*Gan Cao*), 6g, uncooked Radix Albus Paeoniae Lactiflorae (*Bai Shao*), 9g, stir-fried Pericarpium Citri Reticulatae (*Chen Pi*), 6g

Additions & subtractions: For severe qi vacuity, add stir-fried Rhizoma Atractylodis Macrocephalae (*Bai Zhu*), 9g, and Radix Codonopsitis Pilosulae (*Dang Shen*), 9g. For qi vacuity leading to blood stasis with hemiplegia, a dark, purple tongue with static macules and a vacuous pulse, replace *Shen Xiao Huang Qi Tang* with Modified *Bu Yang Huan Wu Tang* (Supplement Yang & Restore Five [Tenths] Decoction): uncooked Radix Astragali Membranacei (*Huang Qi*), 30g, wine mix-fried Radix Angelicae Sinensis (*Dang Gui*), 9g, wine mix-fried Radix Rubrus Paeoniae Lactiflorae (*Chi Shao*), 9g, Lumbricus (*Di Long*), 9g, wine mix-fried Radix Ligustici Wallichii (*Chuan Xiong*), 6g, Semen Pruni Persicae (*Tao Ren*), 6g, and Flos Carthami Tinctorii (*Hong Hua*), 9g.

2. Blood vacuity

Symptoms: Hemilateral numbness, dizziness, vertigo, heart palpitations, insomnia, a lusterless facial complexion, a pale, tender tongue with thin, slightly dry fur, and a fine, weak pulse

Therapeutic principles: Supplement the blood and moisten and nourish the skin

Acupuncture & moxibustion:

Bi Nao (LI 14) *He Gu* (LI 4) *Shou San Li* (LI 10)	Together, these points free the flow of the channels and network vessels when needled with even draining and supplementing method.
Zu San Li (St 36) *San Yin Jiao* (Sp 6) *Xue Hai* (Sp 10)	Together, these points fortify the spleen, supplement the blood, and moisten and nourish the skin when needled with supplementing method.

Additions & subtractions: For blurred vision, add *Gan Shu* (Bl 18). For delayed menstruation with pale, scanty blood, add *Gui Lai* (St 29). For amenorrhea, add *Pi Shu* (Bl 20), *Shen Shu* (Bl 23), and *Gan Shu* (Bl 18). For reduced food intake, add *Gong Sun* (Sp 4). For amnesia, add *Si Shen Cong* (M-HN-1).

Chinese medicinal formula: Modified *Si Wu Tang* (Four Materials Decoction)

Ingredients: Cooked Radix Rehmanniae (*Shu Di*), 12g, uncooked Radix Albus Paeoniae Lactiflorae (*Bai Shao*), 9g, wine mix-fried Radix Angelicae Sinensis (*Dang Gui*), 12g, wine mix-fried Radix Ligustici Wallichii (*Chuan Xiong*), 6g, processed Polygoni Multiflori (*He Shou Wu*), 9g, steamed Fructus Chaenomelis Lagenariae (*Mu Gua*), 6g

Additions & subtractions: For blood vacuity due to spleen vacuity, add rice stir-fried Radix Codonopsitis Pilosulae (*Dang Shen*), 9g, bran stir-fried Rhizoma Atractylodis Macrocephalae (*Bai Zhu*), 6g, and mix-fried Radix Glycyrrhizae (*Gan Cao*), 6g. For habitual constructive and defensive disharmony and blood vacuity with spontaneous perspiration, tendency to contraction of wind cold evils, hemilateral numbness with pain, and back pain, replace *Si Wu Tang* with Modified *Huang Qi Gui Zhi Wu Wu Tang* (Astragalus & Cinnamon Five Materials Decoction): uncooked Radix Astragali Membranacei (*Huang Qi*), 18g, stir-fried Ramulus Cinnamomi Cassiae (*Gui Zhi*), 6g, Radix Albus Paeoniae Lactiflorae (*Bai Shao*), 9g, uncooked Rhizoma Zingiberis (*Sheng Jiang*), 6g, Fructus Zizyphi Jujubae (*Da Zao*), 5 pieces, wine mix-fried Radix Angelicae Sinensis (*Dang Gui*), 9g, Lumbricus (*Di Long*), 6g, and Bombyx Batryticatus (*Jiang Can*), 6g.

3. Wind cold assailing externally

Symptoms: Hemilateral numbness, body aches, headache, aversion to wind cold, no sweating, thin, white tongue fur, and a floating, tight pulse

Therapeutic principles: Course wind and scatter cold, soothe the sinews and quicken the network vessels

Acupuncture & moxibustion:

Wai Guan (TB 5)   Together, these points course wind and scatter cold
Tian Shu (St 25)   when needled with draining method.

Yang Gu (SI 5)   Together, these points soothe the sinews and quicken
Tiao Kou (St 38)   the network vessels when needled with draining
Jie Xi (St 41)   method.

Additions & subtractions: For fever, add *He Gu* (LI 4). For headache, add *Feng Chi* (GB 20). For nasal congestion, add *Yin Xiang* (LI 20).

Chinese medicinal formula: Modified *Huang Qi Gui Zhi Wu Wu Tang* (Astragalus & Cinnamon Five Materials Decoction)

Ingredients: Uncooked Radix Astragali Membranacei (*Huang Qi*), 18g, stir-fried Ramulus Cinnamomi Cassiae (*Gui Zhi*), 9g, Radix Albus Paeoniae Lactiflorae (*Bai Shao*), 9g, uncooked Rhizoma Zingiberis (*Sheng Jiang*), 9g, Fructus Zizyphi Jujubae (*Da Zao*), 5 pieces, Radix Ledebouriellae Divaricatae (*Fang Feng*), 9g, Bombyx Batryticatus (*Jiang Can*), 6g

Additions & subtractions: For wind cold dampness with joint pain and a heavy sensation in the joints, replace *Huang Qi Gui Zhi Wu Wu Tang* with modified *Da Qin Jiao Tang* (Major Gentiana Macrophylla Decoction): Radix Gentianae Macrophyllae (*Qin Jiao*), 9g, uncooked Radix Ligustici Wallichii (*Chuan Xiong*), 6g, wine mix-fried Radix Angelicae Sinensis (*Dang Gui*), 9g, Radix Et Rhizoma Notopterygii (*Qiang Huo*), 9g, Radix Angelicae Pubescentis (*Du Huo*), 9g, uncooked Radix Albus Paeoniae Lactiflorae (*Bai Shao*), 6g, Radix Ledebouriellae Divaricatae (*Fang Feng*), 9g, Herba Asari Cum Radice (*Xi Xin*), 3g, uncooked Rhizoma Atractylodis Macrocephalae (*Bai Zhu*), 6g, Radix Glycyrrhizae (*Gan Cao*), 3g, Lumbricus (*Di Long*), 6g, and Caulis Trachelospermi Jasminoidis (*Luo Shi Teng*), 9g.

4. Liver wind stirring internally

Symptoms: Hemilateral numbness, trembling of the limbs, dizziness, headache, vexation, irascibility, insomnia, profuse dreams, a dark red tongue with reduced or thin, dry, yellow fur, and a bowstring, forceful pulse

Therapeutic principles: Level the liver and extinguish wind, soothe the sinews and quicken the network vessels

Acupuncture & moxibustion:

He Gu (LI 4)
Tai Chong (Liv 3)
Feng Chi (GB 20)
Together, these points level the liver, soothe the sinews, and quicken the network vessels when needled with draining method.

Tai Xi (Ki 3)
San Yin Jiao (Sp 6)
Together, these points nourish yin to moisten wood when needled with supplementing method.

Additions & subtractions: For tinnitus, add *Ting Hui* (GB 2). For afternoon fever, add *Yang Fu* (GB 38). For vexatious heat in the five hearts, add *Xin Shu* (Bl 15). For sore throat, add *Zhao Hai* (Ki 6). For constipation, add *Zhi Gou* (TB 6) and *Shang Ju Xu* (St 37).

Chinese medicinal formula: Modified *Tian Ma Gou Teng Yin* (Gastrodia & Uncaria Drink)

Ingredients: Stir-fried till yellow Rhizoma Gastrodiae Elatae (*Tian Ma*), 9g, Ramulus Uncariae Cum Uncis (*Gou Teng*), 9g, Radix Achyranthis Bidentatae (*Niu Xi*), 9g, Concha Haliotidis (*Shi Jue Ming*), 15g, Ramulus Loranthi Seu Visci (*Sang Ji Sheng*), 9g, Fructus Gardeniae Jasminoidis (*Zhi Zi*), 9g, uncooked Radix Scutellariae Baicalensis (*Huang Qin*), 6g, salt stir-fried Cortex Eucommiae Ulmoidis (*Du Zhong*), 6g, Bulbus Fritillariae Cirrhosae (*Chuan Bei Mu*), 6g, Caulis Bambusae In Taeniis (*Zhu Ru*), 6g, White Flos Chrysanthemi Morifolii (*Ju Hua*), 9g, Fructus Tribuli Terrestris (*Bai Ji Li*), 6g, mix-fried Radix Glycyrrhizae (*Gan Cao*), 3g

Additions & subtractions: For insomnia and profuse dreams, add Sclerotium Pararadicis Poriae Cocos (*Fu Shen*), 9g, and Caulis Polygoni Multiflori (*Ye Jiao Teng*), 12g. For severe headache, add uncooked Bombyx Batryticatus (*Jiang Can*), 9g, and Buthus Martensis (*Quan Xie*), 3g. For liver blood vacuity, add wine mix-fried Radix Angelicae Sinensis (*Dang Gui*), 9g, uncooked Radix Albus Paeoniae Lactiflorae (*Bai Shao*), 9g, and Caulis Milletiae Seu Spatholobi (*Ji Xue Teng*), 15g. For severe liver-kidney yin vacuity, add cooked Radix Rehmanniae (*Shu Di*), 15g, and wine-steamed Fructus Corni Officinalis (*Shan Zhu Yu*), 6g.

5. Dampness & phlegm obstructing the network vessels

Symptoms: Hemilateral numbness with a heavy sensation, clouded, heavy head, dizziness, nausea and vomiting, chest oppression and discomfort, typically an obese constitution, a pale but dark tongue with slippery, moist or white, slimy fur, and a bowstring, slippery pulse

Therapeutic principles: Fortify the spleen and boost the qi, transform phlegm and free the flow of the network vessels

Acupuncture & moxibustion:

Qu Chi (LI 11)	Together, these points free the flow of the network
He Gu (LI 4)	vessels when needled with draining method.

Zu San Li (St 36)	Together, these points fortify the spleen, boost the qi
Feng Long (St 40)	and transform dampness when *Zu San Li* is needled with supplementing method and *Feng Long* is needled with draining method.

Additions & subtractions: For stomach glomus and oppression, add *Zhong Wan* (CV 12). For distention and pain in the abdomen, add *Tian Shu* (St 25). For profuse, clear, thin vaginal discharge, add *Yin Ling Quan* (Sp 9).

Chinese medicinal formula: Modified *Ban Xia Bai Zhu Tian Ma Tang* (Pinellia, Atractylodes & Gastrodia Decoction)

Ingredients: Clear Rhizoma Pinelliae Ternatae (*Ban Xia*), 9g, bran stir-fried Rhizoma Atractylodis Macrocephalae (*Bai Zhu*), 9g, stir-fried Rhizoma Gastrodiae Elatae (*Tian Ma*), 9g, Sclerotium Poriae Cocos (*Fu Ling*), 9g, stir-fried Pericarpium Citri Reticulatae (*Chen Pi*), 9g, uncooked Rhizoma Zingiberis (*Sheng Jiang*), 3g, Fructus Zizyphi Jujubae (*Da Zao*), 2 fruits, mix-fried Radix Glycyrrhizae (*Gan Cao*), 3g, Bombyx Batryticatus (*Jiang Can*), 6g, Buthus Martensis (*Quan Xie*), 6g

Additions & subtractions: For severe spleen qi vacuity, add rice stir-fried Radix Codonopsitis Pilosulae (*Dang Shen*), 9g, and stir-fried Radix Astragali Membranacei (*Huang Qi*), 15g. For severe dizziness, add processed Rhizoma Arsiaematis (*Tian Nan Xing*), 9g, and Rhizoma Typhonii Gigantei (*Bai Fu Zi*), 6g. For obesity, add Folium Nelumbinis Nuciferae (*He Ye*), 9g, and Rhizoma Alismatis (*Ze Xie*), 9g.

17
Hemiplegia *(Ban Shen Bu Sui)*

Hemiplegia refers to the inability to voluntarily move the limbs of one side of the body. In most cases, it is a sequellae of wind stroke. It is often accompanied by deviation of the mouth and eyes on the affected side, wilting muscles, and numbness in the affected limbs over time.

Disease causes, disease mechanisms:

1. Wind striking the channels & network vessels

Wind is the chief of the hundred diseases and often invades the body if the individual has insufficient righteous qi. When a righteous qi vacuity is mixed with deep-lying phlegm, invading wind evils may stir up this phlegm. If this phlegm flows into and obstructs the channels and network vessels, the qi and blood will not be able to flow freely to nourish the limbs. The limbs can only function if they obtain sufficient qi and blood. Therefore, if phlegm deprives the limbs of sufficient nourishment, they may become wilted, weak, and insensitive. Because the channels and network vessels are divided into two halves of the body, wind evils may only stir up phlegm which enters the channels and vessels on one side of the body. In that case, hemiplegia may be seen.

2. Liver yang transforming wind

Ascendant liver yang hyperactivity transforming wind usually develops from yin vacuity of the liver and kidneys in turn due to aging, enduring disease, or excessive sexual activity. If liver yang is so hyperactive that it transforms wind, the wind may stir up deep-lying phlegm. If this internally stirring wind causes phlegm to flow into and create obstruction in the channels and network vessels on one side of the body, hemiplegia may occur.

3. Phlegm fire internally blocking

The phlegm in this disease mechanism is usually engendered by overeating spicy, hot, fried foods which ferment dampness, engender heat, and damage the spleen, thus leading to phlegm formation. The fire mainly comes from mental-emotional disease which gives rise to liver depression which transforms fire. If this fire suddenly bursts forth, it may draft this phlegm upward to harass the heart spirit and confound the clear orifices as well as block the channels and vessels on one side of the body. In that latter case, hemiplegia may occur.

4. Dampness & phlegm internally blocking

Dampness and phlegm may both arise from dietary irregularities which damage the spleen. This may result in the spleen's failure to move and transform fluids which then gather and collect and transform into dampness. If dampness lingers and endures, it may transform into phlegm. Dampness and phlegm are both fluid evils and thus can flow. If these flow upward to confound the clear orifices, clouded spirit will occur. If they flow into and obstruct the channels and network vessels on one side of the body, hemiplegia may occur.

5. Liver kidney yin vacuity

Yin vacuity of the liver and kidneys usually develops from constitutional insufficiency or aging. The liver stores the blood and governs the sinews. The kidneys store the essence and govern the bones. Therefore, if the yin blood of the liver and kidneys becomes vacuous and insufficient, the sinews and the bones may obtain sufficient nourishment. As seen above, the channels and network vessels on the two sides of the body are semi-independent, and it is a clinical fact that the two sides of the body are not equal in all regards. Therefore, if one side of the body is malnourished and the other side is not, over time, hemiplegia may gradually develop.

6. Blood stasis

In most cases of hemiplegia, blood stasis arises due to aging. As one ages, the qi becomes vacuous and can no longer move the blood efficiently. Thus the blood becomes static. In a few cases, it may also be due to external injury severing the channels and vessels. If blood stasis obstructs the channels and network vessels on one side of the body, the muscles and sinews on that side of the body will not obtain sufficient nourishment, thus possibly giving rise to hemiplegia.

Treatment based on pattern discrimination:

1. Wind striking the channels & network vessels

Symptoms: Sudden hemiplegia, insensitivity of the skin, numbness of the hands and feet, sudden deviated mouth and eyes, inhibited speech, drooling, possible fever and aversion to cold, hypertonicity of the limbs, aching joints, thin, white tongue fur, and a floating, slippery pulse. When wind strikes the channels and network vessels (as opposed to the viscera and bowels), there is no loss of consciousness.

Therapeutic principles: Quicken the blood and dispel wind, free the flow of the channels and network vessels

Acupuncture & moxibustion:

Jian Yu (LI 15)	Together, these points dispel wind, quicken the
Qu Chi (LI 11)	blood, and free the flow of the channels and
He Gu (LI 4)	network vessels when needled with draining
Wai Guan (TB 5)	method.

Huan Tiao (GB 30)	Together, these points quicken the blood and free
Yang Ling Quan (GB 34)	the flow of the channels and network vessels
Zu San Li (St 36)	when needled with draining method.
Jie Xi (St 41)	
Kun Lun (Bl 60)	

Remarks: 1. In the early state, only treat the points on the affected side. In enduring cases, both sides should be treated.

2. The above points are mainly located on the yang ming channels with a few from the other yang channels. They are the main points for various patterns of hemiplegia. Select 4-6 of these in each treatment.

Additions & subtractions: For fever, add *Da Zhui* (GV 14). For headache, add *Feng Chi* (GB 20). For body aches, add *Shen Zhu* (GV 12). For aversion to wind, add *Feng Men* (Bl 12).

Chinese medicinal formula: Modified *Da Qin Jiao Tang* (Major Gentiana Macrophylla Decoction)

Ingredients: Radix Gentianae Macrophyllae (*Qin Jiao*), 12g, uncooked Radix Ligustici Wallichii (*Chuan Xiong*), 6g, wine mix-fried Radix Angelicae Sinensis (*Dang Gui*), 9g, Radix Et Rhizoma Notopterygii (*Qiang Huo*), 6g, Radix Angelicae Pubescentis (*Du Huo*), 6g, uncooked Radix Albus Paeoniae Lactiflorae (*Bai Shao*), 6g, Radix Ledebouriellae Divaricatae (*Fang Feng*), 6g, Herba Asari Cum Radice (*Xi Xin*), 3g, Radix Angelicae Dahuricae (*Bai Zhi*), 6g, cooked Radix Rehmanniae (*Shu Di*), 15g, uncooked Rhizoma Atractylodis Macrocephalae (*Bai Zhu*), 6g, Sclerotium Poriae Cocos (*Fu Ling*), 6g, Radix Glycyrrhizae (*Gan Cao*), 3g, Bombyx Batryticatus (*Jiang Can*), 6g, Buthus Martensis (*Quan Xie*), 6g

Additions & subtractions: For heat symptoms, add uncooked Radix Scutellariae Baicalensis (*Huang Qin*), 6g, and uncooked Gypsum Fibrosum (*Shi Gao*), 20g. For fever with aversion to cold, increase the dosage of Notopterygium and Ledebouriella up to 9g. For phlegm dampness, increase the dosage of Atractylodes and Poria up to 9g and add processed Rhizoma Arsiaematis (*Tian Nan Xing*), 9g.

2. Liver yang transforming wind

Symptoms: Sudden onset of hemiplegia, often after an outburst of violent anger and often preceding a sudden loss of consciousness, headache, dizziness and vertigo, tinnitus, blurred vision, a distended feeling in the eyes, heart vexation, irascibility, a red face and ears, a stiff tongue and sluggish speech, deviated mouth and eyes, clouded spirit in severe cases, a red tongue with slimy fur, and a bowstring, slippery pulse

Note: This pattern can also be used for the sequellae of wind striking the viscera and bowels.

Therapeutic principles: Level the liver and subdue yang, flush phlegm and free the flow of the network vessels

Acupuncture & moxibustion: Choose from among Pattern 1 acupuncture points above plus:

Tai Xi (Ki 3)　　　　Together, these points nourish yin and level the liver.
San Yin Jiao (Sp 6)
Tai Chong (Liv 3)

Feng Long (St 40)　　Flushes phlegm when needled with draining method

Additions & subtractions: For vomiting, add *Yong Quan* (Ki 1). For head distention and pain, add *Feng Chi* (GB 20). For a bitter taste in the mouth, heart vexation, yellow tongue fur, and a bowstring, rapid pulse, add *Xing Jian* (Liv 2). For insomnia and profuse dreams, add *Da Dun* (Liv 1).

Chinese medicinal formula: Modified *Tian Ma Gou Teng Yin* (Gastrodia & Uncaria Drink)

Ingredients: Stir-fried till yellow Rhizoma Gastrodiae Elatae (*Tian Ma*), 9g, Ramulus Uncariae Cum Uncis (*Gou Teng*), 9g, Radix Achyranthis Bidentatae (*Niu Xi*), 9g, Concha Haliotidis (*Shi Jue Ming*), 15g, Ramulus Loranthi Seu Visci (*Sang Ji Sheng*), 9g, Fructus Gardeniae Jasminoidis (*Zhi Zi*), 9g, uncooked Radix Scutellariae Baicalensis (*Huang Qin*), 6g, salt stir-fried Cortex Eucommiae Ulmoidis (*Du Zhong*), 6g, white Flos Chrysanthemi Morifolii (*Ju Hua*), 9g, Bombyx Batryticatus (*Jiang Can*), 6g, Buthus Martensis (*Quan Xie*), 6g, Fructus Tribuli Terrestris (*Bai Ji Li*), 6g, mix-fried Radix Glycyrrhizae (*Gan Cao*), 3g

Additions & subtractions: For severe liver yang, add Haemititum (*Dai Zhe Shi*), 30g. For night sweats, add uncooked Radix Albus Paeoniae Lactiflorae (*Bai Shao*), 15g. For numbness of the limbs, add processed Rhizoma Arsiaematis (*Tian Nan Xing*), 9g, and Rhizoma Typhonii Gigantei (*Bai Fu Zi*), 6g; For liver depression, add stir-fried Fructus Meliae Toosendan (*Chuan Lian Zi*), 9g.

3. Phlegm fire internally blocking

Symptoms: Sudden clouding collapse, clouded spirit, hemiplegia, deviated mouth and eyes, closed hands, clenched jaws, a red facial complexion and eyes, hoarse breathing, phlegm rales in the throat, panting, agitation, a red tongue with slimy, yellow fur, and a bowstring, slippery, rapid pulse

Therapeutic principles: Flush phlegm and open the orifices, clear the liver and extinguish wind

Acupuncture & moxibustion: Choose from among Pattern 1 acupuncture points above plus:

Tai Chong (Liv 3) *Xia Xi* (GB 43)	Together, these points clear the liver and extinguish wind when needled with draining method.
Shui Gou (GV 26) *Bai Hui* (GV 20)	Together, these points open the orifices and arouse the spirit when needled with draining method.

Additions & subtractions: For urinary block, add *Zhong Ji* (CV 3). For constipation, add *Nei Ting* (St 44) and *Tian Shu* (St 25). For convulsions, select *He Gu* (LI 4) and *Tai Chong* (Liv 3). For profuse phlegm and somnolence, add *Feng Long* (St 40). For vomiting, add *Zhong Wan* (CV 12). For red face and fever, prick *Shi Xuan* (EX-UE-1) to bleed.

Chinese medicinal formula: Modified *Ling Jiao Gou Teng Tang* (Antelope Horn & Uncaria Decoction)

Ingredients: Cornu Caprae (*Shan Yang Jiao*), 9g, uncooked Folium Mori Albi (*Sang Ye*), 6g, Bulbus Fritillariae Cirrhosae (*Chuan Bei Mu*), 9g, Caulis Bambusae In Taeniis (*Zhu Ru*), 9g, Ramulus Uncariae Cum Uncis (*Gou Teng*), 9g, stir-fried Flos Chrysanthemi Morifolii (*Ju Hua*), 9g, Cinnabar-processed Sclerotium Pararadicis Poriae Cocos (*Fu Shen*), 6g, Concretio Silicea Bambusae (*Tian Zhu Huang*), 6g, bile-processed Rhizoma Arisaematis (*Nan Xing*), 9g, Rhizoma Acori Graminei (*Shi Chang Pu*), 6g

Additions & subtractions: For severe cases, add Buthus Martensis (*Quan Xie*), 3g, and uncooked Bombyx Batryticatus (*Jiang Can*), 6g. For headache, tinnitus, and vertigo, add Spica Prunellae Vulgaris (*Xia Ku Gao*), 9g, and uncooked Concha Haliotidis (*Shi Jue Ming*), 15g. For insomnia, add uncooked Dens Draconis (*Long Chi*), 9g, and Caulis Polygoni Multiflori (*Ye Jiao Teng*), 9g.

4. Dampness & phlegm internally blocking

Symptoms: Sudden collapse, a pale facial complexion with purple lips, hemiplegia, somnolence or clouded sleep, clouded spirit, closed hands, phlegm-drool congestion, a vacuous puffy face, clenched jaws, stillness, lack of warmth in the limbs, glossy, slimy, white tongue fur, and a deep, slippery pulse

Therapeutic principles: Open the orifices, sweep away phlegm, and extinguish wind

Acupuncture & moxibustion: Choose from among Pattern 1 acupuncture points above plus:

Shui Gou (GV 26)   Together, these points open the orifices and arouse the
Bai Hui (GV 20)   spirit when needled with draining method.

Tai Chong (Liv 3)   Together, these points sweep away phlegm and
Feng Long (St 40)   extinguish wind when needled with draining method.

Additions & subtractions: For stiff tongue and sluggish speech, add *Lian Quan* (CV 23). For convulsions of the limbs, select *He Gu* (LI 4).

Chinese medicinal formula: Modified *Dao Tan Tang* (Abduct Phlegm Decoction)

Ingredients: Clear Rhizoma Pinelliae Ternatae (*Ban Xia*), 9g, processed Rhizoma Arisaematis (*Tian Nan Xing*), 9g, Fructus Citri Aurantii (*Zhi Ke*), 6g, Sclerotium Poriae Cocos (*Fu Ling*), 9g, Exocarpium Citri Erythrocarpae (*Ju Hong*), 9g, uncooked Rhizoma Zingiberis (*Sheng Jiang*), 3g, mix-fried Radix Glycyrrhizae (*Gan Cao*), 3g, stir-fried Rhizoma Gastrodiae Elatae (*Tian Ma*), 9g, bran stir-fried Rhizoma Atractylodis Macrocephalae (*Bai Zhu*), 6g, Ramulus Uncariae Cum Uncis (*Gou Teng*), 6g, Buthus Martensis (*Quan Xie*), 3g, uncooked Bombyx Batryticatus (*Jiang Can*), 6g

Additions & subtractions: For nausea and/or vomiting with profuse phlegm, add Flos Inulae Racemosae (*Xuan Fu Hua*), 6g. For fatigue, poor appetite, and loose stools, add rice stir-fried Radix Codonopsitis Pilosulae (*Dang Shen*), 9g. For dizziness or heavy-headedness, add Rhizoma Acori Graminei (*Shi Chang Pu*), 9g. For clouding sleep and clouded spirit, add Lapis Micae Seu Chloriti (*Meng Shi*), 3g (powdered and taken with the strained decoction).

5. Liver kidney yin vacuity

Symptoms: Gradual development of hemiplegia usually seen in elderly patients, low back and knee aching and limpness, loose teeth, hair loss, tinnitus and vertigo, impaired memory, blurred vision, inhibited speech, feeble-mindedness, a somber white facial complexion, a pale white tongue, and a deep, fine, weak pulse

Therapeutic principles: Enrich and supplement the liver and kidneys

Acupuncture & moxibustion: Choose from among Pattern 1 acupuncture points above plus:

San Yin Jiao (Sp 6)	Together, these points enrich and supplement
Tai Xi (Ki 3)	the liver and kidneys when needled with
Guan Yuan (CV 4)	supplementing method.
Si Shen Cong (M-HN-1)	Boosts intelligence

Additions & subtractions: For reduced sleep and profuse dreams, add *Shen Men* (Ht 7). For heart palpitations and vacuity vexation, add *Nei Guan* (Per 6). For night sweats, add *Yin Xi* (Ht 6).

Chinese medicinal formula: Modified *Di Huang Yin Zi* (Rehmannia Decoction)

Ingredients: Cooked Radix Rehmanniae (*Shu Di*), 12g, steamed Fructus Corni Officinalis (*Shan Zhu Yu*), 9g, Herba Dendrobii (*Shi Hu*), 9g, Fructus Schisandrae Chinensis (*Wu Wei Zi*), 6g, Tuber Ophiopogonis Japonici (*Mai Men Dong*), 9g, Radix Morindae Officinalis (*Ba Ji Tian*), 6g, Herba Cistanchis Deserticolae (*Rou Cong Rong*), 9g, bland Radix Lateralis Praeparatus Aconiti Carmichaeli (*Fu Zi*), 6g, Cortex Cinnamomi Cassiae (*Rou Gui*), 3g, Sclerotium Poriae Cocos (*Fu Ling*), 6g, Rhizoma Acori Graminei (*Shi Chang Pu*), 6g, licorice-processed Radix Polygalae Tenuifoliae (*Yuan Zhi*), 6g, Caulis Trachelospermi Jasminoidis (*Luo Shi Teng*), 9g

6. Blood stasis & qi vacuity

Symptoms: Hemiplegia as the sequella of wind stroke, insensitivity of the skin, possible stabbing pain on the affected side of the body, hypertonicity of the sinews, possible deviated mouth and eyes with sluggish speech, a somber white facial complexion, dry, scaly skin, reduced qi and laziness to speak, spontaneous perspiration, fatigued spirit, frequent urination or enuresis, a pale white or dark tongue with possible static macules and spots, and a bowstring, fine or choppy, vacuous pulse

Therapeutic principles: Fortify the spleen and boost the qi, quicken the blood and transform stasis

Acupuncture & moxibustion: Choose from among Pattern 1 acupuncture points above plus:

Qi Hai (CV 6) Supplements the qi when combined with *Zu San Li* and needled with supplementing method

San Yin Jiao (Sp 6) Quickens the blood and transforms stasis when combined with *He Gu* and needled with draining method

Additions & subtractions: For frequent urination, add *Zhong Ji* (CV 3). For deviated mouth and eyes, add *Jia Che* (St 6), *Di Cang* (St 4), and *Si Zhu Kong* (TB 23). For difficult, sluggish speech, add *Lian Quan* (CV 23). For constipation, add *Zhi Gou* (TB 6).

Chinese medicinal formula: Modified *Bu Yang Huan Wu Tang* (Supplement Yang & Restore Five [Tenths] Decoction)

Ingredients: Uncooked Radix Astragali Membranacei (*Huang Qi*), 30g, wine mix-fried Radix Angelicae Sinensis (*Dang Gui*), 9g, wine mix-fried Radix Rubrus Paeoniae Lactiflorae (*Chi Shao*), 9g, Lumbricus (*Di Long*), 6g, wine mix-fried Radix Ligustici Wallichii (*Chuan Xiong*), 9g, Semen Pruni Persicae (*Tao Ren*), 9g, Flos Carthami Tinctorii (*Hong Hua*), 9g, Caulis Trachelospermi Jasminoidis (*Luo Shi Teng*), 9g

18
Paralysis *(Tan Huan)*

Paralysis refers to limpness, weakness, and slackened muscles of the limbs and body which are difficult or even impossible to move. It mainly involves the lower extremities. This disease includes wilting condition or *wei zheng*.

Disease causes, disease mechanisms:

1. Lung-stomach fluid damage

The fluid damage is mainly due to warm heat evils which invade the body and then burn and damage the liquids of the lungs and stomach. The stomach is the sea of water and grains and is the source of the qi and blood. The lungs face the hundreds of vessels and are responsible for distributing the qi and blood. Warm heat evils are yang evils which easily consume and damage the fluids of the lungs and stomach. If the fluids of the lungs and stomach are damaged, the lungs and stomach cannot perform their functions. As a result, less qi and blood will be engendered, and the distribution of what qi and blood there is will not be as efficient, thus leading to insufficient moistening and nourishment to the sinews and muscles. Hence, paralysis or wilting may occur.

2. Liver-kidney yin vacuity

Liver-kidney yin vacuity usually results from constitutional insufficiency, aging, enduring disease, or from excessive sexual activity. The liver stores the blood and governs the sinews, while the kidneys store the essence and govern the bones. Therefore, when liver blood and kidney yin are vacuous and insufficient, the sinews will not be sufficiently moistened and nourished, and the bones will not be banked up strongly. As a result, paralysis or wilting may occur.

3. Cold dampness invading & spreading

Cold dampness usually arises from external contraction of evils, from enduring exposure to cold damp evils such as living and working enduringly in damp surroundings, being caught in rain, etc., or from dietary irregularities which damage the spleen and form accumulation of water dampness in the body. Cold is a yin evil which causes contracture and constriction. Dampness is also a yin evil which is sticky and stagnant by nature. Therefore, both of these can create obstruction when they invade the body. If they invade and spread in the muscles, the muscles will receive less nourishment from qi and blood and thus become withered. If these evils remain undispelled but invade and spread to the sinews, the sinews will be deprived of sufficient nourishment and paralysis may occur.

4. Damp heat invading & spreading

Damp heat may arise from external contraction of damp heat evils, from external contraction of cold dampness which transform heat over time, or from excessive consumption of fried, greasy, sweet foods, or alcohol which ferment dampness and engender heat. Heat is a yang evil which causes slackness of the sinews. Dampness is a yin evil which is sticky and stagnant and thus can cause obstruction, especially when bound with heat. If damp heat invades and spreads into the sinews, the heat will make the sinews slack, while the obstruction will result in less nourishment to the sinews. As a result, paralysis may occur.

5. Qi vacuity of the spleen & stomach

Spleen and stomach qi vacuity resulting in paralysis often develops from constitutional vacuity or enduring disease. The spleen and stomach are the latter heaven root and the source of qi and blood engenderment and transformation whose normal function depends on their qi. Therefore, if the qi of the spleen and stomach is vacuous and weak, less qi and blood will be engendered. Furthermore, the spleen governs the muscles and the four limbs. If less qi and blood are engendered by the spleen and stomach, the muscles may not obtain sufficient nourishment. As a result, paralysis may be seen.

6. Kidney yang vacuity

Kidney yang vacuity may be due to constitutional insufficiency, aging, enduring disease, or from excessive sexual activity. In that case, the kidney qi will be vacuous and the essence will not be sufficiently formed, since qi engenders the essence. Therefore, the bones will not be banked up, leading to paralysis. On the other hand, yang qi is responsible for warming the sinews and muscles. If yang becomes vacuous, it may not be able to warm the sinews and muscles efficiently and paralysis may occur as a result. As it is said, "The unyielding aspect of yang qi nourishes the spirit, while the soft aspect [nourishes] the sinews."

7. Blood stasis obstructing the network vessels

The blood stasis involved in paralysis is usually due to external injury, enduring disease, or from qi stagnation. As is well known, blood stasis can block the channels and network vessels. Qi and blood provide nourishment to the sinews and muscles through the channels and network vessels. If static blood obstructs the network vessels, the qi and blood cannot freely flow to and sufficiently nourish the sinews and muscles. Thus paralysis may occur.

8. Liver depression with blood vacuity

Liver depression usually arises from unfulfilled desires or anger damaging the liver. The liver stores the blood and governs the sinews. Liver depression causes abnormal coursing and discharging of the liver. Therefore, the blood is not efficiently supplied to the sinews and muscles. As it is said:

> The qi moves the blood. If the qi moves, the blood moves. If the qi stops, the blood stops.

If, for any reason, the blood is also vacuous, A) the supply of blood will be further lessened to the sinews and muscles, and B) liver depression will worsen. This is because the liver can only function, *i.e.*, only course and discharge, as long as it receives sufficient nourishment from blood. Therefore, liver depression and blood vacuity mutually reinforce one another. If they are bad enough, paralysis may occur.

Treatment based on pattern discrimination:

1. Lung stomach fluid damage

Symptoms: During or after a fever due to external contraction of evils, limpness and weakness of the upper or lower limbs may appear. The hands cannot hold things or the feet may fail to support the body. In severe cases, paralysis occurs and the muscles gradually wither. Other symptoms include dry skin, heart vexation, thirst, heat in the palms of the hands and soles of the feet, red cheekbones, possible dry cough with no or scanty phlegm, dry throat, nose, and lips, short voidings of dark-colored urine, a red tongue with scanty liquids and yellow fur, and a fine, rapid pulse.

Therapeutic principles: Clear heat and moisten dryness, nourish the lungs and boost the stomach

Acupuncture & moxibustion:

Da Zhui (GV 14) *Qu Chi* (LI 11) *He Gu* (LI 4)	Together, these points clear heat when needled with draining method.
Chi Ze (Lu 5) *Tai Yuan* (Lu 9) *Shang Qiu* (Sp 5)	Together, these points nourish the lungs and moisten dryness when needled with supplementing method.

Note: This prescription is for the early stage of this pattern. After the early stage of this pattern, one should use the followings points:

A) For paralysis of upper limbs, choose 2-3 points from *Da Zhui* (GV 14) and Hua Tuo's paravertebral points located at the levels from T1-T8 and combine these with 2-3 points chosen from among *Jian Yu* (LI 15), *Bi Nao* (LI 14), *Qu Chi* (LI 11), *Shou San Li* (LI 10), *He Gu* (LI 4), and *Wai Guan* (TB 5).

B) For paralysis of lower limbs, choose 2-3 points from among *Ci Liao* (Bl 32), *Zhi Bian* (Bl 34), *Yao Yang Guan* (GV 3), and Hua Tuo's paravertebral points located at the levels of T10-L5 and combine these with 2-3 points chosen from among *Bi Guan* (St 31), *Fu Tu* (St 32), *Liang Qiu* (St 34), *Zu San Li* (St 36), *Shang Ju Xu* (St 37), and *Jie Xi* (St 41).

Additions & subtractions: For cough with scanty phlegm, add *Fei Shu* (Bl 13). For painful urination, add *Zhong Ji* (CV 3) and *Guan Yuan* (CV 4). For fever, add *Wai Guan* (TB 5). For constipation, add *Tian Shu* (St 25). For dry retching and hiccup, add *Ge Shu* (Bl 17).

Chinese medicinal formula: *Qing Zao Jiu Fei Tang* (Clear Dryness & Rescue the Lungs Decoction)

Ingredients: Honey stir-fried Folium Mori Albi (*Sang Ye*), 9g, uncooked Gypsum Fibrosum (*Shi Gao*), 12g, Radix Pseudostellariae Heterophyllae (*Tai Zi Shen*), 9g, black Semen Sesami Indici (*Hei Zhi Ma*), 6g, Gelatinum

Corii Asini (*E Jiao*), 9g, Tuber Ophiopogonis Japonici (*Mai Dong*), 9g, Semen Pruni Armeniacae (*Xing Ren*), 9g, honey stir-fried Folium Eriobotryae Japonicae (*Pi Pa Ye*), 9g, mix-fried Radix Glycyrrhizae (*Gan Cao*), 3g

Additions & subtractions: For severe heat dryness of the lungs, add uncooked Rhizoma Anemarrhenae Asphodeloidis (*Zhi Mu*), 9g. For severe dryness of the stomach, add Rhizoma Polygonati Odorati (*Yu Zhu*), 9g, and Radix Glehniae Littoralis (*Sha Shen*), 9g. For concomitant blood vacuity, add uncooked Radix Rehmanniae (*Sheng Di*), 12g. For concomitant qi vacuity, add uncooked Radix Astragali Membranacei (*Huang Qi*), 15g, and uncooked Radix Codonopsitis Pilosulae (*Dang Shen*), 9g. For constipation with dry stools, add uncooked Radix Et Rhizoma Rhei (*Da Huang*), 6g.

2. Liver kidney yin vacuity

Symptoms: Paralysis develops gradually from limpness and weakness of the upper or, more often, the lower limbs. This is followed by emaciation over time. Low back and spine aching and limpness is present. Numbness, hypertonicity, and twitching of the muscles are possible. Other symptoms include dizziness, tinnitus, seminal emission, tidal fever, night sweats, tidal reddening of the cheekbones, low-grade fever, a dry throat, scanty urination, dry stools, a crimson tongue with scanty fluids, and a bowstring, fine, rapid pulse.

Therapeutic principles: Nourish the liver and supplement the kidneys, enrich yin and clear heat

Acupuncture & moxibustion: Choose the same local points as in Pattern 1 above and combine these with:

Gan Shu (Bl 18) Together, these points supplement and enrich the
Shen Shu (Bl 23) liver and kidneys.
San Yin Jiao (Sp 6)

Additions & subtractions: For sore throat, add *Zhao Hai* (Ki 6). For constipation, add *Tian Shu* (St 25). For premature ejaculation, add *Guan Yuan* (CV 4). For blurred vision, add *Guang Ming* (GB 37). For scanty menstruation, add *Xue Hai* (Sp 10).

Chinese medicinal formula: Modified *Zhi Bai Di Huang Wan* (Anemarrhena & Phellodendron Rehmannia Pills)

Ingredients: Cooked Radix Rehmanniae (*Shu Di*), 18g, steamed Fructus Corni Officinalis (*Shan Zhu Yu*), 9g, stir-fried Radix Dioscoreae Oppositae (*Shan Yao*), 9g, Sclerotium Poriae Cocos (*Fu Ling*), 6g, Cortex Radicis Moutan (*Dan Pi*), 6g, salt mix-fried Rhizoma Alismatis (*Ze Xie*), 6g, salt mix-fried Rhizoma Anemarrhenae Asphodeloidis (*Zhi Mu*), 9g, salt mix-fried Cortex Phellodendri (*Huang Bai*), 9g, Cortex Radicis Acanthopanacis (*Wu Jia Pi*), 9g, Radix Achyranthis Bidentatae (*Niu Xi*), 9g

Additions & subtractions: For both yin and yang vacuity, replace *Zhi Bai Di Huang Wan* with Modified *Hu Qian Wan* (Hidden Tiger Pills): salt mix-fried Cortex Phellodendri (*Huang Bai*), 6g, salt mix-fried Rhizoma Anemarrhenae Asphodeloidis (*Zhi Mu*), 6g, cooked Radix Rehmanniae (*Shu Di*), 12g, Plastrum Testudinis (*Gui Ban*), 15g, Radix Albus Paeoniae Lactiflorae (*Bai Shao*), 9g, wine mix-fried Radix Angelicae Sinensis (*Dang Gui*), 9g, Herba Cynomorii Songarici (*Suo Yang*), 9g, Os Suis (*Zhu Gu*), 12g, Cortex Radicis Acanthopanacis (*Wu Jia Pi*), 12g, salt stir-fried Radix Achyranthis Bidentatae (*Niu Xi*), 9g, Pericarpium Citri Reticulatae (*Chen Pi*), 6g, steamed Fructus Corni Officinalis (*Shan Zhu Yu*), 9g, and salt stir-fried Cortex Eucommiae Ulmoidis (*Du Zhong*), 9g.

3. Cold dampness invading & spreading

Symptoms: Paralysis follows facial edema and encumbered, heavy limbs and leads to clumsy movement and low back and spine aching and limpness. Other symptoms are stomach oppression, abdominal distention, torpid intake, nausea, increased vaginal discharge, slight edema in the dorsum of the feet, an enlarged tongue with teeth-marks on its edges and slimy, white fur, and a slippery, moderate (*i.e.*, slightly slow) pulse

Therapeutic principles: Fortify the spleen and dry dampness, warm and dispel cold evils

Acupuncture & moxibustion: Choose the same local point as in Pattern 1 above and combine these with:

Yin Ling Quan (Sp 9)	Together, these points fortify the spleen, dry
Pi Shu (Bl 20)	dampness, and warm and dispel cold when needled with moxibustion on the heads of the needles.

Additions & subtractions: For itching, add *San Yin Jiao* (Sp 6) and *Xue Hai* (Sp 10). For loose stools, add *Xia Ju Xu* (St 39). For heavy-headedness, add

Feng Long (St 40). For fatigued spirit and fear of cold, moxa *Guan Yuan* (CV 4).

Chinese medicinal formula: *Shi Pi Yin* (Bolster the Spleen Drink)

Ingredients: Ginger mix-fried Cortex Magnoliae Officinalis (*Hou Po*), 9g, uncooked Rhizoma Atractylodis Macrocephalae (*Bai Zhu*), 9g, uncooked Fructus Chaenomelis Lagenariae (*Mu Gua*), 9g, Radix Auklandiae Lappae (*Mu Xiang*), 6g, Semen Alpiniae Katsumadai (*Cao Dou Kou*), 9g, Semen Arecae Catechu (*Bing Lang*), 9g, Radix Lateralis Praeparatus Aconiti Carmichaeli (*Fu Zi*), 6g, Sclerotium Poriae Cocos (*Fu Ling*), 9g, dry Rhizoma Zingiberis (*Gan Jiang*), 6g, mix-fried Radix Glycyrrhizae (*Gan Cao*), 6g

Additions & subtractions: For severe edema with inhibited urination, add Sclerotium Polypori Umbellati (*Zhu Ling*), 9g, and Rhizoma Alismatis (*Ze Xie*), 9g. For severe spleen qi vacuity, add Radix Astragali Membranacei (*Huang Qi*), 18g. For severe encumbered heavy limbs, add uncooked Rhizoma Atractylodis (*Cang Zhu*), 9g.

4. Damp heat invading & spreading

Symptoms: Lower limb limpness and weakness followed by paralysis, burning heat in the limbs which gets better on obtaint of cold, numbness, swollen feet, unsurfaced fever, stomach oppression, torpid intake, a yellow facial complexion, encumbered body, heavy-headedness, a vacuous puffy face, dryness and stickiness in the mouth with a bitter taste, dark-colored urine, a red tongue with slimy, yellow fur, and a soggy, rapid or slippery, rapid pulse

Therapeutic principles: Clear heat and disinhibit dampness

Acupuncture & moxibustion: Choose the same local points as in Pattern 1 above and combine these with:

Yin Ling Quan (Sp 9)	Together, these points clear heat and disinhibit
Yang Ling Quan (GB 34)	dampness when needled with draining method.
Nei Ting (St 44)	

Additions & subtractions: For painful urination, add *Zhong Ji* (CV 3). For constipation, add *Shang Ju Xu* (St 37). For loose stools, add *Xia Ju Xu* (St

39). For chest oppression, add *Dan Zhong* (CV 17). For thick, yellow vaginal discharge, add *Lou Gu* (Sp 7). For jaundice, add *Zhi Yang* (GV 9).

Chinese medicinal formula: Modified *Si Miao Wan* (Four Marvels Pills)

Ingredients: Uncooked Cortex Phellodendri (*Huang Bai*), 9g, Rhizoma Atractylodis (*Cang Zhu*), 9g, Radix Achyranthis Bidentatae (*Niu Xi*), 9g, Semen Coicis Lachryma-jobi (*Yi Yi Ren*), 15g, steamed Fructus Chaenomelis Lagenariae (*Mu Gua*), 9g

Additions & subtractions: For severe paralysis, add Cortex Radicis Acanthopanacis (*Wu Jia Pi*), 12g. For lower limb distention and heaviness, add Radix Stephaniae Tetrandrae (*Han Fang Ji*), 9g, and Radix Angelicae Pubescentis (*Du Huo*), 9g. For redness and swelling of knees and feet, a bitter taste in the mouth, and red urine, add Caulis Akebiae (*Mu Tong*), 3g, Semen Plantaginis (*Che Qian Zi*), 9g, and Fructus Gardeniae Jasminoidis (*Zhi Zi*), 6g. For severe numbness and burning pain in the lower limbs, add Caulis Lonicerae Japonicae (*Ren Dong Teng*), 9g, and Caulis Sargentodoxae (*Hong Teng*), 9g. For edema in the lower limbs, add Sclerotium Polypori Umbellati (*Zhu Ling*), 6g, Rhizoma Alismatis (*Ze Xie*), 6g, and Semen Plantaginis (*Che Qian Zi*), 6g. For concomitant yin vacuity with dry throat and mouth which are worse at night, low back weakness, and vexatious heat in the five hearts, add uncooked Radix Rehmanniae (*Sheng Di*), 12g, Fructus Ligustri Lucidi (*Nu Zhen Zi*), 9g, and Herba Ecliptae Prostratae (*Han Lian Cao*), 9g.

5. Spleen stomach qi vacuity

Symptoms: Gradual development of limpness of the lower limbs followed by paralysis, fatigued limbs, emaciation, reduced qi with laziness to speak, low voice, fatigued spirit and lassitude, a pale white, lusterless facial complexion, dizziness, loose stools, reduced and torpid intake, a pale tongue with thin fur, and a fine, soft pulse

Therapeutic principles: Fortify the spleen and boost the stomach

Acupuncture & moxibustion: Choose the same local points as in Pattern 1 above and combine these with:

Pi Shu (Bl 20)	Together, these points fortify the spleen and boost the
Tai Bai (Sp 3)	stomach when needled with supplementing method.
Wei Shu (Bl 21)	

Additions & subtractions: For somnolence, add *Bai Hui* (GV 20). For abdominal distention, add *Fu Tong Gu* (Ki 20). For dull pain in the stomach which gets better with pressure, add *Zu San Li* (St 36).

Chinese medicinal formula: *Bu Zhong Yi Qi Tang* (Supplement the Center & Boost the Qi Decoction)

Ingredients: Honey mix-fried Radix Astragali Membranacei (*Huang Qi*), 18g, honey stir-fried Radix Codonopsis Pilosulae (*Dang Shen*), 12g, bran stir-fried Rhizoma Atractylodis Macrocephalae (*Bai Zhu*), 12g, honey mix-fried Radix Glycyrrhizae (*Gan Cao*), 6g, stir-fried Radix Angelicae Sinensis (*Dang Gui*), 6g, stir-fried Pericarpium Citri Reticulatae (*Chen Pi*), 6g, Radix Bupleuri (*Chai Hu*), 3g, Rhizoma Cimicifugae (*Sheng Ma*), 3g

Additions & subtractions: For spleen vacuity leading to damp accumulation with loose stools, diarrhea, sliminess in the mouth, and slimy tongue fur, replace *Bu Zhong Yi Qi Tang* with Modified *Shen Ling Bai Zhu San* (Ginseng, Poria & Atractylodes Powder): stir-fried Semen Dolichoris Lablab (*Bai Bian Dou*), 9g, stir-fried Radix Dioscoreae Oppositae (*Shan Yao*), 9g, bran stir-fried Rhizoma Atractylodis Macrocephalae (*Bai Zhu*), 15g, Sclerotium Poriae Cocos (*Fu Ling*), 9g, rice stir-fried Radix Codonopsitis Pilosulae (*Dang Shen*), 12g, stir-fried till yellow Semen Nelumbinis Nuciferae (*Lian Zi*), 9g, Radix Platycodi Grandiflori (*Jie Geng*), 6g, Fructus Amomi (*Sha Ren*), 3g, mix-fried Radix Glycyrrhizae (*Gan Cao*), 6g, and uncooked Radix Astragali Membranacei (*Huang Qi*), 15g. For chest, stomach, and abdominal oppression or distention, nausea, a slimy feeling mouth, and reduced food intake, add Herba Agastachis Seu Pogostemi (*Huo Xiang*), 9g, Herba Eupatorei Fortunei (*Pei Lan*), 9g, and Rhizoma Acori Graminei (*Shi Chang Pu*), 6g. For qi and blood dual vacuity, replace *Bu Zhong Yi Qi Tang* with *Ren Shen Yang Rong Tang* (Ginseng Nourish the Constructive Decoction): Radix Codonopsitis Pilosulae (*Dang Shen*), 12g, uncooked Radix Astragali Membranacei (*Huang Qi*), 15g, uncooked Radix Albus Paeoniae Lactiflorae (*Bai Shao*), 9g, Radix Angelicae Sinensis (*Dang Gui*), 9g, stir-fried Pericarpium Citri Reticulatae (*Chen Pi*), 9g, Cortex Cinnamomi Cassiae (*Rou Gui*), 3g, stir-fried Rhizoma Atractylodis Macrocephalae (*Bai Zhu*), 12g, cooked Radix Rehmanniae (*Shu Di*), 9g, Fructus Schisandrae Chinensis (*Wu Wei Zi*), 9g, licorice-processed Radix Polygalae Tenuifoliae (*Yuan Zhi*), 3g, Sclerotium Poriae Cocos (*Fu Ling*), 9g, and mix-fried Radix Glycyrrhizae (*Gan Cao*), 6g.

6. Kidney yang vacuity

Symptoms: Paralysis, low back and leg aching and limpness, slight edema on the dorsum of the feet, cold limbs, a bright white facial complexion, dizziness and vertigo, tinnitus, fatigue and lack of strength, impotence, seminal emission, hair loss, sweating, a pale tongue, and a weak pulse at the cubit position

Therapeutic principles: Warm and supplement kidney yang

Acupuncture & moxibustion: Choose the same local points as in Pattern 1 above and combine these with:

Ming Men (GV 4)	Together, these points warm and supplement
Shen Shu (Bl 23)	kidney yang when needled with moxibustion on the
Fu Liu (Ki 7)	heads of the needles or when directly moxaed.
Yao Yang Guan (GV 3)	

Additions & subtractions: For abdominal distention and fullness, add *Fu Tong Gu* (Ki 20). For daybreak diarrhea, moxa *Shen Que* (CV 8). For pain in the periumbilical region, moxa *Shen Que* (CV 8). For enuresis, add *Guan Yuan* (CV 4). For clear, thin vaginal discharge, add *San Yin Jiao* (Sp 6).

Chinese medicinal formula: Modified *Lu Jiao Jiao Wan* (Deer Horn Glue Pills)

Chinese medicinal formula: Gelatinum Cornu Cervi (*Lu Jiao Jiao*), 12g, cooked Radix Rehmanniae (*Shu Di*), 9g, salt stir-fried Radix Achyranthis Bidentatae (*Niu Xi*), 9g, Sclerotium Poriae Cocos (*Fu Ling*), 9g, salt mix-fried Semen Cuscutae Chinensis (*Tu Si Zi*), 12g, stir-fried Radix Angelicae Sinensis (*Dang Gui*), 6g, bran stir-fried Rhizoma Atractylodis Macro-cephalae (*Bai Zhu*), 9g, Cortex Eucommiae Ulmoidis (*Du Zhong*), 9g, Radix Dipsaci (*Xu Duan*), 9g, Cortex Radicis Acanthopanacis (*Wu Jia Pi*), 9g, Rhizoma Drynariae (*Gu Sui Bu*), 9g

7. Blood stasis obstructing the network vessels

Symptoms: In most cases, the paralysis follows external injury. Other symptoms are incontinence of the urine and feces, inability to sense pain or itching, edema on the dorsum of the feet, and dry, thin skin. As the condition progresses, there is emaciation of the flesh, scaly skin, lack of warmth in the limbs, stabbing pain in the chest or low back, a red tongue with possible static macules or spots, and a deep, fine, choppy pulse

Therapeutic principles: Quicken the blood and transform stasis, free the flow of the channels and disinhibit the network vessels

Acupuncture & moxibustion: Choose the same local points as in Pattern 1 above and combine these with:

San Yin Jiao (Sp 6)　　Together, these points move the qi and quicken the
He Gu (LI 4)　　blood when needled with draining method.

8. Liver depression with blood vacuity

Symptoms: Emotional lability and/or depression, susceptibility to grief and a tendency to cry for little or no reason, sudden onset of enduring paralysis after strong anger, no emaciation of the flesh of the limbs even though the paralysis endures, lustrous skin, rib-side distention and pain, belching, torpid intake, a bitter taste in the mouth, a pale red tongue, and a bowstring, fine pulse

Remarks: This pattern often describes patients suffering from hysterical paralysis.

Therapeutic principles: Course the liver and nourish the blood

Acupuncture & moxibustion: Choose the same local points as in Pattern 1 above and combine these with:

Tai Chong (Liv 3)　　Together, these points course the liver and rectify
Qi Men (Liv 14)　　the qi when needled with draining method.

Gan Shu (Bl 18)　　Together, these points nourish the blood when
Pi Shu (Bl 20)　　needled with supplementing method.
Wei Shu (Bl 21)

Additions & subtractions: For frequent sighing, add *Ge Shu* (Bl 17). For lower abdominal distention and pain, add *Yin Bao* (Liv 9). For stomachache and acid regurgitation, add *Yang Ling Quan* (GB 34) or *Shang Wan* (CV 13). For irregular menstruation with pale, scanty blood, add *Xue Hai* (Sp 10). For insomnia, add *Xin Shu* (Bl 15). For dizziness, add *Bai Hui* (GV 20).

Chinese medicinal formula: Modified *Xiao Yao San* (Rambling Powder)

Ingredients: Vinegar stir-fried Radix Bupleuri (*Chai Hu*), 6g, bran stir-fried Rhizoma Atractylodis Macrocephalae (*Bai Zhu*), 9g, uncooked Radix Albus Paeoniae Lactiflorae (*Bai Shao*), 9g, wine mix-fried Radix Angelicae Sinensis (*Dang Gui*), 9g, Sclerotium Poriae Cocos (*Fu Ling*), 9g, Pericarpium Citri Reticulatae (*Chen Pi*), 6g, Herba Menthae Haplocalysis (*Bo He*), 3g, Fructus Tritici Aestivi (*Huai Xiao Mai*), 18g, Fructus Zizyphi Jujubae (*Da Zao*), 5 pieces, honey mix-fried Radix Glycyrrhizae (*Gan Cao*), 3g, steamed Fructus Chaenomelis Lagenariae (*Mu Gua*), 9g, salt stir-fried Radix Achyranthis Bidentatae (*Niu Xi*), 9g

Additions & subtractions: For severe emotional disturbance and insomnia with profuse dreams, add stir-fried Semen Zizyphi Spinosae (*Suan Zao Ren*), 9g, and Caulis Polygoni Multiflori (*Ye Jiao Teng*), 12g. For severe blood vacuity, add cooked Radix Rehmanniae (*Shu Di*), 9g. For depressive liver heat, add uncooked Cortex Radicis Moutan (*Dan Pi*), 9g, and uncooked Fructus Gardeniae Jasminoidis (*Zhi Zi*), 9g. For severe liver depression, add vinegar mix-fried Tuber Curcumae (*Yu Jin*), 6g, and Rhizoma Cyperi Rotundi (*Xiang Fu*), 9g. For concomitant spleen qi vacuity, add rice stir-fried Radix Codonopsitis Pilosulae (*Dang Shen*), 9g.

19

Twitching Muscles *(Ji Rou Shun Dong)*

Twitching muscles in Chinese medicine refers to uncontrollable tic of the muscles.

Disease causes, disease mechanisms:

1. Yang vacuity

Yang vacuity in this case usually develops from yang desertion due to great sweating, vomiting, or diarrhea. Yang is supposed to warm the sinews and flesh. Therefore, if yang deserts, yin cold will become exuberant. Cold causes contracture and constriction. This contracture and constriction due to cold may cause twitching of the muscles. In addition, when there is great sweating, vomiting, or diarrhea, body fluids are damaged and become vacuous. If they are vacuous and insufficient, they may be unable to moisten and nourish the sinews and flesh properly. Therefore, the sinews dry and shrink, also giving rise to possible twitching of the muscles.

2. Blood vacuity

Blood vacuity often arises from constitutional insufficiency, spleen-stomach vacuity, bleeding, enduring disease, or from excessive thinking. The blood is supposed to moisten and nourish the sinews and flesh. If, for any reason, the blood becomes vacuous and insufficient, the sinews and flesh may not be sufficiently moistened or nourished. Therefore, they may dry out and shrink, leading to twitching of the muscles.

3. Fright & fear damaging the spirit

Sudden fear or fright may damage the spirit and cause chaos in the qi flow. Movement is a function of the flow of qi. Therefore, if the qi moves chaotically, movement may also become chaotic and uncontrollable. On the other hand, chaotic qi flow may deprive the sinews from receiving adequate nourishment and hence contract. Both of these mechanisms may give rise to what are called in Chinese medicine "fright spasms," a species of twitching muscles.

4. Cold water

Spleen and kidney yang vacuity may result from constitutional insufficiency, overwork taxation, aging, and enduring disease. If, for any of these reasons, spleen and kidney yang become vacuous and weak, yang qi may not move and transform body fluids properly. In that case, water dampness may gather and collect internally. If this accumulated water spills over into the flesh, it may prevent the nourishing of the sinews and flesh. Without this nourishment, the sinews may contract and twitching of the muscles may occur.

Treatment based on pattern discrimination:

I. Yang vacuity

Symptoms: Twitching of the muscles, a bright white facial complexion, fear of cold, sweating, counterflow cold of the limbs, fatigued spirit, lack of strength, a pale tongue with white fur, and a faint pulse

Therapeutic principles: Warm yang and stop twitching

Acupuncture & moxibustion:

A shi points   Free the flow of the network vessels to stop twitching when needled with even draining and supplementing method

Guan Yuan (CV 4)   Together, these points warm yang when moxaed.
Qi Hai (CV 6)
Pi Shu (Bl 20)
Shen Shu (Bl 23)

Additions & subtractions: For dizziness, moxa *Bai Hui* (GV 20). For heart palpitations, add *Nei Guan* (Per 6). For abdominal pain that likes warmth and pressure, add *Shen Que* (CV 8). For reduced food intake, add *Zu San Li* (St 36).

Chinese medicinal formula: *Si Ni Tang* (Four Counterflows Decoction)

Ingredients: Blast-fried Radix Lateralis Praeparatus Aconiti Carmichaeli (*Fu Zi*), 6g, dry Rhizoma Zingiberis (*Gan Jiang*), 9g, mix-fried Radix Glycyrrhizae (*Gan Cao*), 6g

Additions & subtractions: For great sweating leading to yang desertion, add Radix Panacis Quinquefolii (*Xi Yang Shen*), 12g, and uncooked Fructus Schisandrae Chinensis (*Wu Wei Zi*), 9g. For severe counterflow chilling of the limbs, severe fear of cold, a curled-up lying posture, and a faint pulse due to yang and qi desertion, add Red Radix Panacis Ginseng (*Hong Shen*), 15g. For diarrhea, add earth stir-fried Rhizoma Atractylodis Macrocephalae (*Bai Zhu*), 9g.

2. Blood vacuity

Symptoms: Twitching of the muscles, numb or shaking hands and feet, heart palpitations, insomnia, dizziness, blurred vision, a somber white facial complexion, pale lips and nails, a pale tongue, and a fine, forceless pulse

Therapeutic principles: Supplement the blood and stop twitching

Acupuncture & moxibustion:

A shi points	Free the flow of the network vessels to stop twitching
Xin Shu (Bl 15) *Ge Shu* (Bl 17) *Pi Shu* (Bl 20) *Zu San Li* (St 36)	Together, these points supplement the blood when needled with supplementing method.

Additions & subtractions: For scanty menstruation, add *Xue Hai* (St 10). For reduced food intake, add *Zhong Wan* (CV 12). For tinnitus, add *Er Men* (TB 21). For constipation, add *Shang Ju Xu* (St 37) and *San Yin Jiao* (Sp 6).

Chinese medicinal formula: Modified *Si Wu Tang* (Four Materials Decoction)

Ingredients: Cooked Radix Rehmanniae (*Shu Di*), 12g, uncooked Radix Albus Paeoniae Lactiflorae (*Bai Shao*), 12g, wine mix-fried Radix Angelicae Sinensis (*Dang Gui*), 12g, wine mix-fried Radix Ligustici Wallichii (*Chuan Xiong*), 6g, honey stir-fried Radix Astragali Membranacei (*Huang Qi*), 24g

Additions & subtractions: For severe blood vacuity, add processed Polygoni Multiflori (*He Shou Wu*), 9g. For shaking or spasms in the lower limbs, add steamed Fructus Chaenomelis Lagenariae (*Mu Gua*), 9g. For blood vacuity due to spleen vacuity, add rice stir-fried Radix Codonopsitis Pilosulae (*Dang Shen*), 9g, bran stir-fried Rhizoma Atractylodis Macrocephalae (*Bai*

Zhu), 6g, and Fructus Amomi (*Sha Ren*), 6g. For concomitant yin vacuity leading to internal wind with severe shaking of the hands and feet, vertigo, and hot flashes in the face, replace *Si Wu Tang* with modified *E Jiao Ji Zi Huang Tang* (Donkey Skin Glue & Egg Yolk Decoction): Gelatinum Corii Asini (*E Jiao*), 12g, Radix Albus Paeoniae Lactiflorae (*Bai Shao*), 15g, Concha Haliotidis (*Shi Jue Ming*), 18g, Ramulus Uncariae Cum Uncis (*Gou Teng*), 9g, uncooked Radix Rehmanniae (*Sheng Di*), 12g, mix-fried Radix Glycyrrhizae (*Gan Cao*), 6g, Concha Ostreae (*Mu Li*), 15g, Caulis Trachelospermi Jasminoidis (*Luo Shi Teng*), 9g, egg yolks, 2 pieces, and Sclerotium Pararadicis Poriae Cocos (*Fu Shen*), 9g.

3. Fright & fear damaging the spirit

Symptoms: Twitching of the muscles immediately after fright, susceptibility to fright, timidity, heart palpitations, profuse dreams, nightmares with occasional waking up in a fright, insomnia, dizziness, dry throat and mouth, a pale red tongue with scanty fur, and a fine pulse

Therapeutic principles: Settle fright and calm the spirit, nourish blood and quiet the heart

Acupuncture & moxibustion:

Xin Shu (Bl 15) *Shen Men* (Ht 7)	Together, these points calm the spirit and quiet the heart when needled with supplementing method.
Da Ling (Per 7)	Settles fright and rectifies chaotic qi due to fright
San Yin Jiao (Sp 6)	Nourishes the blood and quiets the spirit

Chinese medicinal formula: Modified *Suan Zao Ren Tang* (Zizyphus Spinosa Decoction)

Ingredients: Stir-fried Semen Zizyphi Spinosae (*Suan Zao Ren*), 15g, Radix Albus Paeoniae Lactiflorae (*Bai Shao*), 9g, mix-fried Radix Glycyrrhizae (*Gan Cao*), 6g, Rhizoma Anemarrhenae Asphodeloidis (*Zhi Mu*), 6g, Sclerotium Pararadicis Poriae Cocos (*Fu Shen*), 9g, Radix Ligustici Wallichii (*Chuan Xiong*), 3g, rice stir-fried Radix Codonopsitis Pilosulae (*Dang Shen*), 9g, uncooked Concha Ostreae (*Mu Li*), 20g, Magnetitum (*Ci Shi*), 20g

Additions & subtractions: For severe fright, add Succinum (*Hu Po*), 3g (powdered and taken with the strained decoction). For severe heart vacuity with insomnia, profuse dreams, and impaired memory, add Semen Biotae Orientalis (*Bai Zi Ren*), 9g, and Caulis Polygoni Multiflori (*Ye Jiao Teng*), 12g. For severe heart palpitations, add Arillus Euphoriae Longanae (*Long Yan Rou*), 9g, Semen Biotae Orientalis (*Bai Zi Ren*), 9g, and Radix Salviae Miltiorrhizae (*Dan Shen*), 6g. For severe blood vacuity, add wine mix-fried Radix Angelicae Sinensis (*Dang Gui*), 9g, and cooked Radix Rehmanniae (*Shu Di*), 9g.

4. Cold water

Symptoms: Severe twitching of the muscles, palpitations below the heart, dizziness, pain and heaviness of the four limbs, fear of cold, abdominal pain, a pale tongue with white fur, and a deep pulse

Therapeutic principles: Warm yang and disinhibit water

Acupuncture & moxibustion:

Guan Yuan (CV 4)	Together, these points warm the spleen and kidneys
Qi Hai (CV 6)	to disinhibit dampness when moxaed and needled
Zu San Li (St 36)	with supplementing method.
Yin Ling Quan (Sp 9)	Together, these points disinhibit water when
San Jiao Shu (CV 22)	needled with draining method.

Additions & subtractions: For coughing, add *Feng Chi* (Bl 12) and *Fei Shu* (Bl 13). For diarrhea, add *Shen Que* (CV 8). For vomiting, add *Shang Wan* (CV 13). For edema, add *Dao Shui* (St 28).

Chinese medicinal formula: *Zhen Wu Tang* (True Warrior Decoction)

Ingredients: Bland Radix Lateralis Praeparatus Aconiti Carmichaeli (*Fu Zi*), 9g, uncooked Rhizoma Atractylodis Macrocephalae (*Bai Zhu*), 9g, Radix Albus Paeoniae Lactiflorae (*Bai Shao*), 6g, uncooked Rhizoma Zingiberis (*Sheng Jiang*), 9g, Sclerotium Poriae Cocos (*Fu Ling*), 9g

Additions & subtractions: For edema and inhibited urination, add Sclerotium Polypori Umbellati (*Zhu Ling*), 9g, stir-fried Ramulus Cinnamomi Cassiae (*Gui Zhi*), 9g, and Semen Plantaginis (*Che Qian Zi*), 12g. For severe yang vacuity, add Cortex Cinnamomi Cassiae (*Rou Gui*), 3g. For diarrhea, add dry Rhizoma Zingiberis (*Gan Jiang*), 6g. For vomiting, subtract Aconite and increase the dosage of Ginger up to 15g. For coughing and/or panting with thin, clear phlegm, add dry Rhizoma Zingiberis (*Gan Jiang*), 6g, Fructus Schisandrae Chinensis (*Wu Wei Zi*), 9g, and Herba Asari Cum Radice (*Xi Xin*), 3g. For dizziness, add lime-processed Rhizoma Pinelliae Ternatae (*Ban Xia*), 9g, and Rhizoma Gastrodiae Elatae (*Tian Ma*), 9g. For heart palpitations and a regularly interrupted pulse, add Radix Salviae Miltiorrhizae (*Dan Shen*), 9g, and mix-fried Radix Glycyrrhizae (*Gan Cao*), 9g.

20
Generalized Pain *(Shen Tong)*

This refers to pain all over the body. For pain confined to specific areas of the body, please see the relevant chapters in previous volumes of this series.

Disease causes, disease mechanisms:

In Chinese medicine, the single most important and definitive statement about pain is:

If there is pain, there is no free flow. If there is free flow, there is no pain.

Therefore, all pain is due to some mechanism adversely affecting the free and easy flow of the qi and blood, and the mechanisms for generalized pain are no exception to this rule.

1. Wind cold fettering the exterior

When external evils attack the exterior, these evils cause replete congestion in the exterior. Cold's nature is contracting and constricting. Therefore when wind combines with cold evils and invades the body it may cause the channels and network vessels to also become contracted and constricted. As a result, the qi and blood cannot flow freely through the channels and network vessels, thus leading to pain. If these wind cold evils are widely dispersed throughout the body, then generalized pain may occur.

2. Dampness fixed in the flesh exterior

Dampness causing generalized pain usually is the result of enduring exposure to external damp evils, such as living in a damp environment. Dampness is a yin evil which is sticky and stagnant. When it invades the body, it commonly fixes in the flesh exterior where it inhibits the flow of the qi and blood. Because the qi and blood are no longer freely flowing, there is pain. If these damp evils are widely dispersed throughout the body, generalized pain may occur.

3. Damp heat

Damp heat causing generalized pain may arise from either external contraction of damp heat evils or from excessive consumption of fatty, sweet, oily foods which ferment and engender damp heat. If damp heat penetrates the vessels and blocks the flow of qi and blood there, pain may occur. If this damp heat is widely dispersed throughout the body, generalized pain may occur.

4. Stasis obstructing the vessels & network vessels

More often than not, this disease mechanism of generalized pain develops from enduring impediment conditions, from qi disease that enters the blood, or from irregularities of the qi and blood flow due to enduring disease. As it is said, "Enduring disease enters the network vessels, and enduring disease must cause stasis." If the evils of enduring disease enter the blood causing stasis and block the network vessels, the flow of the qi and blood will become inhibited. Because of this inhibition and lack of free flow of the qi and blood, there is pain. If blood stasis is widely dispersed about the body, generalized pain may occur.

5. Blood or qi & blood vacuity

Qi and blood vacuity may be due to childbirth, constitutional insufficiency, enduring or serious disease, great loss of blood, overthinking, or over-work taxation. Qi commands, *i.e.,* moves the blood, while blood is responsible for filling up the network vessels in order to nourish the body. If, for any reason, the qi becomes vacuous and weak and, therefore, fails to move the blood, or the blood becomes vacuous and insufficient and, therefore, does not fill the network vessels, qi and blood will not flow freely and thus pain is likely to occur. Since qi and/or blood vacuities are systemic rather than localized conditions, such qi and blood vacuity often leads to generalized as opposed to localized pain.

6. Yang vacuity

Yang vacuity may be due to constitutional yang vacuity, aging, enduring disease, or overwork taxation. In addition, yang vacuity may be divided into spleen yang vacuity, kidney yang vacuity, and spleen-kidney yang vacuity. If there is spleen yang vacuity, the spleen will fail to engender qi and blood to nourish the channels and vessels. If there is kidney yang vacuity, the body is not warmed and internal cold will be engendered. Since cold's nature is contracting and constricting, this internal cold may congeal the blood and prevent it from flowing freely. If there is spleen-kidney yang vacuity, there will be both insufficient qi and blood to fill and nourish the channels and network vessels, and vacuity cold contracting the vessels and constricting their flow. Hence, yang vacuity often gives rise to generalized pain.

Treatment based on pattern discrimination:

I. Wind cold fettering the exterior

Symptoms: Body aches, especially in the joints, aversion to cold, fever, no sweating, nasal congestion, headache, itchy throat, cough, thin, white tongue fur, and a floating, tight pulse

Therapeutic principles: Course wind and dispel cold, promote sweating and resolve the exterior

Acupuncture & moxibustion:

Wai Guan (TB 5)	Together, these points course wind, scatter cold,
Feng Men (Bl 12)	and resolve the exterior when needled with
He Gu (LI 4)	draining method.
Da Zhui (GV 14)	Together, these points free the flow of the
Yao Yang Guan (GV 3)	governing vessel, move yang, and stop pain when
	needled with draining method.

Additions & subtractions: For high fever, prick *Wei Zhong* (Bl 40) to bleed. For severe coughing, add *Fei Shu* (Bl 13). For sore throat, add *Shao Shang* (Lu 11).

Chinese medicinal formula: *Ma Huang Tang* (Ephedra Decoction)

Ingredients: Uncooked Herba Ephedrae (*Ma Huang*), 9g, uncooked Ramulus Cinnamomi Cassiae (*Gui Zhi*), 6g, Semen Pruni Armeniacae (*Xing Ren*), 6g, Radix Glycyrrhizae (*Gan Cao*), 5g

Additions & subtractions: For pain combined with a heavy sensation, add uncooked Rhizoma Atractylodis (*Cang Zhu*), 9g. For severe pain in the nape of the neck and upper back, add uncooked Radix Puerariae (*Ge Gen*), 9g. For severe pain in the upper part of the body, add Radix Et Rhizoma

Notopterygii (*Qiang Huo*), 9g. For severe pain in the lower part of the body, add Radix Angelicae Pubescentis (*Du Huo*), 9g. For concomitant interior heat with heart vexation, thirst, and a higher fever, add uncooked Gypsum Fibrosum (*Shi Gao*), 20g.

2. Dampness fixed in the flesh exterior

Symptoms: Generalized pain, heavy limbs, distention in the head with a feeling as if the head were swathed, possible aversion to cold and fever, no sweating, slimy, white tongue fur, and a soggy pulse

Therapeutic principles: Resolve the exterior and dispel dampness

Acupuncture & moxibustion:

Zhi Gou (TB 6) *He Gu* (LI 4)	Together, these points free the flow of yang and resolve the exterior when needled with draining method.
Da Zhui (GV 14) *Tao Dao* (GV 13) *Yin Ling Quan* (Sp 9)	Together, these points move yang and eliminate dampness when needled with even draining and supplementing method.

Additions & subtractions: For aversion to cold and fever, add *Feng Men* (Bl 12) and *Wai Guan* (TB 5). For nausea, add *Zhong Wan* (CV 12). For chest oppression, add *Dan Zhong* (CV 17).

Chinese medicinal formula: *Ma Xing Yi Gan Tang* ((Ephedra, Armeniaca, Coix & Licorice Decoction)

Ingredients: Uncooked Herba Ephedrae (*Ma Huang*), 6g, Semen Pruni Armeniacae (*Xing Ren*), 6g, mix-fried Radix Glycyrrhizae (*Gan Cao*), 6g, uncooked Semen Coicis Lachryma-jobi (*Yi Yi Ren*), 30g

Additions & subtractions: For severe body pain, replace *Ma Xing Yi Gan Tang* with *Qiang Huo Sheng Shi Tang* (Notopterygium Overcome Dampness Decoction): Radix Et Rhizoma Notopterygii (*Qiang Huo*), 9g, Radix Angelicae Pubescentis (*Du Huo*), 9g, Radix Et Rhizoma Ligustici Chinensis (*Gao Ben*), 6g, Radix Ledebouriellae Divaricatae (*Fang Feng*), 9g, Radix Ligustici Wallichii (*Chuan Xiong*), 6g, Fructus Viticis (*Man Jing Zi*), 6g, and Radix Glycyrrhizae (*Gan Cao*), 3g.

3. Damp heat

Symptoms: Body aching with fever, heavy limbs, sweating resulting in abatement of the fever but, when the sweating stops, the fever increases again, thirst without a desire to drink large amounts, short voidings of dark-colored urine, slimy, yellow tongue fur, and a moderate (*i.e.*, slightly slow) pulse

Therapeutic principles: Clear heat and disinhibit dampness

Acupuncture & moxibustion:

Zhong Ji (CV 3) *Zhi Gou* (TB 6) *Nei Ting* (St 44)	Together, these points clear heat and disinhibit dampness when needled with draining method.
San Yin Jiao (Sp 6) *Yin Ling Quan* (Sp 9)	Together, these points clear and eliminate damp heat and disinhibit urination when needled with draining method.

Chinese medicinal formula: Uncooked Radix Scutellariae Baicalensis (*Huang Qin*), 9g, Talcum (*Hua Shi*), 9g, Cortex Sclerotii Poriae Cocos (*Fu Ling Pi*), 9g, Pericarpium Arecae Catechu (*Da Fu Pi*), 6g, Fructus Cardamomi (*Bai Dou Kou*), 6g, Medulla Tetrapanacis Papyriferi (*Tong Cao*), 3g, Sclerotium Polypori Umbellati (*Zhu Ling*), 9g

4. Stasis obstructing the channels & network vessels

Symptoms: Enduring generalized pricking pain which inhibits turning over, a dark tongue with static macules or spots, and a deep, choppy pulse

Therapeutic principles: Quicken the blood and dispel stasis, free the flow of the network vessels and stop pain

Acupuncture & moxibustion:

Ge Shu (Bl 17) *Xue Hai* (Sp 10)	Together, these points quicken the blood and transform stasis when needled with draining method.
He Gu (LI 4) *San Yin Jiao* (Sp 6)	Together, these points move the qi and quicken the blood when needled with draining method.

Wei Zhong (Bl 40)   Frees the flow of the network vessels and stops pain when pricked to bleed

Additions & subtractions: For heart palpitations, add *Nei Guan* (Per 6). For scanty menstruation with dark-colored blood and clots, add *Gui Lai* (St 29) and *Tai Chong* (Liv 3). For reduced qi and spontaneous perspiration, add *Qi Hai* (CV 6).

Chinese medicinal formula: *Shen Tong Zhu Yu Tang* (Body Pain Dispel Stasis Decoction)

Ingredients: Wine mix-fried Radix Ligustici Wallichii (*Chuan Xiong*), 9g, Semen Pruni Persicae (*Tao Ren*), 9g, Flos Carthami Tinctorii (*Hong Hua*), 9g, Radix Et Rhizoma Notopterygii (*Qiang Huo*), 9g, stir-fried Resina Olibani (*Ru Xiang*), 6g, wine mix-fried Radix Angelicae Sinensis (*Dang Gui*), 9g, Rhizoma Cyperi Rotundi (*Xiang Fu*), 6g, Radix Cyathulae (*Chuan Niu Xi*), 9g, Lumbricus (*Di Long*), 9g, Radix Gentianae Macrophyllae (*Qin Jiao*), 6g, vinegar stir-fried Feces Trogopterori Seu Pteromi (*Wu Ling Zhi*), 6g, Radix Glycyrrhizae (*Gan Cao*), 3g

Additions & subtractions: For blood stasis due to wind damp, add Radix Angelicae Pubescentis (*Du Huo*), 9g, Radix Clematidis Chinensis (*Wei Ling Xian*), 9g, and Radix Ledebouriellae Divaricatae (*Fang Feng*), 9g. For blood stasis due to qi vacuity, add rice stir-fried Radix Codonopsitis Pilosulae (*Dang Shen*), 9g, and honey stir-fried Radix Astragali Membranacei (*Huang Qi*), 12g. For blood stasis due to trauma, add Resina Myrrhae (*Mo Yao*), 6g.

5. Blood vacuity

Symptoms: Body aches, dizziness, a pale facial complexion, heart palpitations, pale lips, gums, and nails, scanty menstruation, impaired memory, possible insomnia or profuse dreams, a pale tongue with scanty fur, and a fine pulse

Therapeutic principles: Nourish and harmonize the blood

Acupuncture & moxibustion:

Ge Shu (Bl 17)   Together, these points nourish the blood and
Gan Shu (Bl 18)   supplement the spleen and liver when needled
Pi Shu (Bl 20)   with supplementing method.

San Yin Jiao (Sp 6) *Xue Hai* (Sp 10)	Together, these points harmonize the blood when needled with even supplementing and draining method.

Chinese medicinal formula: *Si Wu Tang* (Four Materials Decoction)

Ingredients: Cooked Radix Rehmanniae (*Shu Di*), 12g, uncooked Radix Albus Paeoniae Lactiflorae (*Bai Shao*), 12g, wine mix-fried Radix Angelicae Sinensis (*Dang Gui*), 9g, wine mix-fried Radix Ligustici Wallichii (*Chuan Xiong*), 6g

Additions & subtractions: For severe blood vacuity, add processed Polygoni Multiflori (*He Shou Wu*), 9g. For blood vacuity allowing the penetration of cold into the network vessels with aversion to cold, cold hands and feet, and a deep, fine pulse, replace *Si Wu Tang* with Modified *Dang Gui Si Ni Tang* (Dang Gui Four Counterflows Decoction): wine mix-fried Radix Angelicae Sinensis (*Dang Gui*), 12g, stir-fried Ramulus Cinnamomi Cassiae (*Gui Zhi*), 9g, wine mix-fried Radix Albus Paeoniae Lactiflorae (*Bai Shao*), 9g, Herba Asari Cum Radice (*Xi Xin*), 3g, Medulla Tetrapanacis Papyriferi (*Tong Cao*), 3g, mix-fried Radix Glycyrrhizae (*Gan Cao*), 3g, and Fructus Zizyphi Jujubae (*Da Zao*), 3 fruits. For concomitant liver-kidney yin vacuity, add processed Polygoni Multiflori (*He Shou Wu*), 9g, Ramulus Loranthi Seu Visci (*Sang Ji Sheng*), 9g, and Radix Achyranthis Bidentatae (*Niu Xi*), 9g. For concomitant blood stasis, add Semen Pruni Persicae (*Tao Ren*), 9g, and Flos Carthami Tinctorii (*Hong Hua*), 6g. For concomitant liver depression with menstrual irregularities, dysmenorrhea, rib-side pain, and breast distention, add vinegar stir-fried Radix Bupleuri (*Chai Hu*), 6g, Rhizoma Cyperi Rotundi (*Xiang Fu*), 9g, and Herba Menthae Haplocalysis (*Bo He*), 3g.

6. Qi & blood vacuity

Symptoms: Generalized pain which is worsened by overwork and over-thinking, dizziness, heart palpitations, shortness of breath, fatigue, lack of strength, reduced food intake, loose stools, a lusterless facial complexion, white lips and nails, a pale tongue with thin, white fur, and a fine, weak pulse

Therapeutic principles: Supplement the qi and nourish the blood

Acupuncture & moxibustion:

Ge Shu (Bl 17) *Gan Shu* (Bl 18) *Pi Shu* (Bl 20)	Together, these points supplement and nourish the blood when needled with supplementing method.

San Yin Jiao (Sp 6)	Together, these points supplement the spleen to
Zu San Li (St 36)	engender the qi and blood when needled with supplementing method.

Chinese medicinal formula: *Ba Zhen Tang* (Eight Pearls Decoction)

Ingredients: Cooked Radix Rehmanniae (*Shu Di*), 9g, Radix Albus Paeoniae Lactiflorae (*Bai Shao*), 9g, wine mix-fried Radix Angelicae Sinensis (*Dang Gui*), 9g, wine mix-fried Radix Ligustici Wallichii (*Chuan Xiong*), 6g, stir-fried Radix Codonopsitis Pilosulae (*Dang Shen*), 9g, bran stir-fried Rhizoma Atractylodis Macrocephalae (*Bai Zhu*), 9g, Sclerotium Poriae Cocos (*Fu Ling*), 6g, mix-fried Radix Glycyrrhizae (*Gan Cao*), 3g

Additions & subtractions: For constructive and defensive disharmony with numbness, weakness and pain in the limbs, spontaneous perspiration, fatigue, shortness of breath, a pale tongue, and a faint, choppy or floating pulse, add stir-fried Ramulus Cinnamomi Cassiae (*Gui Zhi*), 9g, uncooked Rhizoma Zingiberis (*Sheng Jiang*), 12g, and Fructus Zizyphi Jujubae (*Da Zao*), 5 fruits. For a cold sensation in the limbs, add stir-fried Ramulus Cinnamomi Cassiae (*Gui Zhi*), 9g, and Herba Asari Cum Radice (*Xi Xin*), 3g. If there is blood stasis with a purple tongue and slight cyanosis of the fingers, add wine mix-fried Radix Salviae Miltiorrhizae (*Dan Shen*), 9g, and Flos Carthami Tinctorii (*Hong Hua*), 6g. For severe pain, add Caulis Milletiae Seu Spatholobi (*Ji Xue Teng*), 30g. For severe qi vacuity, add uncooked Radix Astragali Membranacei (*Huang Qi*), 15g.

7. Yang vacuity

Symptoms: Body aches, fear of cold, chilled limbs, joint pain, fatigue, a bright white facial complexion, torpid intake, loose stools, fatigued spirit, low back aching and heaviness, clear urine, a pale, fat tongue with glossy, white fur, and a deep, weak pulse

Therapeutic principles: Warm the channels and invigorate yang

Acupuncture & moxibustion:

Zhong Wan (CV 12)	Together, these points warm yang and supplement
Shen Que (CV 8)	the spleen and kidneys when moxaed.
Qi Hai (CV 6)	
Guan Yuan (CV 4)	
Zu San Li (St 36)	

Chinese medicinal formula: Modified *Fu Zi Tang* (Aconite Decoction)

Ingredients: Blast-fried Radix Lateralis Praeparatus Aconiti Carmichaeli (*Fu Zi*), 12g, Sclerotium Poriae Cocos (*Fu Ling*), 9g, rice stir-fried Radix Codonopsitis Pilosulae (*Dang Shen*), 6g, uncooked Radix Albus Paeoniae Lactiflorae (*Bai Shao*), 9g, stir-fried Ramulus Cinnamomi Cassiae (*Gui Zhi*), 6g, Radix Et Rhizoma Notopterygii (*Qiang Huo*), 6g, Radix Angelicae Pubescentis (*Du Huo*), 6g

21
Heavy Body *(Shen Zhong)*

Heavy body refers to generalized heaviness which is often accompanied by difficult or inhibited movement of the limbs. It is also known as heaviness of the four limbs. Hemilateral heaviness and difficulty moving due to wind stroke is not included under this category.

Disease causes, disease mechanisms:

1. Dampness fixed in the fleshy exterior

Dampness causing bodily heaviness usually arises from enduring exposure to water dampness, such as working in the water, repeatedly being caught in the rain, or from living in a damp environment. Dampness is a yin evil which is sticky, stagnant, heavy, and fixed by nature. If dampness invades the body and fixes in the fleshy exterior, the tissues will be filled with more fluid than usual and therefore they will be heavier. Thus a feeling of heaviness of the body may occur.

2. Wind & water binding with each other

Wind is a yang evil which usually attacks the upper body first. The lungs are located in the upper burner and are thus susceptible to attack by wind evils. The lungs are the upper source of water which are supposed to free the flow of the water passageways. If wind invades the lungs and inhibits the lungs' diffusion and descending, water may collect and remain in the fleshy exterior. If this invading wind binds with this collected water in the fleshy exterior, there will be more fluids in the tissue than normal and thus the tissues will be heavier, therefore giving rise to a feeling of heaviness of the body.

3. Summerheat dampness

Invasion of summerheat dampness occurs during the season of summer when there is enduring exposure to summerheat. Dampness often invades the body along with summerheat since long-summer corresponds to earth which, in turn, corresponds to dampness. Because of this dampness, there are more fluids in the tissues than normal and therefore these tissues are heavier than normal. This may be experienced by a subjective sensation of bodily heaviness.

4. Yang vacuity with water flooding

Yang vacuity usually develops from overwork taxation, aging, or enduring disease which damage spleen and kidney yang. The spleen is responsible for the movement and transformation of fluids in the body, while the kidneys govern all the water of the body. It is the yang qi of these two viscera which is mainly responsible for the movement and transformation of water in the body. Therefore, if yang qi becomes vacuous and weak, water dampness will collect internally. If this accumulated water dampness spills over and floods into the fleshy skin, the tissues will contain more fluids than normal and thus also be heavier. This may then be experienced as a feeling of bodily heaviness.

5. Central qi fall

Central qi vacuity commonly arises from internal damage due to overwork taxation, dietary irregularities, or from enduring disease. The spleen qi is responsible for upbearing the clear and transforming dampness. If, for any reason, the spleen qi becomes vacuous and weak, the central qi may fall downwards. In that case, fluids will gather and collect, transforming into dampness. On the one hand, this dampness results in more fluids in the tissues which are consequently heavier than normal. On the other hand, this qi vacuity leads to lack of strength. Therefore, either or both of these disease mechanisms may cause a subjective sensation of bodily heaviness.

Treatment based on pattern discrimination:

1. Dampness fixed in the fleshy exterior

Symptoms: A heavy, aching body with difficulty turning over, pain especially in the shoulders, upper back, spine, and lower back, fever, aversion to cold, headache, head distention as if swathed, chest oppression, torpid intake, thin, slimy, white tongue fur, and a soggy, moderate (*i.e.*, slightly slow) pulse

Therapeutic principles: Eliminate dampness and resolve the exterior

Acupuncture & moxibustion: Please see Pattern 2 in the preceding chapter.

Additions & subtractions: For fever and fatigued body, add *Yang Fu* (GB 38). For body aches, add *Shen Zhu* (GV 12). For nausea, add *Gong Sun* (Sp 4). For panting, add *Lie Que* (Lu 7).

Chinese medicinal formula: *Qiang Huo Sheng Shi Tang* (Notopterygium Overcome Dampness Decoction)

Ingredients: Radix Et Rhizoma Notopterygii (*Qiang Huo*), 9g, Radix Angelicae Pubescentis (*Du Huo*), 9g, Radix Et Rhizoma Ligustici Chinensis (*Gao Ben*), 6g, Radix Ledebouriellae Divaricatae (*Fang Feng*), 6g, Radix Ligustici Wallichii (*Chuan Xiong*), 6g, Fructus Viticis (*Man Jing Zi*), 6g, Radix Glycyrrhizae (*Gan Cao*), 3g

Additions & subtractions: For severe heaviness of the body, add Radix Clematidis Chinensis (*Wei Ling Xian*), 9g, and Rhizoma Atractylodis (*Cang Zhu*), 9g. For cold limbs, add stir-fried Ramulus Cinnamomi Cassiae (*Gui Zhi*), 9g. For severe heaviness of the lower limbs, add Cortex Radicis Acanthopanacis (*Wu Jia Pi*), 9g. For severe heaviness of the upper limbs, add stir-fried Ramulus Cinnamomi Cassiae (*Gui Zhi*), 9g. For wind damp transforming into heat with heat impediment, *i.e.*, severe pain, swelling, and a hot sensation in the joints which are ameliorated by cold and worsened by heat, severe restriction of movement, occasional fever, vexatious heat and thirst, red urine, constipation, a red tongue with dry, yellow fur, and a slippery, rapid pulse, temporarily replace *Qiang Huo Sheng Shi Tang* by Modified *Bai Hu Jia Gui Zhi Tang* (White Tiger Plus Cinnamon Decoction): uncooked Gypsum Fibrosum (*Shi Gao*), 20g, uncooked Rhizoma Anemarrhenae Asphodeloidis (*Zhi Mu*), 9g, Semen Oryzae Sativae (*Geng Mi*), 12g, Radix Glycyrrhizae (*Gan Cao*), 6g, Ramulus Cinnamomi Cassiae (*Gui Zhi*), 6g, Ramulus Mori Albi (*Sang Zhi*), 9g, Caulis Lonicerae Japonicae (*Ren Dong Teng*), 9g, uncooked Cortex Phellodendri (*Huang Bai*), 9g, and Caulis Sargentodoxae (*Hong Teng*), 6g.

2. Wind & water binding with each other

Symptoms: Heavy body, puffy edema in the face and eyelids or generalized edema, aversion to wind and fear of cold, fever, headache, aching joints, cough, sore throat, scanty urination, thin, white tongue fur, and a floating pulse

Therapeutic principles: Diffuse the lungs and disinhibit water

Acupuncture & moxibustion:

He Gu (LI 4) *Da Zhui* (GV 14) *Tian Fu* (Lu 3)	Together, these points diffuse the lungs and dis-inhibit water when needled with draining method.
Shui Gou (GV 26) *Shui Fen* (CV 9)	Together, these points disinhibit water when needled with draining method.

Additions & subtractions: For heart vexation and scanty urination, add *Zhi Gou* (TB 6) and *San Jiao Shu* (Bl 22). For body aches and aversion to cold, add *Wai Guan* (TB 5). For generalized edema and inhibited urination, add *Yin Ling Quan* (Sp 9) and *San Yin Jiao* (Sp 6). For aversion to wind and profuse sweating, moxa *Qi Hai* (CV 6).

Chinese medicinal formula: *Yue Bi Jia Zhu Tang* (Maidservant from Yue Plus Atractylodes Decoction)

Ingredients: Honey stir-fried Herba Ephedrae (*Ma Huang*), 9g, uncooked Rhizoma Atractylodis Macrocephalae (*Bai Zhu*), 12g, uncooked Gypsum Fibrosum (*Shi Gao*), 18g, uncooked Rhizoma Zingiberis (*Sheng Jiang*), 6g, Fructus Zizyphi Jujubae (*Da Zao*), 5 fruits, Radix Glycyrrhizae (*Gan Cao*), 6g

Additions & subtractions: For severe heavy body, replace Atractylodes Macrocephala with Rhizoma Atractylodis (*Cang Zhu*), 9g. For severe edema with inhibited urine, add Rhizoma Alismatis (*Ze Xie*), 9g, and Semen Plantaginis (*Che Qian Zi*), 9g. For severe aversion to wind and cold, add Herba Schizonepetae Tenuifoliae (*Jing Jie*), 9g, and Radix Et Rhizoma Notopterygii (*Qiang Huo*), 9g. For cold limbs, add stir-fried Ramulus Cinnamomi Cassiae (*Gui Zhi*), 9g.

3. Summerheat dampness

Symptoms: Heavy body, encumbered limbs, fever, headache, thirst, spontaneous perspiration, torpid intake, chest oppression, loose stools, short voidings of dark-colored urine, slimy tongue fur, and a rapid, vacuous pulse

Therapeutic principles: Clear summerheat and eliminate dampness, fortify the spleen and boost the qi

Acupuncture & moxibustion:

Wai Guan (TB 5) *He Gu* (LI 4)	Together, these points clear summerheat and drain heat when needled with draining method.
Yin Ling Quan (Sp 9) *San Yin Jiao* (Sp 6)	Together, these points eliminate dampness when needled with draining method.
Zu San Li (St 36) *Wei Shu* (Bl 21)	Together, these points boost the qi and fortify the spleen when needled with supplementing method.

Chinese medicinal formula: Modified *Qing Shu Yi Qi Tang* (Clear Summerheat & Boost the Qi Decoction)

Ingredients: Rhizoma Coptidis Chinensis (*Huang Lian*), 6g, Folium Bambusae (*Zhu Ye*), 6g, Folium Nelumbinis Nuciferae (*He Ye*), 9g, Herba Dendrobii (*Shi Hu*), 3g, Tuber Ophiopogonis Japonici (*Mai Men Dong*), 6g, uncooked Rhizoma Anemarrhenae Asphodeloidis (*Zhi Mu*), 9g, Semen Oryzae Sativae (*Geng Mi*), 12g, Pericarpium Citrulli Vulgaris (*Xi Gua Pi*), 24g, Radix Glycyrrhizae (*Gan Cao*), 3g, Herba Eupatorei Fortunei (*Pei Lan*), 12g, Rhizoma Atractylodis (*Cang Zhu*), 9g

Additions & subtractions: For summerheat dampness with short, yellow or dark urination, nausea, vomiting, stomach and abdominal glomus and distention, slimy, yellow tongue fur, and a soggy pulse, replace *Qing Shu Yi Qi Tang* with *Lian Po Yin* (Coptis & Magnolia Drink): ginger mix-fried Cortex Magnoliae Officinalis (*Hou Po*), 6g, uncooked Rhizoma Coptidis Chinensis (*Huang Lian*), 6g, Rhizoma Acori Graminei (*Shi Chang Pu*), 6g, ginger stir-fried Rhizoma Pinelliae Ternatae (*Ban Xia*), 6g, clear Semen Praeparatus Sojae (*Dan Dou Chi*), 9g, Fructus Gardeniae Jasminoidis (*Zhi Zi*), 9g, and Rhizoma Phragmitis Communis (*Lu Gen*), 9g. For torpid intake, add stir-fried Massa Medica Fermentata (*Shen Qu*), 9g. For severely damaged qi, add Radix Panacis Quinquefolii (*Xi Yang Shen*), 6g, and uncooked Fructus Schisandrae Chinensis (*Wu Wei Zi*), 9g. For severely damaged fluids, increase the dosage of Dendrobium and Ophiopogon up to 9-12g. For severe heat, add uncooked Gypsum Fibrosum (*Shi Gao*), 24g.

4. Yang vacuity with water flooding

Symptoms: Heavy body, edema in the lower extremities, a sallow yellow or somber, lusterless facial complexion, torpid intake, loose stools, fatigued spirit, cold limbs, low back aching and heaviness, short voidings of urine, possible abdominal pain with diarrhea, a pale, fat tongue with glossy, white fur, and a fine, moderate (*i.e.*, slightly slow), deep pulse

Therapeutic principles: Warm yang and transform water

Acupuncture & moxibustion:

Qi Hai (CV 6) *Guan Yuan* (CV 4)	Together, these points warm yang when moxaed.
Shui Fen (CV 9) *Yin Ling Quan* (Sp 9) *San Yin Jiao* (Sp 6)	Together, these points disinhibit water and disperse edema when needled with draining method.
Zu San Li (St 36)	Supplements the qi and moves water when needled with supplementing method

Additions & subtractions: For heart palpitations, add *Nei Guan* (Per 6). For shortage of qi, add *Dan Zhong* (CV 17). For stomach and abdominal distention and oppression, add *Zhong Wan* (CV 12). For dizziness, tinnitus, impotence, and premature ejaculation, add *Shen Shu* (Bl 23) and *Zhi Shi* (Bl 52).

Chinese medicinal formula: Modified *Shi Pi Yin* (Bolster the Spleen Decoction)

Ingredients: Uncooked Rhizoma Atractylodis Macrocephalae (*Bai Zhu*), 15g, Cortex Sclerotii Poriae Cocos (*Fu Ling Pi*), 9g, Pericarpium Arecae Catechu (*Da Fu Pi*), 9g, Semen Alpiniae Katsumadai (*Cao Dou Kou*), 6g, ginger mix-fried Cortex Magnoliae Officinalis (*Hou Po*), 6g, Radix Lateralis Praeparatus Aconiti Carmichaeli (*Fu Zi*), 6g, dry Rhizoma Zingiberis (*Gan Jiang*), 6g, Sclerotium Polypori Umbellati (*Zhu Ling*), 12g, mix-fried Radix Glycyrrhizae (*Gan Cao*), 3g

Additions & subtractions: For severe edema and inhibited urination, add Rhizoma Alismatis (*Ze Xie*), 9g, and Semen Plantaginis (*Che Qian Zi*), 9g. For qi vacuity, add uncooked Radix Astragali Membranacei (*Huang Qi*), 15g, and Radix Codonopsitis Pilosulae (*Dang Shen*), 9g. For severe yang vacuity, add Cortex Cinnamomi Cassiae (*Rou Gui*), 3g. For diarrhea, replace Alpinia Katsumadai with Semen Myristicae Fragrantis (*Rou Dou Kou*).

5. Central qi fall

Symptoms: Heavy body, fatigued limbs, fatigue, shortage of qi, reduced food intake, stomach and abdominal distention and oppression, loose stools, a pale tongue with thin, white fur, and a deep, weak pulse

Therapeutic principles: Upbear the clear and downbear the turbid, transform qi and disinhibit water

Acupuncture & moxibustion:

Bai Hui (GV 20) *Zu San Li* (St 36) *Qi Hai* (CV 6)	Together, these points supplement the qi to help upbear the clear and downbear the turbid when needled with supplementing method.
Yin Ling Quan (Sp 9) *San Yin Jiao* (Sp 6)	Together, these points disinhibit water when needled with even supplementing and draining method.

Chinese medicinal formulas: For predominant central qi fall: Modified *Bu Zhong Yi Qi Tang* (Supplement the Center & Boost the Qi Decoction)

Ingredients: Honey mix-fried Radix Astragali Membranacei (*Huang Qi*), 15g, stir-fried Radix Codonopsis Pilosulae (*Dang Shen*), 9g, bran stir-fried Rhizoma Atractylodis Macrocephalae (*Bai Zhu*), 9g, mix-fried Radix Glycyrrhizae (*Gan Cao*), 6g, stir-fried Pericarpium Citri Reticulatae (*Chen Pi*), 6g, stir-fried Radix Bupleuri (*Chai Hu*), 5g, honey mix-fried Rhizoma Cimicifugae (*Sheng Ma*), 5g, Sclerotium Poriae Cocos (*Fu Ling*), 9g, Rhizoma Acori Graminei (*Shi Chang Pu*), 6g, Rhizoma Atractylodis (*Cang Zhu*), 9g

For predominant spleen-stomach vacuity with damp accumulation: Modified *Shen Ling Bai Zhu San* (Ginseng, Poria & Atractylodes Powder)

Ingredients: Stir-fried Semen Dolichoris Lablab (*Bai Bian Dou*), 9g, earth stir-fried Radix Dioscoreae Oppositae (*Shan Yao*), 9g, earth stir-fried Rhizoma Atractylodis Macrocephalae (*Bai Zhu*), 9g, Sclerotium Poriae Cocos (*Fu Ling*), 9g, rice stir-fried Radix Codonopsitis Pilosulae (*Dang Shen*), 9g, stir-fried till yellow Semen Nelumbinis Nuciferae (*Lian Zi*), 6g, Rhizoma Acori Graminei (*Shi Chang Pu*), 6g, Semen Coicis Lachryma-jobi (*Yi Yi Ren*), 9g, Fructus Amomi (*Sha Ren*), 6g, mix-fried Radix Glycyrrhizae (*Gan Cao*), 3g

Additions & subtractions: For poor appetite, add stir-fried Fructus Germinatus Hordei Vulgaris (*Mai Ya*), 9g, and Semen Raphani Sativi (*Lai Fu Zi*), 6g. For severe damp accumulation, add ginger mix-fried Cortex Magnoliae Officinalis (*Hou Po*), 9g. For worse loose stools on eating even slightly oily food, add stir-fried Fructus Crataegi (*Shan Zha*), 12g. For spleen yang vacuity, add bland Radix Lateralis Praeparatus Aconiti Carmichaeli (*Fu Zi*), 6g, and dry Rhizoma Zingiberis (*Gan Jiang*), 6g. For abdominal distention, add Radix Auklandiae Lappae (*Mu Xiang*), 9g. For profuse vaginal discharge, add Semen Euryalis Ferocis (*Qian Shi*), 9g, and Semen Ginkgonis Bilobae (*Bai Guo*), 9g. For dual vacuity of the qi and blood with, in addition to the main symptoms, heart palpitations, dizziness and pale lips and nails, replace *Bu Zhong Yi Qi Tang* or *Shen Ling Bai Zhu San* with Modified *Chun Ze Tang* (Spring Marsh Decoction): bran stir-fried Rhizoma Atractylodis Macrocephalae (*Bai Zhu*), 9g, stir-fried Ramulus Cinnamomi Cassiae (*Gui Zhi*), 6g, Radix Panacis Ginseng (*Ren Shen*), 3g, honey mix-fried Radix Astragali Membranacei (*Huang Qi*), 15g, wine mix-fried Radix Angelicae Sinensis (*Dang Gui*), 9g, cooked Radix Rehmanniae (*Shu Di*), 12g, Sclerotium Poriae Cocos (*Fu Ling*), 9g, and Rhizoma Atractylodis (*Cang Zhu*), 6g.

22

Generalized Pruritus *(Shen Yang)*

This refers to generalized itching of the skin which the patient tries to relieve by scratching. It is a subjective symptom with no primary skin lesions or damage. Itching that is confined to a certain area or due to some primary skin damage is not included in this chapter.

Disease causes, disease mechanisms:

1. Wind cold

This pattern is usually seen in individuals with habitual bodily yang vacuity and are, therefore, susceptible to wind cold invasion. As it is said in Chinese medicine, "Wind is a yang evil and is swift and changeable," while, "Cold is a yin evil that causes contraction." Therefore, when wind cold evils invade the body of a habitually yang vacuous person, their weak righteous qi cannot dispel these evils by sweating. However, if these invading wind cold evils are not very strong, they cannot force their way into the interior to transform into heat. In that case, such invading wind cold evils may remain in the exterior and fight with the vacuous defensive yang. The weak defensive yang may force the wind evils outward only to be followed by these wind evils forcing their way back inward. As a result, this wind moves in and out through the interstices, vibrating the body hairs and causing itching.

2. Exuberant wind

Spring is the season when wind is abundant and easily attacks. If such invading exuberant wind transforms into heat in the exterior, depressive heat may force the qi to move frenetically, and wind is nothing other than frenetically stirring qi. Therefore, it forces the qi in and out through the interstices leading to generalized pruritus. Often, externally contracted wind evils combine with internally engendered dampness. In that case, generalized pruritus may be accompanied by water-filled vesicles or oozing.

3. Heat in the blood

The heat in the blood often develops from excesses of the five "minds" or emotions which transforms heat or from excessive consumption of spicy, fried foods. It may also be due to the bodily exuberance of qi and blood found in the young or adolescents. Qi is yang and, therefore, warm by nature. Hence, if there is exuberance of qi, there is an easy predisposition to transform heat. When heat in the blood itself becomes exuberant enough, this heat may engender wind, and "Exuberant wind causes itching." Therefore, generalized pruritus may occur.

4. Blood vacuity

This pattern is mainly seen in the elderly whose yin and blood have gradually become vacuous and insufficient. The blood is supposed to nourish the skin. Therefore, if the blood becomes vacuous, first, the skin will receive insufficient nourishment. Thus it becomes dry and begins to desquamate. Secondly, wind will be engendered. This is because blood is the mother of qi, and internally stirring wind is nothing other than frenetically moving qi. This is what is meant by the saying, "Vacuous blood forms wind." Because wind is a yang evil, it moves upward and outward. Hence, wind moves back and forth in the skin, vibrating the body hairs and causing itching. As a result, generalized pruritus may occur since "Exuberant wind causes itching."

Treatment based on pattern discrimination:

1. Wind cold

Symptoms: This pattern mainly occurs in autumn. In most case, the itching affects the head, chest, neck, and hands. Exposure to cold typically makes the itching worse, while obtaint of warmth or sweating can improve it. Other symptoms include a pale tongue with white fur and a floating, moderate or floating, tight pulse.

Therapeutic principles: Course wind, dispel cold, and stop itching

Acupuncture & moxibustion:

Feng Chi (GB 20)	Together, these points course wind and stop itching
He Gu (LI 4)	when needled with draining method.
Feng Shi (GB 31)	

Da Zhui (GV 14)   Arouses yang, dispels cold, and stops itching when moxaed strongly

Additions & subtractions: For headache, add *Tai Yang* (M-HN-5). For nasal congestion, add *Shang Xing* (GV 23). For repeated contraction of common cold, moxa *Zu San Li* (St 36).

Chinese medicinal formula: *Gui Zhi Ma Huang Ge Ban Tang* (Cinnamon & Ephedra Half & Half Decoction)

Ingredients: Uncooked Ramulus Cinnamomi Cassiae (*Gui Zhi*), 9g, uncooked Herba Ephedrae (*Ma Huang*), 9g, Radix Albus Paeoniae Lactiflorae (*Bai Shao*), 9g, Semen Pruni Armeniacae (*Xing Ren*), 6g, mix-fried Radix Glycyrrhizae (*Gan Cao*), 6g, uncooked Rhizoma Zingiberis (*Sheng Jiang*), 6g, Fructus Zizyphi Jujubae (*Da Zao*), 3 pieces

2. Exuberant wind

Symptoms: This pattern mainly occurs in spring. There is generalized pruritus with possible red color of the itchy skin. The itching may move from one location to another and is without fixed site. Pruritus may be incessant, and the skin becomes thick with crusts or vesicles. Heat typically makes the itching worse, while cold can improve it. In addition, there are thirst, heart vexation, a red tongue tip with thin, yellow fur, and a floating, rapid or bowstring pulse.

Therapeutic principles: Course wind and dispel evils, clear heat and stop itching

Acupuncture & moxibustion:

He Gu (LI 4)   Together these points course wind and clear the
Feng Chi (GB 20)   heat when needled with draining method.

Qu Chi (LI 11)   Together these points clear heat and harmonize the
Xue Hai (Sp 10)   blood to stop itching when needled with draining
     method.

Additions & subtractions: For wind heat transforming into heat toxins, add *Ling Tai* (GV 10). For vesicles or oozing, add *Yin Ling Quan* (Sp 9) and *San Yin Jiao* (Sp 6). For heart vexation, add *Da Ling* (Per 7).

Chinese medicinal formula: *Wu Shao Qu Feng Tang* (Zaocys Dhumnades Expel Wind Decoction)

Ingredients: Zaocys Dhumnades (*Wu Shao She*), 3g (powdered and taken with the strained decoction), Periostracum Cicadae (*Chan Tui*), 12g, Herba Schizonepetae Tenuifoliae (*Jing Jie*), 12g, Radix Ledebouriellae Divaricatae (*Fang Feng*), 9g, Radix Et Rhizoma Notopterygii (*Qiang Huo*), 6g, Rhizoma Coptidis Chinensis (*Huang Lian*), 3-6g, Radix Scutellariae Baicalensis (*Huang Qin*), 3-6g, Flos Lonicerae Japonicae (*Jin Yin Hua*), 15g, Fructus Forsythiae Suspensae (*Lian Qiao*), 9g, Radix Angelicae Dahuricae (*Bai Zhi*), 9g, Radix Glycyrrhizae (*Gan Cao*), 6g

3. Wind dampness

Symptoms: This pattern mainly affects the young or adolescent in the autumn. The itching is severe, and blisters or papules may appear after scratching. The blisters or papules will ooze when opened by scratching. Other symptoms include slimy, white or thin, yellow tongue fur and a slippery, rapid pulse.

Therapeutic principles: Dispel wind, eliminate dampness, and stop itching

Acupuncture & moxibustion:

Feng Chi (GB 20)	Together, these points dispel wind and stop itching
Feng Shi (GB 31)	when needled with draining method.

Li Gou (Liv 5)	Together, these points eliminate dampness and
Yin Ling Quan (Sp 9)	stop itching when needled with draining method.
San Yin Jiao (Sp 6)	

Additions & subtractions: For poor appetite, add *Jian Li* (CV 13). For profuse vaginal discharge, add *Dai Mai* (GB 26).

Chinese medicinal formula: Modified *Quan Chong Fang* (Scorpion Formula)

Ingredients: Buthus Martensis (*Quan Xie*), 3g (powdered and taken with the strained decoction), Spina Gleditschiae Chinensis (*Zao Jiao Ci*), 9g, Fructus Tribuli Terrestris (*Bai Ji Li*), 9g, Radix Clematidis Chinensis (*Wei Ling Xian*), 9g, Radix Sophorae Flavescentis (*Ku Shen*), 9g, Cortex Radicis Dictamni Dasycarpi (*Bai Xian Pi*), 9g, Rhizoma Atractylodis (*Cang Zhu*), 9g

4. Heat in the blood

Symptoms: This pattern often occurs in the young and middle-aged. The generalized itching is severe, and worse in summer or on exposure to warmth, while it is better in winter or on obtaint of cold. Scratching leads to easy bleeding. Other symptoms include thirst, heart vexation, a crimson tongue with no or thin, yellow fur, and a bowstring, rapid or slippery, rapid pulse.

Therapeutic principles: Cool the blood and clear heat, extinguish wind and stop itching

Acupuncture & moxibustion:

He Gu (LI 4)	Together, these points eliminate wind and stop
Feng Chi (GB 20)	itching when needled with draining
Qu Chi (LI 11)	method.
Li Gou (Liv 5)	Together, these points clear heat, cool the blood,
Xue Hai (Sp 10)	and stop itching when needled with draining
San Yin Jiao (Sp 6)	method.

Additions & subtractions: For insomnia, add *Shen Men* (Ht 7). For nose-bleeding, add *Shang Xing* (GV 23). For profuse menstruation, add *Xing Jian* (Liv 2) and *Da Dun* (Liv 1).

Chinese medicinal formula: *Zhi Yang Xi Feng Tang* (Stop Itching & Extinguish Wind Decoction)

Ingredients: Uncooked Radix Rehmanniae (*Sheng Di*), 15g, Radix Scrophulariae Ningpoensis (*Xuan Shen*), 12g, uncooked Radix Angelicae Sinensis (*Dang Gui*), 9g, Cortex Radicis Moutan (*Dan Pi*), 9g, Radix Rubrus Paeoniae Lactiflorae (*Chi Shao*), 12g, Fructus Tribuli Terrestris (*Bai Ji Li*), 9g, Concha Ostreae (*Mu Li*), 15g, Radix Glycyrrhizae (*Gan Cao*), 6g

5. Blood vacuity

Symptoms: This pattern is usually seen in the aged or those with habitual bodily weakness. The condition is typically worse in autumn and winter but better in spring and summer. The itching is not very severe, and scratching often gives rise to desquamation, dry skin, possible crusts, or white flakes. Other symptoms include a lusterless facial complexion, heart palpitations, insomnia, dizziness, blurred vision, a pale tongue, and a bowstring, fine pulse

Therapeutic principles: Nourish the blood and moisten dryness, dispel wind and stop itching

Acupuncture & moxibustion:

Xin Shu (Bl 15) *Ge Shu* (Bl 17) *Pi Shu* (Bl 20)	Together, these points nourish the blood and moisten dryness when needled with supplementing method.
Xue Hai (Sp 10) *Qu Chi* (LI 11)	Together, these points dispel wind and stop itching when needled with draining method.

Additions & subtractions: For constipation, add *Shang Ju Xu* (St 37). For heart vexation, add *Tai Xi* (Ki 3) and *Yin Xi* (Ht 6).

Chinese medicinal formula: Modified *Yang Xue Run Fu Tang* (Nourish Blood & Moisten the Skin Decoction)

Ingredients: Uncooked Radix Rehmanniae (*Sheng Di*), 12g, cooked Radix Rehmanniae (*Shu Di*), 12g, uncooked Radix Angelicae Sinensis (*Dang Gui*), 9g, uncooked Radix Astragali Membranacei (*Huang Qi*), 15g, Tuber Ophiopogonis Japonici (*Mai Men Dong*), 6g, Tuber Asparagi Cochinensis (*Tian Men Dong*), 6g, Semen Pruni Persicae (*Tao Ren*), 6g, Flos Carthami Tinctorii (*Hong Hua*), 6g, Herba Schizonepetae Tenuifoliae (*Jing Jie*), 9g, Fructus Tribuli Terrestris (*Bai Ji Li*), 9g, Radix Scutellariae Baicalensis (*Huang Qin*), 6g

Remarks: When treating skin diseases, one should always keep in mind the following diagnostic principles: Red skin usually means blood heat. Dry skin usually means blood vacuity. Oozing and water-filled vesicles usually indicate dampness. And itching, especially if it moves from place to place, usually indicates wind. Thus the major causative factors of skin diseases of all types are nothing other than wind, dampness, blood heat, and blood dryness, and the relative proportions of these in any case can usually be determined by inspection and analysis of the lesions themselves.

23

Generalized Shaking *(Shen Zhen Yao)*

This refers to trembling of the whole body. When severe, this shaking can even cause the patient to fall down. For head shaking, see Chapter 2 in Volume 1 of this series. For tremors of the hands, see Chapter 26 in Volume 4. And for shaking feet, see Chapter 34 in Volume 4.

Disease causes, disease mechanisms:

1. Liver wind stirring internally

This pattern is mainly seen in the individuals who suffer from mental-emotional disease, such as anger, and have a tendency towards hyper-activity of liver yang. Hyperactivity of liver yang gives rise to heat, and heat may transform wind. Therefore, the *Nei Jing (Inner Classic)* says: "All wind with shaking and dizzy vision is ascribed to the liver." All movement is a function of the movement of qi, and internally stirring of wind is nothing other than chaotically and frenetically moving qi. Therefore, if liver wind stirs internally, there may be shaking of the body.

2. Vacuous yang failing to control

Yang vacuity here usually develops from profuse sweating or postpartum vacuity of both the qi and blood. In this case, yang deserts the body with profuse sweating. Yang is supposed to warm and free the flow of the blood. If yang becomes vacuous enough, it may fail to control the blood vessels, thus giving rise to malnourishment of the sinews. Thus the sinews contract, giving rise to shaking of the body.

Treatment based on pattern discrimination:

1. Liver wind stirring internally

Symptoms: Uncontrollable shaking of the body which gets better or worse depending on changes in the emotions, numbness of the extremities, dizziness, heart vexation, irascibility, a red tongue with thin, dry fur, and a bowstring, tense, forceful pulse

Therapeutic principles: Level the liver and extinguish wind

Acupuncture & moxibustion:

Feng Fu (GV 16) *Feng Chi* (GB 20) *Tai Chong* (Liv 3)	Together, these points level the liver and extinguish wind to stop shaking when needled with draining method.
Shen Zhu (GV 12) *Xuan Zhong* (GB 39) *Yang Ling Quan* (GB 34)	Together, these points soothe the sinews when needled with even draining and supplementing method.
San Yin Jiao (Sp 6)	Nourishes yin to lead yang downward when needled with supplementing method

Additions & subtractions: For tinnitus, add *Ting Hui* (GB 2). For a bitter taste in the mouth, add *Xing Jian* (Liv 2). For headache, add *Hou Ding* (GV 19) or *Shuai Gu* (GB 8).

Chinese medicinal formula: Modified *Tian Ma Gou Teng Yin* (Gastrodia & Uncaria Drink)

Ingredients: Stir-fried till yellow Rhizoma Gastrodiae Elatae (*Tian Ma*), 9g, Ramulus Uncariae Cum Uncis (*Gou Teng*), 9g, Radix Achyranthis Bidentatae (*Niu Xi*), 9g, Concha Haliotidis (*Shi Jue Ming*), 15g, Ramulus Loranthi Seu Visci (*Sang Ji Sheng*), 9g, Fructus Gardeniae Jasminoidis (*Zhi Zi*), 9g, uncooked Radix Scutellariae Baicalensis (*Huang Qin*), 6g, salt stir-fried Cortex Eucommiae Ulmoidis (*Du Zhong*), 6g, Fructus Tribuli Terrestris (*Bai Ji Li*), 6g, Scolopendra Subspinipes (*Wu Gong*), 3g (powdered and taken with the strained decoction), Buthus Martensis (*Quan Xie*), 3g (powdered and taken with the strained decoction), uncooked Radix Albus Paeoniae Lactiflorae (*Bai Shao*), 9g, mix-fried Radix Glycyrrhizae (*Gan Cao*), 3g

2. Vacuous yang failing to control

Symptoms: Shaking of the body which gets worse on exposure to cold and better on obtaint of warmth and which can be controlled by oneself in minor cases, cold body and chilled limbs, possible abdominal pain and vomiting, possible diarrhea of clear grains, possible falling on the ground due to shaking in very severe cases, a pale tongue with thin, glossy fur, and a deep, tight pulse

Therapeutic principles: Warm yang to stop shaking

Acupuncture & moxibustion:

Qiang Jian (GV 18) *Shen Zhu* (GV 12) *Tao Dao* (GV 13) *Da Zhui* (GV 14)	Together, these points warm yang to stop shaking when needled with moxibustion on the heads of the needles.
Zu San Li (St 36) *Xuan Zhong* (GB 39)	Together, these points soothe the sinews and stop shaking when needled with even draining and supplementing method.

Additions & subtractions: For shaking due to profuse sweating after labor, add *Xue Hai* (Sp 10) and *San Yin Jiao* (Sp 6). For shortage of qi and laziness to speak, add *Qi Hai* (CV 6). For heart palpitations, add *Nei Guan* (Per 6). For diarrhea of clear grains, moxa *Guan Yuan* (CV 4). For abdominal pain, moxa *Shen Que* (CV 8). For nausea and vomiting, add *Zhong Wan* (CV 12).

Chinese medicinal formulas: For predominant spleen yang vacuity: *Ling Gui Zhu Gan Tang* (Poria, Cinnamon, Atractylodes & Licorice Decoction)

Ingredients: Sclerotium Poriae Cocos (*Fu Ling*), 12g, stir-fried Ramulus Cinnamomi Cassiae (*Gui Zhi*), 9g, uncooked Rhizoma Atractylodis Macrocephalae (*Bai Zhu*), 6g, mix-fried Radix Glycyrrhizae (*Gan Cao*), 6g

For predominant kidney yang vacuity: *Zhen Wu Tang* (True Warrior Decoction)

Ingredients: Bland Radix Lateralis Praeparatus Aconiti Carmichaeli (*Fu Zi*), 9g, uncooked Rhizoma Atractylodis Macrocephalae (*Bai Zhu*), 9g, Radix Albus Paeoniae Lactiflorae (*Bai Shao*), 6g, uncooked Rhizoma Zingiberis (*Sheng Jiang*), 9g, Sclerotium Poriae Cocos (*Fu Ling*), 9g

For shaking of the body after childbirth: *Dang Gui Sheng Jiang Yang Rou Tang* (Angelica, Ginger & Mutton Decoction)

Ingredients: Radix Angelicae Sinensis (*Dang Gui*), 9g, uncooked Rhizoma Zingiberis (*Sheng Jiang*), 15g, lamb, 100g

Remarks: This last formula should be cooked and eaten once a day as a soup or stew. Garlic, onions, salt, pepper, clove, etc. can be added to make it taste better.

24

Generalized Jaundice *(Quan Shen Fa Huang)*

Generalized jaundice refers to yellowing of the whites of the eyes and the skin. Usually, the yellowing starts from the whites of the eyes and then gradually develops on the skin of the whole body.

Disease causes, disease mechanisms:

1. Damp heat

Damp heat causing jaundice usually results from external contraction of damp heat evils, excessive consumption of alcohol and fatty, sweet foods, or constitutional excess of dampness. Whether externally invading or internally engendered, damp heat fumes and steams within the body. If damp heat fumes and steams in the liver and gallbladder, the bile, which is yellow in color, will be forced out. If the bile flows up into the eyes along the liver channel, the whites of the eyes will become yellow. When the bile flows into the flesh, the skin will become yellow. If it flows into the bladder, the urine will turn yellow.

2. Contraction of epidemic toxins

Epidemic toxins are very strong evils which can suddenly cause severe disease. They easily enter the constructive and blood divisions and create exuberant heat. This exuberant heat may force out the bile which then flows into the flesh causing jaundice.

3. Cold dampness

The cold dampness that causes jaundice usually develops from constitutional yang vacuity of the spleen and stomach, dietary irregularities, enduring disease which damages spleen yang, or from excessive administration of bitter, cold medicinals. If the spleen yang becomes vacuous, first, cold will result since, "Yang vacuity causes internal cold." Secondly, the spleen will fail to move and transform water dampness, thus giving rise to damp accumulation. If this cold and dampness combine and obstruct the middle burner, they may block the flow of bile. In that case, the bile will over-flow into the flesh, thus leading to jaundice.

4. Liver depression & blood stasis

This disease mechanism often develops from enduring liver qi stagnation. However, it may also play a role in lingering and enduring jaundice. In that case, damp heat suppresses and inhibits the qi mechanism. The liver governs free coursing, and the normal discharge of the bile depends upon the normal free coursing of the liver. If blood becomes static within the liver, the free coursing of the liver will be affected and, therefore, the discharge of the bile will be inhibited. Hence the bile will overflow into the flesh, giving rise to jaundice.

5. Spleen vacuity & blood insufficiency

Spleen vacuity may arise from excessive thinking, constitutional insufficiency, overwork taxation, dietary irregularities, enduring disease, or due to childbirth. The spleen is the latter heaven source of qi and blood engenderment and transformation. If the spleen becomes vacuous and weak, it may not transform and engender the qi and the blood sufficiently. The flesh corresponds to earth and yellow is the color of earth. The skin and flesh are nourished by the blood which is red in color. If the flesh is deprived of blood, its rosy red color is missing and, instead, only a lusterless yellow is left.

Treatment based on pattern discrimination:

1. Damp heat with predominant heat

Symptoms: Yang jaundice with bright-colored yellowing of the whites of the eyes and body, fever, thirst, heart vexation, stomach and abdominal distention and fullness, reduced food intake, aversion to oily, greasy, fatty foods, nausea, vomiting, short voidings of dark yellow urine, dry stools and constipation, a red tongue with slimy, yellow fur, and a slippery, rapid pulse

Therapeutic principles: Clear heat and disinhibit dampness

Acupuncture & moxibustion:

Ri Yue (GB 24) Together, these points clear and disinhibit damp heat
Tai Chong (Liv 3) in the liver-gallbladder when needled with draining
Nei Ting (St 44) method.
Yang Ling Quan (GB 34)
Zu San Li (St 36)

Zhi Yang (GV 9)   Frees the flow of yang, drains heat, and eliminates jaundice when needled with draining method

Additions & subtractions: For a bitter taste in the mouth, add *Xia Xi* (GB 43). For heart vexation and insomnia, add *Jian Shi* (Per 5).

Chinese medicinal formula: Modified *Yin Chen Hao Tang* (Artemisia Capillaris Decoction)

Ingredients: Herba Artemisiae Capillaris (*Yin Chen Hao*), 30g, Fructus Gardeniae Jasminoidis (*Zhi Zi*), 15g, cooked Radix Et Rhizoma Rhei (*Da Huang*), 9g, Cortex Phellodendri (*Huang Bai*), 9g

Additions & subtractions: For severe dry stools and constipation, replace cooked with uncooked Rhubarb and add Mirabilitum (*Mang Xiao*), 3g (powdered and taken with the strained decoction). For severely inhibited, dark urination, add Rhizoma Alismatis (*Ze Xie*), 9g, Semen Plantaginis (*Che Qian Zi*), 9g, and Sclerotium Polypori Umbellati (*Zhu Ling*), 9g. For severe nausea or vomiting of bitter fluids, add ginger mix-fried Rhizoma Coptidis Chinensis (*Huang Lian*), 6g, and ginger mix-fried Caulis Bambusae In Taeniis (*Zhu Ru*), 12g. For rib-side pain, add Radix Bupleuri (*Chai Hu*), 9g, Tuber Curcumae (*Yu Jin*), 9g, and Fructus Meliae Toosendan (*Chuan Lian Zi*), 9g. For severe stomach and abdominal distention and fullness, add ginger mix-fried Cortex Magnoliae Officinalis (*Hou Po*), 9g, Fructus Immaturus Citri Aurantii (*Zhi Shi*), 9g, stir-fried Fructus Crataegi (*Shan Zha*), 9g, and stir-fried Fructus Germinatus Hordei Vulgaris (*Mai Ya*), 9g.

2. Damp heat with predominant dampness

Symptoms: Yang jaundice with not as bright yellowing of the whites of the eyes and body, unsurfaced fever, heavy-headedness, encumbered body, thirst without drinking a lot, reduced appetite, aversion to oily, greasy, fatty foods, nausea, vomiting, chest and stomach oppression and fullness, fatigued body, lack of strength, short voidings of yellow urine, difficult defecation of loose stools, thick, slimy, yellow tongue fur, and a soggy, moderate (*i.e.,* slightly slow) or slippery, bowstring pulse

Therapeutic principles: Disinhibit dampness and transform turbidity, clear heat and abate jaundice

Acupuncture & moxibustion:

Yang Ling Quan (GB 34) *Yin Ling Quan* (Sp 9) *Tai Chong* (Liv 3) *Zu San Li* (St 36)	Together, these points clear and disinhibit dampness and heat and abate jaundice when needled with draining method.
Qiu Xu (GB 40)	Drains damp heat and eliminates jaundice when needled with draining method

Chinese medicinal formula: Modified *Yin Chen Wu Ling Tang* (Artemisia Capillaris Five [Ingredients] Poria Decoction)

Ingredients: Herba Artemisiae Capillaris (*Yin Chen Hao*), 30g, Rhizoma Alismatis (*Ze Xie*), 9g, Sclerotium Poriae Cocos (*Fu Ling*), 15g, Sclerotium Polypori Umbellati (*Zhu Ling*), 9g, uncooked Rhizoma Atractylodis Macrocephalae (*Bai Zhu*), 9g, Ramulus Cinnamomi Cassiae (*Gui Zhi*), 6g, Radix Scutellariae Baicalensis (*Huang Qin*), 6g

Additions & subtractions: For nausea and vomiting, add ginger stir-fried Rhizoma Pinelliae Ternatae (*Ban Xia*), 9g, and uncooked Pericarpium Citri Reticulatae (*Chen Pi*), 9g. For abdominal distention, add Pericarpium Arecae Catechu (*Da Fu Pi*), 9g, and Radix Auklandiae Lappae (*Mu Xiang*), 9g. For turbidity accumulating in the center with loss of taste or a sweet taste in the mouth, nausea, stomach fullness, loose stools, and greyish white tongue fur, replace *Yin Chen Wu Ling Tang* with *Yin Chen Wei Ling Tang* (Artemisia Capillaris Stomach Poria Decoction): Herba Artemisiae Capillaris (*Yin Chen Hao*), 30g, uncooked Rhizoma Atractylodis (*Cang Zhu*), 9g, uncooked Cortex Magnoliae Officinalis (*Hou Po*), 9g, uncooked Pericarpium Citri Reticulatae (*Chen Pi*), 9g, bran stir-fried Rhizoma Atractylodis Macrocephalae (*Bai Zhu*), 9g, stir-fried Ramulus Cinnamomi (*Gui Zhi*), 6g, Sclerotium Polypori Umbellati (*Zhu Ling*), 6g, Sclerotium Poriae Cocos (*Fu Ling*), 9g, Rhizoma Alismatis (*Ze Xie*), 6g, and mix-fried Radix Glycyrrhizae (*Gan Cao*), 6g.

3. Damp heat with a simultaneous exterior pattern

Symptoms: Yang jaundice, early stage of jaundice, slightly yellow eyes and possibly body, aversion to cold, fever, heavy-headedness, generalized body pain, fatigue, stomach oppression, yellow urine, thin, slimy tongue fur, and a floating, bowstring or floating, rapid pulse

Therapeutic principles: Resolve the exterior, clear heat, and disinhibit dampness

Acupuncture & moxibustion:

Wai Guan (TB 5) *He Gu* (LI 4)	Together, these points resolve the exterior.
Yang Ling Quan (GB 34) *Qiu Xu* (GB 40) *Tai Chong* (Liv 3)	Together, these points clear and disinhibit dampness and heat and abate jaundice when needled with draining method.

Chinese medicinal formula: Modified *Ma Huang Lian Qiao Xiao Dou Tang* (Ephedra, Forsythia & Aduki Bean Decoction)

Ingredients: Uncooked Herba Ephedrae (*Ma Huang*), 6g, Fructus Forsythiae Suspensae (*Lian Qiao*), 9g, Semen Phaseoli Calcarati (*Chi Xiao Dou*), 15g, Cortex Radicis Mori Albi (*Sang Bai Pi*), 9g, Semen Pruni Armeniacae (*Xing Ren*), 6g, Radix Isatidis Seu Baphicacanthi (*Ban Lan Gen*), 15g, Herba Artemisiae Capillaris (*Yin Chen Hao*), 18g

Additions & subtractions: For severe aversion to cold without sweating, add uncooked Ramulus Cinnamomi Cassiae (*Gui Zhi*), 9g. For severely inhibited, yellow urination, add Talcum (*Hua Shi*), 9g, Semen Plantaginis (*Che Qian Zi*), 9g, and Sclerotium Rubrum Poriae Cocos (*Chi Fu Ling*), 9g. For vexatious thirst, add uncooked Gypsum Fibrosum (*Shi Gao*), 20g.

4. Damp heat in the liver gallbladder

Symptoms: Yang jaundice with severe, sudden right rib-side pain. After the pain, the jaundice appears. There is accompanying abdominal cramps if pressure is placed on the gallbladder area. Other symptoms include possible high fever with shivering or aversion to cold, vomiting, nausea, burping and belching, abdominal fullness and distention, aversion to oily, greasy, fried, and fatty food, dryness and a bitter taste in the mouth, constipation, short voiding of dark-colored urine, a red tongue with yellow fur, and a bowstring, slippery pulse

Note: This pattern corresponds to cholecystitis accompanied by jaundice in Western medicine.

Therapeutic principles: Clear the liver and disinhibit the gallbladder, transform dampness and abate jaundice

Acupuncture & moxibustion:

Xing Jian (Liv 2) *Qi Men* (Liv 14) *Xia Xi* (GB 43) *Ri Yue* (GB 24)	Together, these points clear the liver and disinhibit the gallbladder, transform dampness and abate jaundice.

Additions & subtractions: For severe pain, add *He Gu* (LI 4). For severe jaundice, add *Zhi Yang* (GV 9). For high fever, add *Qu Chi* (LI 11). For vomiting, add *Nei Guan* (Per 6). For cholelithiasis, add *Dan Nang Xue* (M-LE-6).

Chinese medicinal formula: Modified *Yin Chen Hao Tang* (Artemisia Capillaris Decoction) plus *Da Chai Hu Tang* (Major Bupleurum Decoction)

Ingredients: Herba Artemisiae Capillaris (*Yin Chen Hao*), 30g, Fructus Gardeniae Jasminoidis (*Zhi Zi*), 9g, cooked Radix Et Rhizoma Rhei (*Da Huang*), 9g, Radix Scutellariae Baicalensis (*Huang Qin*), 9g, uncooked Radix Bupleuri (*Chai Hu*), 9g, ginger stir-fried Rhizoma Pinelliae Ternatae (*Ban Xia*), 9g, Radix Auklandiae Lappae (*Mu Xiang*), 6g, Tuber Curcumae (*Yu Jin*), 9g, Semen Plantaginis (*Che Qian Zi*), 9g, Radix Albus Paeoniae Lactiflorae (*Bai Shao*), 9g

Additions & subtractions: For cholelithiasis, use a different modification of *Yin Chen Hao Tang* plus *Da Chai Hu Tang*: Herba Artemisiae Capillaris (*Yin Chen Hao*), 30g, Herba Lysimachiae (*Jin Qian Cao*), 30g, Fructus Gardeniae Jasminoidis (*Zhi Zi*), 9g, cooked Radix Et Rhizoma Rhei (*Da Huang*), 9g, Radix Scutellariae Baicalensis (*Huang Qin*), 9g, uncooked Radix Bupleuri (*Chai Hu*), 9g, Radix Auklandiae Lappae (*Mu Xiang*), 6g, Radix Et Rhizoma Polygoni Cuspidati (*Hu Zhang*), 9g, Radix Albus Paeoniae Lactiflorae (*Bai Shao*), 9g, Fructus Immaturus Citri Aurantii (*Zhi Shi*), 9g. For cholelithiasis with fever, add Flos Lonicerae Japonicae (*Jin Yin Hua*), 15g, and Fructus Forsythiae Suspensae (*Lian Qiao*), 9g, to the preceding formula. For cholelithiasis with vomiting, add ginger stir-fried Rhizoma Pinelliae Ternatae (*Ban Xia*), 9g, and ginger stir-fried Caulis Bambusae In Taeniis (*Zhu Ru*), 9g, to the preceding formula.

5. Contraction of epidemic toxins

Symptoms: Acute jaundice with sudden onset and fast development, golden yellowing of the whites of the eyes and body, high fever, thirst, vexation and agitation, possible clouded spirit and delirium, possible nose-bleeding, bleeding gums, hematemesis, or hemafecia, static macules in the skin, a crimson red tongue with slimy, yellow fur and reduced liquids, and a rapid pulse

Therapeutic principles: Clear heat and resolve toxins, cool the blood, open the orifices, and disinhibit the gallbladder

Acupuncture & moxibustion:

Shao Fu (Ht 8)   Together, these points clear heat and cool the blood
Xing Jian (Liv 2)   when needled with draining method.
Xia Xi (GB 43)

Da Zhui (GV 14)   Together, these points clear heat, resolve toxins,
Qu Ze (Per 3)   and open the orifices when pricked to bleed.
Wei Zhong (Bl 40)

Dan Shu (Bl 19)   Together, these points clear and disinhibit damp
Yang Ling Quan   heat in the liver-gallbladder when needled with draining
(GB 34)   method.

Additions & subtractions: For clouded spirit and delirium, prick *Shui Gou* (GV 26) to bleed. For rib-side pain and abdominal fullness, add *Zhang Men* (Liv 13). For nosebleed, add *Shang Xing* (GV 23). For hematemesis, add *Xi Men* (Per 4) and *Liang Qiu* (St 34). For constipation, add *Nei Ting* (St 44). For frequent vomiting, add *Nei Guan* (Per 6).

Chinese medicinal formula: Modified *Xi Jiao San* (Rhinoceros Horn Powder)

Ingredients: Cornu Bubali (*Shui Niu Jiao*), 20g, uncooked Rhizoma Coptidis Chinensis (*Huang Lian*), 6g, uncooked Radix Scutellariae Baicalensis (*Huang Qin*), 9g, Rhizoma Cimicifugae (*Sheng Ma*), 6g, uncooked Fructus Gardeniae Jasminoidis (*Zhi Zi*), 9g, Herba Artemisiae Capillaris (*Yin Chen Hao*), 30g, ginger mix-fried Cortex Magnoliae Officinalis (*Hou Po*), 9g, Folium Daqingye (*Da Qing Ye*), 12g, Flos Lonicerae Japonicae (*Jin Yin Hua*), 18g, Fructus Forsythiae Suspensae (*Lian Qiao*), 9g, Radix Scrophulariae Ningpoensis (*Xuan Shen*), 15g, Cortex Radicis Moutan (*Dan Pi*), 9g, uncooked Radix Rehmanniae (*Sheng Di*), 15g

Additions & subtractions: Without bleeding, subtract Scrophularia, Moutan, and uncooked Rehmannia. For severe bleeding, add Cacumen Biotae Orientalis (*Ce Bai Ye*), 9g, and Herba Agrimoniae Pilosae (*Xian He Cao*), 9g. For inhibited urination, add Semen Plantaginis (*Che Qian Zi*), 9g, Rhizoma

Imperatae Cylindricae (*Bai Mao Gen*), 9g, and Pericarpium Arecae Catechu (*Da Fu Pi*), 9g. For high fever with delirium, add the ready-made medicine *An Gong Niu Huang Wan* (Quiet the Palace Bezoar Pills).

Note: Another possible substitution for Rhinoceros Horn in this case is to use the "three yellows": Radix Scutellariae Baicalensis (*Huang Qin*), Rhizoma Coptidis Chinensis (*Huang Lian*), and Cortex Phellodendri (*Huang Bai*).

6. Cold dampness

Symptoms: Yin jaundice with dull-colored yellowing of the eyes and body, torpid, reduced food intake, stomach and abdominal oppression and distention, encumbered, heavy limbs, fatigued spirit, cold body and chilled limbs, a bland taste in the mouth and no thirst, inhibited urination, loose stools, slimy, white tongue fur, and a soggy, moderate (*i.e.*, slightly slow) or deep, slow pulse

Therapeutic principles: Warm and transform cold dampness coupled with fortifying the spleen and harmonizing the stomach

Acupuncture & moxibustion:

Pi Shu (Bl 20)	Together, these points warm the center, fortify the
Wei Shu (Bl 21)	spleen, and transform cold dampness when needled
Zhong Wan (CV 12)	with moxibustion on the heads of the needles.
Zu San Li (St 36)	
Guan Yuan (CV 4)	Boosts fire to engender earth when moxaed
San Jiao Shu (Bl 22)	Together, these points free the flow of the triple
San Yin Jiao (Sp 6)	burner and disinhibit dampness when needled with
	draining method.

Additions & subtractions: For nausea and vomiting, add *Nei Guan* (Per 6). For rib-side distention, add *Qi Men* (Liv 14). For profuse, clear vaginal discharge, add *Dai Mai* (GB 26).

Chinese medicinal formula: Modified *Yin Chen Si Ni Tang* (Artemisia Capillaris Four Counterflows Decoction)

Ingredients: Herba Artemisiae Capillaris (*Yin Chen Hao*), 30g, dry Rhizoma Zingiberis (*Gan Jiang*), 6g, bland Radix Lateralis Praeparatus Aconiti

Carmichaeli (*Fu Zi*), 6g, uncooked Rhizoma Atractylodis Macrocephalae (*Bai Zhu*), 9g, uncooked Rhizoma Atractylodis (*Cang Zhu*), 9g, Sclerotium Poriae Cocos (*Fu Ling*), 9g, mix-fried Radix Glycyrrhizae (*Gan Cao*), 6g

Additions & subtractions: For itching, add Radix Gentianae Macrophyllae (*Qin Jiao*), 9g, and Fructus Kochiae Scopariae (*Di Fu Zi*), 9g. For abdominal distention with thick tongue fur, subtract Atractylodes and Licorice and add Herba Agastachis Seu Pogostemi (*Huo Xiang*), 9g, Fructus Cardamomi (*Bai Dou Kou*), 6g, and Cortex Magnoliae Officinalis (*Hou Po*), 9g. For inhibited urination, add Sclerotium Polypori Umbellati (*Zhu Ling*), 9g, and Rhizoma Alismatis (*Ze Xie*), 9g. For predominant fatigue, reduced appetite, and loose stools which suggest spleen vacuity, replace *Yin Chen Si Ni Tang* with Modified *Xiang Sha Liu Jun Zi Tang* (Aucklandia & Amomum Six Gentlemen Decoction): rice stir-fried Radix Codonopsitis Pilosulae (*Dang Shen*), 9g, bran stir-fried Rhizoma Atractylodis Macrocephalae (*Bai Zhu*), 9g, Sclerotium Poriae Cocos (*Fu Ling*), 9g, mix-fried Radix Glycyrrhizae (*Gan Cao*), 3g, stir-fried Pericarpium Citri Reticulatae (*Chen Pi*), 9g, uncooked Radix Auklandiae Lappae (*Mu Xiang*), 6g, Fructus Amomi (*Sha Ren*), 6g, and Herba Artemisiae Capillaris (*Yin Chen Hao*), 18g.

7. Liver depression & blood stasis

Symptoms: Yin jaundice with dull yellowing of the body, a blue-green, purple, or soot black facial complexion, possible lumps below the rib-side which is painful and uncomfortable, possible lower abdominal distention and pain but uninhibited urination, possible spider-like, fine, red vessels in the skin, possible low-grade fever, possible black stools, a dark, purple tongue with possible static macules or spots, and a bowstring, choppy or fine, choppy pulse

Therapeutic principles: Quicken the blood and transform the stasis, soften the hard and disperse binding

Acupuncture & moxibustion:

Tai Chong (Liv 3)	Together, these points course the liver and move
Qi Men (Liv 14)	the qi to disperse binding when needled with
Gan Shu (Bl 18)	draining method.
Yang Ling Quan (GB 34)	Together, these points disinhibit the gallbladder and abate jaundice when needled with
Dan Shu (Bl 19)	draining method.

Ge Shu (Bl 17)	Together, these points quicken the blood, transform
Da Bao (Sp 21)	stasis, and soften the hard when needled with
Xue Hai (Sp 10)	draining method.

Additions & subtractions: For dull pain in the rib-side, add *Zhang Men* (Liv 13). For stabbing pain in the chest and rib-side which refuses pressure, add *He Gu* (LI 4) and *San Yin Jiao* (Sp 6).

Chinese medicinal formula: Modified *Ge Xia Zhu Yu Tang* (Below the Diaphragm Dispel Stasis Decoction)

Ingredients: Vinegar mix-fried Feces Trogopterori Seu Pteromi (*Wu Ling Zhi*), 9g, wine mix-fried Radix Angelicae Sinensis (*Dang Gui*), 9g, wine mix-fried Radix Ligustici Wallichii (*Chuan Xiong*), 6g, Semen Pruni Persicae (*Tao Ren*), 6g, Flos Carthami Tinctorii (*Hong Hua*), 6g, uncooked Cortex Radicis Moutan (*Dan Pi*), 6g, wine mix-fried Radix Rubrus Paeoniae Lactiflorae (*Chi Shao*), 9g, uncooked Radix Albus Paeoniae Lactiflorae (*Bai Shao*), 9g, wine mix-fried Radix Linderae Strychnifoliae (*Wu Yao*), 6g, wine mix-fried Rhizoma Corydalis Yanhusuo (*Yan Hu Suo*), 9g, vinegar mix-fried Rhizoma Cyperi Rotundi (*Xiang Fu*), 9g, uncooked Fructus Citri Aurantii (*Zhi Ke*), 9g, Herba Artemisiae Capillaris (*Yin Chen Hao*), 30g

Additions & subtractions: For severe accumulation lumps below the rib-side (including hepatomegaly and/or splenomegaly), subtract Lindera, Cyperus, and Moutan and add Pericarpium Citri Reticulatae Viride (*Qing Pi*), 9g, Rhizoma Sparganii (*San Leng*), 6g, and Rhizoma Curcumae Zedoariae (*E Zhu*), 6g. For concomitant blood vacuity, subtract Lindera and Moutan and add cooked Radix Rehmanniae (*Shu Di*), 9g.

8. Spleen vacuity & blood insufficiency

Symptoms: Yin or sallow jaundice with pale, lusterless yellowing of the face, eyes, and body, yellow urine, possible lack of yellowing of the eyes and urine, dull pain in the abdomen, weak limbs, fatigued spirit, heart palpitations, insomnia, dizziness, pale nails, shortness of breath, reduced food intake, loose stools, a pale tongue with thin fur, and a soggy, fine pulse

Therapeutic principles: Fortify the spleen and harmonize the stomach, boost the qi and supplement the blood

Acupuncture & moxibustion:

Ge Shu (Bl 17)	Together, these points fortify the spleen and harmonize
Gan Shu (Bl 18)	the stomach, boost the qi and supplement the blood
Pi Shu (Bl 20)	when needled with supplementing method.
Wei Shu (Bl 21)	

Zu San Li (St 36)	Together, these points fortify the spleen, regulate the
Tai Chong (Liv 3)	liver, and abate jaundice when needled with even
	supplementing and draining method.

Chinese medicinal formula: Modified *Xiao Jian Zhong Tang* (Minor Fortify the Center Decoction)

Ingredients: Maltose (*Yi Tang*), 25g, stir-fried Ramulus Cinnamomi Cassiae (*Gui Zhi*), 9g, Radix Albus Paeoniae Lactiflorae (*Bai Shao*), 15g, mix-fried Radix Glycyrrhizae (*Gan Cao*), 6g, uncooked Rhizoma Zingiberis (*Sheng Jiang*), 9g, Fructus Zizyphi Jujubae (*Da Zao*), 5 pieces, Herba Artemisiae Capillaris (*Yin Chen Hao*), 30g, stir-fried Radix Codonopsitis Pilosulae (*Dang Shen*), 9g, vinegar stir-fried Radix Bupleuri (*Chai Hu*), 6g

Additions & subtractions: For severe qi vacuity, add honey stir-fried Radix Astragali Membranacei (*Huang Qi*), 15g. For severe blood vacuity, add honey stir-fried Radix Astragali Membranacei (*Huang Qi*), 15g, and Radix Angelicae Sinensis (*Dang Gui*), 9g. For abdominal distention, add ginger mix-fried Cortex Magnoliae Officinalis (*Hou Po*), 9g, stir-fried Pericarpium Citri Reticulatae (*Chen Pi*), 6g, and Sclerotium Poriae Cocos (*Fu Ling*), 9g. For damp accumulation, subtract Maltose and add bran stir-fried Rhizoma Atractylodis Macrocephalae (*Bai Zhu*), 12g. For spleen vacuity coupled with kidney yin vacuity, replace *Xiao Jian Zhong Tang* with Modified *Liu Wei Di Huang Wan* (Six Flavors Rehmannia Pills): cooked Radix Rehmanniae (*Shu Di*), 12g, steamed Fructus Corni Officinalis (*Shan Zhu Yu*), 9g, stir-fried Radix Dioscoreae Oppositae (*Shan Yao*), 12g, Sclerotium Poriae Cocos (*Fu Ling*), 12g, Cortex Radicis Moutan (*Dan Pi*), 6g, Rhizoma Alismatis (*Ze Xie*), 6g, salt stir-fried Fructus Gardeniae Jasminoidis (*Zhi Zi*), 6g, rice stir-fried Radix Codonopsitis Pilosulae (*Dang Shen*), 9g, honey mix-fried Radix Astragali Membranacei (*Huang Qi*), 15g, and Herba Artemisiae Capillaris (*Yin Chen Hao*), 18g.

Remarks: 1. Acupuncture and moxibustion are very effective for jaundice.

2. Strict sterilization procedures should be observed with hepatitis patients receiving acupuncture to prevent cross-contamination.

3. Patients with contagious hepatitis due to epidemic evils should be quarantined for 30-40 days.

4. Another cause of jaundice which is rarely seen in Western countries is due to hookworm larva. This is called *huang pang* in Chinese, "yellow obesity." The main symptoms of this condition are yellowing and swelling of the face, jaundice of the whole body with white lines, itchy, red papule on the skin, increased appetite, abdominal distention after eating, a predilection for eating strange things, such as uncooked cereals, tea, and charcoal, fatigue, weakness of limbs, a pale tongue, and a soggy pulse. The treatment is Modified *Huang Bing Jiang Fan Wan* (Yellow Disease Crimson Alumen Pills): processed Alumen (*Ming Fan*), 1g (powdered and taken with the strained decoction), ginger mix-fried Cortex Magnoliae Officinalis (*Hou Po*), 9g, uncooked Rhizoma Atractylodis (*Cang Zhu*), 6g, uncooked Pericarpium Citri Reticulatae (*Chen Pi*), 6g, mix-fried Radix Glycyrrhizae (*Gan Cao*), 6g, Semen Arecae Catechu (*Bing Lang*), 9g, Radix Stemonae (*Bai Bu*), 9g, Fructus Carpesii Seu Daucusi (*He Shi*), 9g, Sclerotium Omphaliae Lapidescentis (*Lei Wan*), 6g, and Semen Torreyae Grandis (*Fei Zi*), 12g.

5. Roundworms in the biliary tract resulting in cholecystitis may also cause jaundice. The main symptoms of this condition are acute attacks of severe upper abdominal pain, jaundice after attack of abdominal pain, nausea, vomiting, possible vomiting of roundworms, and return to apparently normal health after attack. In this case, treatment should be addressed at the root, *i.e.*, treating the parasites, and not the jaundice. The most commonly used formula for this condition is *Wu Mei Wan* (Mume Pills): Fructus Pruni Mume (*Wu Mei*), 9g, Herba Asari Cum Radice (*Xi Xin*), 1-3g, dry Rhizoma Zingiberis (*Gan Jiang*), 6g, Fructus Zanthoxyli Bungeani (*Chuan Jiao*), 3-6g, Ramulus Cinnamomi Cassiae (*Gui Zhi*), 6g, Radix Lateralis Praeparatus Aconiti Carmichaeli (*Fu Zi*), 6g, Rhizoma Coptidis Chinensis (*Huang Lian*), 6g, Cortex Phellodendri (*Huang Bai*), 6g, Radix Codonopsitis Pilosulae (*Dang Shen*), 9g, and Radix Angelicae Sinensis (*Dang Gui*), 9g. This treatment is efficient for calming the roundworms and stopping the pain but is insufficient for killing the ascarids.

6. Chinese medicinals are very effective for treating either hepatitis A, B or C. Some are specific for regulating transaminase. These include Fructus Schisandrae Chinensis (*Wu Wei Zi*), Radix Istadis Seu Baphicacanthi (*Ban Lan Gen*), Herba Artemisiae Capillaris (*Yin Chen Hao*), Radix Rubrus

Paeoniae Lactiflorae (*Chi Shao*), Concretio Silicea Bambusae (*Tian Zhu Huang*), Radix Glycyrrhizae (*Gan Cao*), Herba Sedi Sarmentosi (*Chui Pen Cao*), Radix Angelicae Sinensis (*Dang Gui*), Herba Patriniae Heterophyllae Cum Radice (*Bai Jiang Cao*), Radix Et Rhizoma Polygoni Cuspidati (*Hu Zhang*), Rhizoma Coptidis Chinensis (*Huang Lian*), Cortex Phellodendri (*Huang Bai*), and Radix Gentianae Scabrae (*Long Dan Cao*). Some are specific for lowering the γ-glutamyl transpepsidase (GGT). These include Radix Angelicae Sinensis (*Dang Gui*), Fructus Schisandrae Chinensis (*Wu Wei Zi*), Radix Gentianae Scabrae (*Long Dan Cao*), Herba Patriniae Heterophyllae Cum Radice (*Bai Jiang Cao*), Radix Glycyrrhizae (*Gan Cao*), Radix Istadis Seu Baphicacanthi (*Ban Lan Gen*), Fructus Forsythiae Suspensae (*Lian Qiao*), Radix Salviae Miltiorrhizae (*Dan Shen*), Ganoderma (*Ling Zhi*), Endothelium Corneum Gigeriae Galli (*Ji Nei Jin*), and Radix Bupleuri (*Chai Hu*). Some are specific for protecting or regenerating the liver cells. These include Radix Angelicae Sinensis (*Dang Gui*), cooked Radix Rehmanniae (*Shu Di*), Radix Salviae Miltiorrhizae (*Dan Shen*), Fructus Lycii Chinensis (*Gou Qi Zi*), Rhizoma Atractylodis Macrocephalae (*Bai Zhu*), Radix Astragali Membranacei (*Huang Qi*), Radix Codonopsitis Pilosulae (*Dang Shen*), Ganoderma (*Ling Zhi*), Radix Bupleuri (*Chai Hu*), Herba Artemisiae Capillaris (*Yin Chen Hao*), Radix Et Rhizoma Polygoni Cuspidati (*Hu Zhang*), Rhizoma Alismatis (*Ze Xie*), Herba Patriniae Heterophyllae Cum Radice (*Bai Jiang Cao*), and Fructus Forsythiae Suspensae (*Lian Qiao*). And some are specific for preventing fibrosis of the liver. These include Rhizoma Sparganii (*San Leng*), Rhizoma Curcumae Zedoariae (*E Zhu*), Squama Manitis Pentadactylis (*Chuan Shan Jia*), Carapax Amydae Sinensis (*Bie Jia*), Fructus Crataegi (*Shan Zha*), Radix Salviae Miltiorrhizae (*Dan Shen*), Radix Bupleuri (*Chai Hu*), and Radix Glycyrrhizae (*Gan Cao*).

25
Purple Macules on the Skin *(Pi Fu Zi Ban)*

This refers to purple discoloration of the skin. This discoloration is spot-like or macular in shape, but flat and non-palpable.

Disease causes, disease mechanisms:

I. Blood heat

Frenetic blood heat usually results from deep-lying heat in the blood division coupled with invasion of wind evils or eating "emitting substances" such as seafood, milk, egg, etc., to which the individual's body is allergic. "Wind and fire may mutually fan." This means that wind and fire mutually exacerbate each other. When heat becomes exuberant, it may cause the blood to frenetically flow out of its vessels or flow into and congest in the fine network vessels, thus leading to blood stasis in the vessels or the skin. Static blood is "dead blood" and often takes a purple color. Therefore, purple macules may appear on the skin.

2. Damp heat pouring downward

Damp heat pouring downward can result from external contraction of damp heat evils, a predilection for fatty, sweet food or alcohol, or from enduring damp accumulation which transforms heat. If damp heat pours downward and blocks the network vessels, the movement of qi and blood will be inhibited. As a result, the blood will congest in the network vessels, and blood stasis may occur, thus giving rise to purple macules on the skin.

3. Spleen qi failing to contain the blood

The spleen is responsible for keeping the blood inside the vessels. This function of the spleen depends on its qi. Excessive thought, overwork taxation, and enduring disease may all render the spleen qi vacuous. If the spleen qi becomes so vacuous that it cannot contain the blood, the blood will flow out of its vessels. The blood can only flow as long as it remains within the vessels. Therefore, extravasated blood is static blood, and static blood is typically purple in color when visible. If this static blood occurs in the skin, purple macules may occur. In addition, if spleen qi vacuity endures for a long time, it may evolve into yang vacuity of the spleen and kidneys. In that case, vacuity cold may add yet another mechanism for the formation of blood stasis.

4. Yin vacuity & fire effulgence

Yin vacuity can result from aging, enduring disease, unrestrained sexual activity, or from frequent and enduring administration of exterior-resolving and/or yang-invigorating medicinals which excessively damage and consume liver and kidney yin. Yin is supposed to check yang. Therefore, if yin becomes vacuous, yang typically becomes hyperactive, thus giving rise to effulgent fire. This effulgent fire may force the blood to move frenetically outside its vessels which then engenders blood stasis. Because visible static blood is often purple in color, purple macules may occur.

5. Cold congelation & blood stasis

Cold congelation may be the result of constitutional yang vacuity or external contraction of cold evils. "Cold is a yin evil which causes contracture and constriction." If cold evils contract and constrict the blood vessels of the skin, they may cause blood stasis. Since visible static blood is typically purple in color, purple macules may occur.

6. Blood stasis

In fact, blood stasis is the sole proximate cause of this condition. In addition to the above disease mechanisms, blood stasis may be due to qi vacuity, blood vacuity, and qi stagnation. Blood stasis due to any of these occurring in the skin may give rise to purple macules.

Treatment based on pattern discrimination:

1. Blood heat

Symptoms: This pattern appears more in juveniles and the young than in any other age groups. There is often sudden onset. The purple macules may occur in any part of the body but most often symmetrically on the medial side of the lower legs. Itching in the diseased area is possible. The purple part may protrude slightly in the form of miliary rash or the macules may be as big as coins. The purple discoloration may disappear in 2-3 weeks, and reoccurrences often happen in batches. Other symptoms may include fever, which may worsen at night, possible delirium in severe cases, heart vexation, sore throat, thirst, occasional fatigue and lack of strength, possible nose-bleeding, hematuria, hemafecia, or hematemesis, a red tongue with thin, yellow fur, and a slippery, rapid or fine, rapid pulse.

Therapeutic principles: Clear heat and cool the blood, quicken the blood and disperse macules

Acupuncture & moxibustion:

Nei Ting (St 44)	Together, these points clear heat in the lungs and
Yu Ji (Lu 10)	stomach when needled with draining method.

Shao Fu (Ht 8)	Together, these points clear heat in the blood when
Xue Hai (Sp 10)	needled with draining method.
Da Du (Sp 2)	
Da Zhui (GV 14)	

Additions & subtractions: For purple macules all over the body, blue-green, swollen legs, and ulcerated gums with incessant bleeding, all of which suggest accumulated heat in the yang ming, add *Qu Chi* (LI 11), *He Gu* (LI 4) and *Li Dui* (St 45) to clear heat and resolve toxins, cool the blood and transform macules.

Chinese medicinal formula: Modified *Xi Jiao Di Huang Tang* (Rhinoceros Horn & Rehmannia Decoction)

Ingredients: Cornu Bubali (*Shui Niu Jiao*), 20g, uncooked Radix Rehmanniae (*Sheng Di*), 30g, uncooked Radix Rubrus Paeoniae Lactiflorae (*Chi Shao*), 12g, Cortex Radicis Moutan (*Dan Pi*), 12g, uncooked Gypsum Fibrosum (*Shi Gao*), 18g, Radix Scrophulariae Ningpoensis (*Xuan Shen*), 9g, Herba Violae Yedoensitis Cum Radice (*Zi Hua Di Ding*), 9g, Radix Glycyrrhizae (*Gan Cao*), 6g

Additions & subtractions: For high fever, add Rhizoma Coptidis Chinensis (*Huang Lian*), 6g, Radix Scutellariae Baicalensis (*Huang Qin*), 9g, and Fructus Gardeniae Jasminoidis (*Zhi Zi*), 9g. For spirit confusion and delirium, add the ready-made medicine *An Gong Niu Huang Wan* (Quiet the Palace Bezoar Pills).

2. Damp heat pouring downward

Symptoms: This pattern is often seen in young women. The purple macules mostly appear on the lower legs and thighs. They are usually accompanied by plum pit sized, hard lumps which are painful when touched but leave no marks after disappearing. Swelling is possible around these lumps. Painful joints may also be present. Other symptoms include heavy, encumbered limbs whose bending and stretching are inhibited, a sticky sliminess in the mouth, uneasy defecation, a red tongue with slimy, yellow fur, and a slippery, rapid pulse.

Remarks: This pattern corresponds to erythema nodosum in Western medicine.

Therapeutic principles: Clear heat and disinhibit dampness, quicken the blood and free the flow of the network vessels

Acupuncture & moxibustion:

Xing Jian (Liv 2) *Xia Xi* (GB 43) *Yang Ling Quan* (GB 34)	Together, these points clear and disinhibit dampness and heat in the liver-gallbladder when needled with draining method.
San Yin Jiao (Sp 6) *Xue Hai* (Sp 10) *He Gu* (LI 4)	Together, these points disinhibit dampness and quicken the blood when needled with draining method.

Additions & subtractions: For sticky, slimy, fishy, foul vaginal discharge, add *Yin Ling Quan* (Sp 9). For poor appetite, add *Zhong Wan* (CV 12). For heart vexation, add *Yin Xi* (Ht 6). For painful urination, add *Zhong Ji* (CV 3).

Chinese medicinal formula: Modified *Gan Lu Xiao Du Dan* (Sweet Dew Disperse Toxins Elixir)

Ingredients: Talcum (*Hua Shi*), 15g, Herba Artemisiae Capillaris (*Yin Chen Hao*), 12g, uncooked Radix Scutellariae Baicalensis (*Huang Qin*), 6g, Rhizoma Acori Graminei (*Shi Chang Pu*), 9g, Bulbus Fritillariae Cirrhosae (*Chuan Bei Mu*), 6g, Caulis Akebiae (*Mu Tong*), 3g, Herba Agastachis Seu Pogostemi (*Huo Xiang*), 9g, Fructus Forsythiae Suspensae (*Lian Qiao*), 9g, Herba Menthae Haplocalysis (*Bo He*), 3g, Fructus Cardamomi (*Bai Dou Kou*), 6g, Radix Rubrus Paeoniae Lactiflorae (*Chi Shao*), 12g

Additions & subtractions: For severe painful and swollen joints, replace *Gan Lu Xiao Du Dan* with Modified *Juan Bi Tang* (Alleviate Impediment Decoction): Radix Et Rhizoma Notopterygii (*Qiang Huo*), 9g, Radix Angelicae Pubescentis (*Du Huo*), 9g, Ramulus Cinnamomi Cassiae (*Gui*

Zhi), 6g, Radix Gentianae Macrophyllae (*Qin Jiao*), 9g, wine mix-fried Radix Angelicae Sinensis (*Dang Gui*), 9g, wine mix-fried Radix Ligustici Wallichii (*Chuan Xiong*), 6g, Caulis Lonicerae Japonicae (*Ren Dong Teng*), 9g, Ramulus Mori Albi (*Sang Zhi*), 9g, stir-fried Resina Olibani (*Ru Xiang*), 6g, Radix Stephaniae Tetrandrae (*Han Fang Ji*), 9g, and Fructus Chaenomelis Lagenariae (*Mu Gua*), 9g. For swollen, red, painful, hot joints, replace *Gan Lu Xiao Du Dan* with Modified *Bai Hu Jia Gui Zhi Tang* (White Tiger Plus Cinnamon Decoction): uncooked Gypsum Fibrosum (*Shi Gao*), 20g, uncooked Rhizoma Anemarrhenae Asphodeloidis (*Zhi Mu*), 9g, Semen Oryzae Sativae (*Geng Mi*), 12g, Radix Glycyrrhizae (*Gan Cao*), 6g, Ramulus Cinnamomi Cassiae (*Gui Zhi*), 6g, Ramulus Mori Albi (*Sang Zhi*), 9g, Caulis Lonicerae Japonicae (*Ren Dong Teng*), 9g, Radix Rubrus Paeoniae Lactiflorae (*Chi Shao*), 9g, and Caulis Sargentodoxae (*Hong Teng*), 6g.

3. Spleen qi failing to contain the blood

Symptoms: In this pattern, there is often a long disease course and frequent reoccurrences. The diseased skin is flat and discolored dark purple which worsens with taxation. Skin lesions are possible in the diseased area. Other symptoms may include a sallow yellow or somber white, lusterless facial complexion, reduced food intake, fatigue, shortness of breath, laziness to speak, heart palpitations, loose stools, a pale tongue, and a fine, weak pulse, especially in the bar position.

Therapeutic principles: Supplement the spleen, boost the qi, and lead the blood back to the vessels

Acupuncture & moxibustion:

Pi Shu (Bl 20)   Together, these points supplement the spleen and boost
Ge Shu (Bl 17)   the qi when needled with supplementing method.
Zu San Li (St 36)

Qi Hai (CV 6)   Together, these points warm yang and boost the qi
Shen Que (CV 8) when moxaed.

Additions & subtractions: For nose-bleeding, moxa *Shang Xing* (GV 23). For hemafecia, add moxibustion to *Ge Shu* after needling. For uterine bleeding, add *Da He* (Ki 12). For rectal prolapse, add *Cheng Shan* (Bl 57).

Chinese medicinal formula: Modified *Gui Pi Tang* (Return the Spleen Decoction)

Ingredients: Radix Codonopsitis Pilosulae (*Dang Shen*), 9g, honey stir-fried Radix Astragali Membranacei (*Huang Qi*), 15g, bran stir-fried Rhizoma Atractylodis Macrocephalae (*Bai Zhu*), 9g, stir-fried Radix Angelicae Sinensis (*Dang Gui*), 9g, Arillus Euphoriae Longanae (*Long Yan Rou*), 9g, Sclerotium Poriae Cocos (*Fu Ling*), 9g, Radix Auklandiae Lappae (*Mu Xiang*), 3g, Fructus Lycii Chinensis (*Gou Qi Zi*), 9g, Radix Salviae Miltiorrhizae (*Dan Shen*), 9g, mix-fried Radix Glycyrrhizae (*Gan Cao*), 6g, Herba Agrimoniae Pilosae (*Xian He Cao*), 15g

Additions & subtractions: For impaired memory, heart palpitations, and insomnia, add stir-fried Semen Zizyphi Spinosae (*Suan Zao Ren*), 9g, and licorice-processed Radix Polygalae Tenuifoliae (*Yuan Zhi*), 9g. For diarrhea, add stir-fried Semen Nelumbinis Nuciferae (*Lian Zi*), 9g, and earth stir-fried Radix Dioscoreae Oppositae (*Shan Yao*), 9g. For profuse menstruation, add carbonized Fibra Stipulae Trachycarpi (*Zong Lu Tan*), 3g, Crinis Carbonisatus (*Xue Yu Tan*), 3g, and Radix Pseudoginseng (*San Qi*), 3g, all powdered and taken with the strained decoction.

4. Spleen kidney yang vacuity

Symptoms: In most cases presenting this pattern, purple macules occur repeatedly on the lower limbs. The diseased skin may manifest a miliary rash or macules the size of small coins. The color of the macules is often pale purple, and the macules usually do not connect. Other symptoms include cold limbs, fear of cold, fatigued spirit, loose stools, a sallow yellow facial complexion, dull pain in the abdomen which likes warmth and pressure, a bland taste in the mouth, long voidings of clear urine, worsening of symptoms with cold and overwork taxation, a pale tongue, and a deep, fine pulse.

Therapeutic principles: Supplement the kidneys and fortify the spleen, supplement fire to warm earth

Acupuncture & moxibustion:

Da Zhui (GV 14)	Together, these points warm and free the flow of
Ming Men (GV 4)	yang when needled with moxibustion on the heads
Guan Yuan (CV 4)	of the needles.
Zu San Li (St 36)	

202

Pi Shu (Bl 20)	Together, these points warm the center and fortify
Zhong Wan (CV 12)	the spleen when needled with moxibustion on the heads of the needles.

Additions & subtractions: For daybreak diarrhea, moxa *Shen Que* (CV 8). For puffy edema, add *Shui Fen* (CV 9). For shortness of breath and laziness to speak, add *Dan Zhong* (CV 17). For dull pain in the lower abdomen, needle *Huang Shu* (Ki 16) with moxibustion on the heads of the needles.

Chinese medicinal formula: Modified *You Gui Wan* (Restore the Right [Kidney] Pills)

Ingredients: Caulis Millettiae Seu Spatholobi (*Ji Xue Teng*), 15g, cooked Radix Rehmanniae (*Shu Di*), 12g, stir-fried Radix Dioscoreae Oppositae (*Shan Yao*), 9g, steamed Fructus Corni Officinalis (*Shan Zhu Yu*), 9g, stir-fried Semen Cuscutae Chinensis (*Tu Si Zi*), 9g, Fructus Lycii Chinensis (*Gou Qi Zi*), 6g, salt stir-fried Cortex Eucommiae Ulmoidis (*Du Zhong*), 9g, Radix Lateralis Praeparatus Aconiti Carmichaeli (*Fu Zi*), 6g, Cortex Cinnamomi Cassiae (*Rou Gui*), 3g, Gelatinum Cornu Cervi (*Lu Jiao Jiao*), 6g, stir-fried Radix Angelicae Sinensis (*Dang Gui*), 6g

Additions & subtractions: For dual vacuity of yin and yang, add Herba Ecliptae Prostratae (*Han Lian Cao*), 9g, and Fructus Ligustri Lucidi (*Nu Zhen Zi*), 9g. For seminal emission, loose stools, or vaginal discharge, add salt mix-fried Fructus Psoraleae Corylifoliae (*Bu Gu Zhi*), 9g, and Semen Euryalis Ferocis (*Qian Shi*), 9g. For diarrhea with undigested food, add Semen Myristicae Fragrantis (*Rou Dou Kou*), 6g, wine-steamed Fructus Schisandrae Chinensis (*Wu Wei Zi*), 9g, and salt mix-fried Fructus Psoraleae Corylifoliae (*Bu Gu Zhi*), 9g. For torpid intake, nausea, and vomiting, add dry Rhizoma Zingiberis (*Gan Jiang*), 6g. For low back and knee soreness and weakness, add wine mix-fried Radix Dipsaci (*Xu Duan*), 9g, and Radix Morindae Officinalis (*Ba Ji Tian*), 9g.

5. Yin vacuity & effulgent fire

Symptoms: Point or spot-like purple macules on the skin which come and go accompanied by bleeding gums, nose-bleeding, profuse menstruation, dizziness, heart vexation, red cheekbones, heat in the five hearts, throat and mouth dryness, tidal hectic fever, night sweats, a red tongue with scanty fur, and a fine, rapid pulse

Therapeutic principles: Enrich yin and downbear fire, quiet the network vessels and stop bleeding

Acupuncture & moxibustion:

He Gu (LI 4) *Qu Chi* (LI 11)	Together, these point clear heat when needled with draining method.
Wei Zhong (Bl 40) *Xue Hai* (Sp 10)	Together, these points clear heat from the blood when *Xue Hai* is bled.
Tai Xi (Ki 3) *San Yin Jiao* (Sp 6) *Ge Shu* (Bl 17)	Together, these points supplement blood and enrich yin when needled with supplementing method.

Additions & subtractions: If there are night sweats, add *Yin Xi* (Ht 6). If there is nose-bleeding or bleeding gums, add *Nei Ting* (St 44). If there is heat in the five hearts, add *Qu Zi* (Per 3). If there is dry throat and/or constipation, add *Zhao Hai* (Ki 6).

Chinese medicinal formula: Modified *Qian Gen San* (Rubia Powder)

Ingredients: Radix Rubiae Cordifoliae (*Qian Cao Gen*), 12g, Cacumen Biotae Orientalis (*Ce Bai Ye*), 9g, Cortex Phellodendri (*Huang Bai*), 6g, uncooked Radix Rehmanniae (*Sheng Di*), 15g, Gelatinum Corii Asini (*E Jiao*), 9g, Herba Ecliptae Prostratae (*Han Lian Cao*), 9g, Fructus Ligustri Lucidi (*Nu Zhen Zi*), 9g, Radix Angelicae Sinensis (*Dang Gui*), 9g, Rhizoma Anemarrhenae Asphodeloidis (*Zhi Mu*), 9g

Additions & subtractions: If night sweats are severe, add Fructus Levis Tritici Aestivi (*Fu Xiao Mai*), 18g, and Concha Ostreae (*Mu Li*), 12g. If throat and mouth dryness are severe, add Fructus Schisandrae Chinensis (*Wu Wei Zi*), 9g, and Tuber Ophiopogonis Japonici (*Mai Dong*), 12g. If menstruation is profuse and contains clots, add Cortex Radicis Lycii Chinensis (*Di Gu Pi*), 9g, and Cortex Radicis Moutan (*Dan Pi*), 9g. If there is concomitant spleen qi vacuity, add Radix Astragali Membranacei (*Huang Qi*), 15g, Radix Pseudostellariae Heterophyllae (*Tai Zi Shen*), 12g, and Radix Dioscoreae Oppositae (*Shan Yao*), 9g. If there is concomitant liver depression, add Fructus Meliae Toosendan (*Chuan Lian Zi*), 12g. For more severe blood stasis, add Radix Salviae Miltiorrhizae (*Dan Shen*), 9g, and Semen Pruni Persicae (*Tao Ren*), 9g.

6. Cold congelation & blood stasis

Symptoms: The purple macules usually appear on the face, nose, ears, and dorsal part of the hands and feet and mainly affect young women. They get worse in winter and improve in summer. Other symptoms include a pale tongue with static macules and a deep, fine, slow pulse.

Therapeutic principles: Warm the channels and scatter cold, quicken the blood, and transform macules

Acupuncture & moxibustion:

Ge Shu (Bl 17) *Xue Hai* (Sp 6)	Together, these points quicken the blood and transform macules when needled with draining method.
San Yin Jiao (Sp 6) *Pi Shu* (Bl 20) *Fei Shu* (Bl 13)	Together, these points warm and free the flow of the channels when moxaed.

Additions & subtractions: For localized cold pain, moxa the *a shi* points. For cold pain in the abdomen, moxa *Shen Que* (CV 8). For cold pain in the lower back, moxa *Yao Yang Guan* (GV 3). For painful menstruation, add *Zhong Ji* (CV 3) and *Di Ji* (Sp 8). For cold pain in the lower abdomen, add *Qu Quan* (Liv 8) or *Li Gou* (Liv 5).

Chinese medicinal formula: Modified *Dang Gui Si Ni Tang* (Dang Gui Four Counterflows Decoction)

Ingredients: Wine mix-fried Radix Angelicae Sinensis (*Dang Gui*), 12g, Ramulus Cinnamomi Cassiae (*Gui Zhi*), 9g, Radix Albus Paeoniae Lactiflorae (*Bai Shao*), 9g, Herba Asari Cum Radice (*Xi Xin*), 3g, mix-fried Radix Glycyrrhizae (*Gan Cao*), 6g, Radix Cyathulae (*Chuan Niu Xi*), 9g, Caulis Milletiae Seu Spatholobi (*Ji Xue Teng*), 15g, Flos Carthami Tinctorii (*Hong Hua*), 6g

Additions & subtractions: For severe blood vacuity, add cooked Radix Rehmanniae (*Shu Di*), 15g, and Caulis Milletiae Seu Spatholobi (*Ji Xue Teng*), 12g. For severe cold, add Radix Lateralis Praeparatus Aconiti Carmichaeli (*Fu Zi*), 6g, and processed Fructus Evodiae Rutecarpae (*Wu Zhu Yu*), 3g. For qi vacuity, add Radix Astragali Membranacei (*Huang Qi*), 15g, and Radix Codonopsitis Pilosulae (*Dang Shen*), 9g.

8. Blood stasis

Symptoms: Purple macules may be congenital or start during puberty and develop slowly. A family history is often present. The color of the affected skin may be purple, brown, or bluish purple, and the skin is flat. The macules commonly appear on the chest, upper back, lower back, abdomen, limbs, cheeks, temples, forehead, or eyelids. Hair does grow through these macules. In addition, there may be static macules on the tongue and a choppy pulse or other such symptoms of blood stasis.

Therapeutic principles: Quicken the blood, transform stasis and disperse macules

Acupuncture & moxibustion:

He Gu (LI 4) *Ge Shu* (Bl 17) *San Yin Jiao* (Sp 6) *Xue Hai* (Sp 10)	Together, these points quicken the blood, transform stasis, and disperse macules when needled with draining method.
Tai Chong (Liv 3) *Zhi Gou* (TB 6)	Together, these points move the qi to help transform stasis when needled with draining method.

Chinese medicinal formula: Modified *Tong Qiao Huo Xue Tang* (Free the Orifices & Quicken the Blood Decoction)

Ingredients: Wine mix-fried Radix Rubrus Paeoniae Lactiflorae (*Chi Shao*), 9g, wine mix-fried Radix Ligustici Wallichii (*Chuan Xiong*), 6g, wine mix-fried Radix Angelicae Sinensis (*Dang Gui*), 9g, Flos Carthami Tinctorii (*Hong Hua*), 6g, uncooked Semen Pruni Persicae (*Tao Ren*), 9g, uncooked Radix Rehmanniae (*Sheng Di*), 9g, uncooked Rhizoma Zingiberis (*Sheng Jiang*), 3g, Fructus Zizyphi Jujubae (*Da Zao*), 3 pieces

Additions & subtractions: For any bleeding, add Radix Pseudoginseng (*San Qi*), 3g (powdered and taken with the strained decoction), Pollen Typhae (*Pu Huang*), 9g, and Radix Rubi Cordifoliae (*Qian Cao*), 9g. For concomitant qi vacuity, add honey mix-fried Radix Codonopsitis Pilosulae (*Dang Shen*), 9g, honey mix-fried Radix Astragali Membranacei (*Huang Qi*), 12g, and bran stir-fried Rhizoma Atractylodis Macrocephalae (*Bai Zhu*), 9g. For concomitant blood vacuity, add wine mix-fried Radix Angelicae Sinensis (*Dang Gui*), 9g, and uncooked Radix Albus Paeoniae Lactiflorae (*Bai Shao*), 9g.

26
Edema *(Fu Zhong)*

Edema refers to swelling of the body due to water accumulation. If an indentation is left after pushing down on the affected area with the fingertip, this is referred to as pitting edema.

Disease causes, disease mechanisms:

The basic disease mechanism of edema is water dampness accumulating in the body. Water metabolism in Chinese medicine mainly involves the three viscera of the lungs, spleen, and kidneys. The lungs are the upper source of water. The spleen governs the movement and transformation of water dampness. And the kidneys governs the fluids of the entire body. Damage to the function of any of the viscera may lead to edema. In addition, qi also plays an important role in the formation of edema since it is qi which moves and transforms body fluids.

1. External evils invading the lungs

Out of all the external evils, wind cold and wind heat are the most likely to cause edema. When wind cold invades the lungs, it fetters the exterior and depresses the lung qi, thus inhibiting the lungs' diffusion. When wind heat invades the lungs, it may congest in the lungs and affect their depurative downbearing. The lungs are the upper source of water, responsible for regulating the free flow of water through its passageways. If the lungs are damaged by external evils, they may fail their duty of depurative downbearing and will not promote the free flow of water through its passageways. This leads to accumulation of water dampness in the body and thus edema.

2. Water dampness encumbering the spleen

Water dampness encumbering the spleen usually develops from constitutional spleen qi vacuity coupled with enduring exposure to dampness, such as getting caught in the rain, working in water or living in a damp environment. The spleen is responsible for moving and transforming water dampness. If the spleen becomes encumbered by dampness, water dampness will gather and collect internally. If this accumulated water dampness spills over into the flesh, edema may occur.

3. Damp heat

Damp heat mainly results from external contraction of evils or excessive consumption of alcohol, fatty meats, fine grains, rich-flavored foods, and sweet, fatty foods. The kidneys govern fluids and the two yin, while the bladder stores the urine. If damp heat pours downward into the lower burner, first, the qi transformation of the bladder is affected. Secondly, the kidneys may lose the control over the steaming and vaporizing of fluids. This leads to water dampness accumulation internally. Again, if this water dampness spills over into the flesh, edema may occur.

4. Lung qi vacuity cold

Lung qi vacuity may be due to enduring cough or asthma, constitutional insufficiency, or from spleen qi vacuity which fails to engender metal. The lungs are the upper source of water which are responsible for regulating the free flow of water through its passageways. If there is lung qi vacuity cold, first, the qi will fail to transform liquids which accumulate in the upper part of the body, while secondly, the lungs may fail their depurative downbearing and will not regulate the free flow of the water passageways. This combination of mechanisms leads to water dampness accumulating in the body. If this water dampness spills over into the space between the skin and flesh, edema will appear.

5. Spleen yang vacuity

This pattern usually develops from enduring replete patterns of edema which eventually damage spleen yang. Overwork taxation and other enduring diseases can also contribute to spleen yang vacuity as can simple aging. Spleen yang's function is to warm and transform water dampness. Therefore, if spleen yang becomes vacuous, water dampness may accumulate internally. If this accumulated water spills over into the flesh, edema may occur.

6. Kidney yang vacuity

Kidney yang vacuity causing edema may result from constitutional insufficiency and/or enduring disease. The kidneys are the water viscera governing the fluids of the entire body. The kidneys help water metabolism in two ways. First, the kidneys govern the two yin, controlling the qi transformation of the bladder, and the opening and closing of the bladder. Secondly, kidney yang is the original yang which controls the steaming and vaporizing of fluids. Therefore, if kidney yang becomes vacuous, the waterways in the lower burner may A) become blocked, and B) the fluids may not be steamed and vaporized. As a result, water dampness may accumulate internally and flood into the flesh, leading to edema.

7. Dual vacuity of qi & blood

Dual vacuity of the qi and blood can develop from spleen-stomach vacuity, enduring disease, childbirth, and overwork taxation. Qi is responsible for moving the fluids, and the blood is responsible for nourishing the viscera so that the viscera can function efficiently to metabolize fluids. Therefore, if, for any reason, the qi and the blood both become vacuous, fluids may accumulate and transform into water evil. If this water evil spills over into the space between the skin and flesh, edema may occur.

8. Qi stagnation & water collecting

The liver governs coursing and discharge. If emotional disturbance and frustration cause lack of coursing and discharge, this will lead to liver depression and qi stagnation. This, in turn, will affect the movement of the qi. If the qi stagnates, fluids will accumulate since it is the qi which moves fluids in the body. In addition, the liver corresponds to wood, and the spleen, to earth. When the liver becomes depressed, its qi becomes replete. When liver wood is replete, it may counterflow horizontally and assail spleen earth, thus affecting the spleen's movement and transformation. Therefore, water may accumulate for either of these two reasons. If this accumulation spills over into the flesh, edema may occur.

Treatment based on pattern discrimination:

1. Wind cold invading the lungs

Symptoms: Sudden onset of edema which first appears in the eyelids and is then followed by edema in the limbs and eventually the whole body, aversion to wind and cold, possible fever, aching joints, short voidings of urine, thin, white tongue fur, and a floating pulse

Therapeutic principles: Course and dispel wind cold, diffuse the lungs and disinhibit water

Acupuncture & moxibustion:

Lie Que (Lu 7) *He Gu* (LI 4) *Chi Ze* (Lu 5) *Fei Shu* (Bl 13)	Together, these points diffuse the lungs and resolve the exterior to regulate and free the flow of the water passageways when needled with draining method.
San Yin Jiao (Sp 6) *Yin Ling Quan* (Sp 9)	Together, these points free the flow of qi of the three burners and fortify the spleen to disinhibit water when needled with draining method.

Additions & subtractions: For aversion to wind and spontaneous perspiration, add *Feng Men* (Bl 12) and *Zu San Li* (St 36). If the exterior has been resolved but edema remains, add *Shui Fen* (CV 9) and *Shui Dao* (St 28) to dry dampness. For fever, add *Da Zhui* (GV 14).

Chinese medicinal formula: *Ma Huang Jia Zhu Tang* (Ephedra Plus Atractylodes Decoction)

Ingredients: Uncooked Herba Ephedrae (*Ma Huang*), 9g, uncooked Ramulus Cinnamomi Cassiae (*Gui Zhi*), 6g, Semen Pruni Armeniacae (*Xing Ren*), 9g, mix-fried Radix Glycyrrhizae (*Gan Cao*), 3g, uncooked Rhizoma Atractylodis Macrocephalae (*Bai Zhu*), 9g

Additions & subtractions: For severe edema, add Cortex Sclerotii Poriae Cocos (*Fu Ling Pi*), 9g, and Pericarpium Arecae Catechu (*Da Fu Pi*), 9g. For severe aversion to cold and fever, add Folium Perillae Frutescentis (*Zi Su Ye*), 9g, and Radix Et Rhizoma Notopterygii (*Qiang Huo*), 9g. For coughing and/or wheezing, add Semen Lepidii Seu Descurainiae (*Ting Li Zi*), 9g, and Fructus Perillae Frutescentis (*Su Zi*), 9g.

2. Wind heat harassing the lungs

Symptoms: Sudden onset of edema in the eyelids and face, fever, aversion to wind, sweating, thirst, coughing, red, sore throat, short voidings of urine, slightly red tongue edges and tip with thin, yellow fur, and a floating, rapid pulse

Therapeutic principles: Diffuse the lungs, clear heat, and disinhibit water

Acupuncture & moxibustion:

Fei Shu (Bl 13)	Together, these points diffuse the lungs and clear
Feng Men (Bl 12)	heat to disinhibit water when needled with
Chi Ze (Lu 5)	draining method.
He Gu (LI 4)	

Wei Yang (Bl 39)	Together, these points clear heat when needled with
Yu Ji (Lu 10)	draining method.

Additions & subtractions: For high fever, add *Da Zhui* (GV 14). For sore throat, prick *Shao Shang* (Lu 11) to bleed. For vexatious heat and voiding of scanty urine, add *San Jiao Shu* (Bl 22).

Chinese medicinal formula: Modified *Yue Bi Jia Zhu Tang* (Maidservant from Yue Plus Atractylodes Decoction)

Ingredients: Honey stir-fried Herba Ephedrae (*Ma Huang*), 9g, uncooked Rhizoma Atractylodis Macrocephalae (*Bai Zhu*), 12g, uncooked Gypsum Fibrosum (*Shi Gao*), 25g, uncooked Rhizoma Zingiberis (*Sheng Jiang*), 6g, Fructus Zizyphi Jujubae (*Da Zao*), 4 fruits, Radix Glycyrrhizae (*Gan Cao*), 3g

Additions & subtractions: For severe heat, add Fructus Forsythiae Suspensae (*Lian Qiao*), 9g, Rhizoma Imperatae Cylindricae (*Bai Mao Gen*), 9g, and Semen Phaseoli Calcarati (*Chi Xiao Dou*), 12g. For sore throat, add Radix Istadis Seu Baphicacanthi (*Ban Lan Gen*), 9g, Rhizoma Belamcandae Chinensis (*She Gan*), 9g, and Fructus Arctii Lappae (*Niu Bang Zi*), 9g. For exuberant heat damaging fluids, add Rhizoma Phragmitis Communis (*Lu Gen*), 9g, and Rhizoma Anemarrhenae Asphodeloidis (*Zhi Mu*), 9g. For phlegm heat obstructing the lungs, replace *Yue Bi Jia Zhu Tang* with modified *Qing Jin Hua Tan Tang* (Clear Metal & Transform Phlegm Decoction): uncooked Radix Scutellariae Baicalensis (*Huang Qin*), 6g, uncooked Rhizoma Anemarrhenae Asphodeloidis (*Zhi Mu*), 9g, Rhizoma Phragmitis Communis (*Lu Gen*), 9g, honey stir-fried Cortex Radicis Mori Albi (*Sang Bai Pi*), 9g, uncooked Pericarpium Citri Reticulatae (*Chen Pi*), 6g, honey stir-fried Radix Platycodi Grandiflori (*Jie Geng*), 6g, Semen Trichosanthis Kirlowii (*Gua Lou Ren*), 6g, Sclerotium Poriae Cocos (*Fu Ling*), 12g, and Semen Benincasae Hispidae (*Dong Gua Zi*), 9g.

3. Water dampness encumbering the spleen

Symptoms: Edema starting from the limbs with a slow onset and long disease course, more severe edema in the abdominal area and limbs, heavy, fatigued body, chest oppression, nausea, a bland taste in the mouth, short voidings of clear urine, slimy, white tongue fur, and a deep, moderate or deep, slow pulse

Therapeutic principles: Fortify the spleen and transform dampness, free the flow of yang and disinhibit water

Acupuncture & moxibustion:

Tai Bai (Sp 3) *Zu San Li* (St 36) *Yin Ling Quan* (Sp 9) *Wai Guan* (TB 5)	Together, these points fortify the spleen, free the flow of yang, and disinhibit water.
Zhang Men (Liv 13) *Xia Wan* (CV 10)	Together, these points warm the center and transform dampness when moxaed indirectly on a slice of ginger.

Additions & subtractions: For fatigued spirit, moxa *San Yin Jiao* (Sp 6). For torpid intake, add *Jian Li* (CV 11). For severe edema and panting, add *Fei Shu* (Bl 13) and *Shui Fen* (CV 9).

Chinese medicinal formula: Modified *Wei Ling Tang* (Stomach Poria Decoction) plus *Wu Pi Yin* (Five Skins Decoction)

Ingredients: Uncooked Rhizoma Atractylodis (*Cang Zhu*), 6g, uncooked Cortex Magnoliae Officinalis (*Hou Po*), 6g, uncooked Pericarpium Citri Reticulatae (*Chen Pi*), 9g, mix-fried Radix Glycyrrhizae (*Gan Cao*), 3g, uncooked Rhizoma Atractylodis Macrocephalae (*Bai Zhu*), 6g, uncooked Cortex Zingiberis (*Sheng Jiang Pi*), 9g, honey stir-fried Cortex Radicis Mori Albi (*Sang Bai Pi*), 9g, Pericarpium Arecae Catechu (*Da Fu Pi*), 9g, Cortex Sclerotii Poriae Cocos (*Fu Ling Pi*), 9g, Rhizoma Alismatis (*Ze Xie*), 9g

Additions & subtractions: For diarrhea, add Sclerotium Polypori Umbellati (*Zhu Ling*), 9g. For stomach or abdominal distention, add Fructus Cardamomi (*Bai Dou Kou*), 6g. For a cold sensation in the stomach or abdomen, add dry Rhizoma Zingiberis (*Gan Jiang*), 6g, and Semen Myristicae Fragrantis (*Rou Dou Kou*), 6g. For nausea or vomiting, add Herba Agastachis Seu Pogostemi (*Huo Xiang*), 9g, and ginger stir-fried Rhizoma Pinelliae Ternatae (*Ban Xia*), 9g.

4. Damp heat

Symptoms: Edema of the face and feet or generalized edema in severe cases, reduced food intake, vexatious heat in the five hearts, unsurfaced fever, thirst, short voidings of inhibited urine, turbid yellow urine, slimy, yellow tongue fur, and a rapid pulse

Therapeutic principles: Clear heat and eliminate dampness, disinhibit water and disperse swelling

Acupuncture & moxibustion:

San Jiao Shu (Bl 22)
Zhong Ji (CV 3)
San Yin Jiao (Sp 6)
Yin Ling Quan (Sp 9)

Together, these points free the flow of qi of the three burners and disinhibit water when needled with draining method.

Nei Ting (St 44) Clears heat

Chinese medicinal formula: Modified *Tong Ling San* (Akebia & Poria Powder)

Ingredients: Caulis Akebiae (*Mu Tong*), 5g, Sclerotium Poriae Cocos (*Fu Ling*), 9g, Sclerotium Polypori Umbellati (*Zhu Ling*), 9g, uncooked Rhizoma Atractylodis Macrocephalae (*Bai Zhu*), 6g, Rhizoma Alismatis (*Ze Xie*), 9g, Semen Plantaginis (*Che Qian Zi*), 9g, Herba Artemisiae Capillaris (*Yin Chen Hao*), 6g, Cortex Phellodendri (*Huang Bai*), 6g

Additions & subtractions: For turbid urine and low back pain, subtract Atractylodes and add Rhizoma Dioscoreae Hypoglaucae (*Bei Xie*), 12g, and Radix Sophorae Flavescentis (*Ku Shen*), 6g. For heat damaging the network vessels with bloody urine, add Rhizoma Imperatae Cylindricae (*Bai Mao Gen*), 12g, uncooked Radix Rehmanniae (*Sheng Di*), 15g, and Herba Cephalanoploris Segeti (*Xiao Ji*), 9g.

5. Lung qi vacuity cold

Symptoms: Facial edema or edema of the four limbs in severe cases, shortness of breath, weakness, fatigue, low voice, fear of cold, cough with a weak sound, thin, clear phlegm, a pale facial complexion, a pale tongue with white fur, and a weak, fine pulse

Therapeutic principles: Warm yang and scatter cold, diffuse the lungs and disinhibit water

Acupuncture & moxibustion:

Da Zhui (GV 14) *Fei Shu* (Bl 13) *Feng Men* (Bl 12)	Together, these points warm and diffuse the lungs to disinhibit water when moxaed.
He Gu (LI 4) *Zu San Li* (St 36)	Together, these points replenish the exterior and supplement earth to engender metal when needled with supplementing method.

Chinese medicinal formula: Modified *Ling Gan Wu Wei Jia Jiang Xin Ban Xia Xing Ren Tang* (Poria, Licorice, Schisandra, Ginger, Asari, Pinellia & Armeniaca Decoction)

Ingredients: Sclerotium Poriae Cocos (*Fu Ling*), 9g, mix-fried Radix Glycyrrhizae (*Gan Cao*), 6g, uncooked Fructus Schisandrae Chinensis (*Wu Wei Zi*), 9g, uncooked Radix Astragali Membranacei (*Huang Qi*), 15g, dry Rhizoma Zingiberis (*Gan Jiang*), 6g, Herba Asari Cum Radice (*Xi Xin*), 3g, clear Rhizoma Pinelliae Ternatae (*Ban Xia*), 9g, Semen Pruni Armeniacae (*Xing Ren*), 9g

Additions & subtractions: For lung-spleen qi vacuity with generalized edema, spontaneous perspiration, inhibited urination, fear of cold, loose stools, and reduced appetite, replace *Ling Gan Wu Wei Jia Jiang Xin Ban Xia Xing Ren Tang* with Modified *Si Jun Zi Tang* (Four Gentlemen Decoction) plus *Fang Ji Huang Qi Tang* (Stephania & Astragalus Decoction): rice stir-fried Radix Codonopsitis Pilosulae (*Dang Shen*), 6g, uncooked Atractylodis Macrocephalae (*Bai Zhu*), 9g, Sclerotium Poriae Cocos (*Fu Ling*), 9g, mix-fried Radix Glycyrrhizae (*Gan Cao*), 3g, uncooked Radix Astragali Membranacei (*Huang Qi*), 15g, Radix Stephaniae Tetrandrae (*Han Fang Ji*), 12g, and Rhizoma Alismatis (*Ze Xie*), 9g.

6. Spleen stomach qi vacuity

Symptoms: Facial edema or edema of the four limbs which comes and goes with no apparent reason, reduced appetite, fatigue, weakness of the limbs, shortness of breath, a pale, lusterless facial complexion, loose stools, abdominal distention, a pale tongue with white fur, and a weak, fine pulse

Therapeutic principles: Supplement and boost the spleen and stomach, transform dampness and disperse swelling

Acupuncture & moxibustion:

Pi Shu (Bl 20)	Together, these points supplement and boost the
Wei Shu (Bl 21)	spleen and stomach and transform dampness when
Zu San Li (St 36)	moxaed and needled with supplementing method.

Yin Ling Quan (Sp 9)	Together, these points fortify the spleen and
San Yin Jiao (Sp 6)	disinhibit water when needled with even
	supplementing and draining method.

Chinese medicinal formula: *Shen Ling Bai Zhu San* (Ginseng, Poria & Atractylodes Powder)

Ingredients: Stir-fried Semen Dolichoris Lablab (*Bai Bian Dou*), 9g, earth stir-fried Radix Dioscoreae Oppositae (*Shan Yao*), 9g, uncooked Rhizoma Atractylodis Macrocephalae (*Bai Zhu*), 12g, Sclerotium Poriae Cocos (*Fu Ling*), 12g, rice stir-fried Radix Codonopsitis Pilosulae (*Dang Shen*), 6g, stir-fried till yellow Semen Nelumbinis Nuciferae (*Lian Zi*), 6g, Radix Platycodi Grandiflori (*Jie Geng*), 3g, Semen Coicis Lachryma-jobi (*Yi Yi Ren*), 12g, Fructus Amomi (*Sha Ren*), 6g, mix fried Radix Glycyrrhizae (*Gan Cao*), 3g

Additions & subtractions: For severe edema, subtract Platycodon and Licorice and add uncooked Radix Astragali Membranacei (*Huang Qi*), 15g, and Sclerotium Polypori Umbellati (*Zhu Ling*), 9g. For severe damp accumulation, add ginger mix-fried Cortex Magnoliae Officinalis (*Hou Po*), 9g, and replace Atractylodes with bran stir-fried Rhizoma Atractylodis (*Cang Zhu*). For abdominal distention, add Radix Auklandiae Lappae (*Mu Xiang*), 9g, and stir-fried Pericarpium Citri Reticulatae (*Chen Pi*), 6g. For frequent loose stools with a sagging sensation in the rectum due to central qi fall, replace *Shen Ling Bai Zhu San* with *Bu Zhong Yi Qi Tang* (Supplement the Center & Boost the Qi Decoction): honey mix-fried Radix Astragali Membranacei (*Huang Qi*), 18g, honey stir-fried Radix

Codonopsitis Pilosulae (*Dang Shen*), 9g, uncooked Rhizoma Atractylodis Macrocephalae (*Bai Zhu*), 12g, honey mix-fried Radix Glycyrrhizae (*Gan Cao*), 3g, stir-fried Radix Angelicae Sinensis (*Dang Gui*), 3g, stir-fried Pericarpium Citri Reticulatae (*Chen Pi*), 6g, Radix Bupleuri (*Chai Hu*), 3g, and Rhizoma Cimicifugae (*Sheng Ma*), 3g.

7. Spleen yang vacuity

Symptoms: Lingering edema which is more severe below the waist, pitting edema, fatigued spirit, fear of cold, cold limbs, reduced food intake, no thirst, loose stools, short voidings of clear urine, a pale tongue with thin, white, watery, glossy fur, and a deep, moderate pulse

Therapeutic principles: Warm and move spleen yang, transform dampness and disinhibit water

Acupuncture & moxibustion:

Pi Shu (Bl 20) *Shen Shu* (Bl 23) *Ming Men* (GV 4)	Together, these points warm and move spleen yang to transform dampness when moxaed.
San Jiao Shu (Bl 22)	Frees the flow of yang when moxaed
Yin Ling Quan (Sp 9) *Zu San Li* (St 36)	Together, these points fortify the spleen and disinhibit water when needled with draining method.

Additions & subtractions: For dizziness, vertigo, and vomiting of clear, thin drool, moxa *Guan Yuan* (CV 4). For heart palpitations and panting, add *Xin Shu* (Bl 15) and *Fei Shu* (Bl 13). For profuse, clear, thin vaginal discharge, add *Dai Mai* (GB 26). For abdominal distention, add *Gong Sun* (Sp 4).

Chinese medicinal formula: *Shi Pi Yin* (Bolster the Spleen Drink)

Ingredients: Ginger mix-fried Cortex Magnoliae Officinalis (*Hou Po*), 6g, uncooked Rhizoma Atractylodis Macrocephalae (*Bai Zhu*), 9g, uncooked Fructus Chaenomelis Lagenariae (*Mu Gua*), 6g, Radix Auklandiae Lappae (*Mu Xiang*), 3g, Semen Alpiniae Katsumadai (*Cao Dou Kou*), 9g, Semen Arecae Catechu (*Bing Lang*), 9g, Radix Lateralis Praeparatus Aconiti Carmichaeli (*Fu Zi*), 6g, Sclerotium Poriae Cocos (*Fu Ling*), 12g, dry Rhizoma Zingiberis (*Gan Jiang*), 6g, mix-fried Radix Glycyrrhizae (*Gan Cao*), 3g

Additions & subtractions: For severe edema, add Rhizoma Alismatis (*Ze Xie*), 9g, Sclerotium Polypori Umbellati (*Zhu Ling*), 9g, and stir-fried Ramulus Cinnamomi Cassiae (*Gui Zhi*), 6g. For fatigue and weakness of the limbs, add uncooked Radix Astragali Membranacei (*Huang Qi*), 15g, and Radix Codonopsitis Pilosulae (*Dang Shen*), 9g. For severe fear of cold, add stir-fried Ramulus Cinnamomi Cassiae (*Gui Zhi*), 9g.

8. Kidney yang vacuity

Symptoms: Whole body edema which starts from the waist and feet and is more severe below the waist and especially on the inner ankles, low back and knees aching, limpness, and heaviness, damp, cold scrotum, fear of cold, cold limbs, short voidings of clear urine or frequent urination, urination of clear urine at night, a pale, enlarged tongue with thin, white fur, and a deep, fine, weak pulse

Therapeutic principles: Warm the kidneys, transform qi, and disinhibit water

Acupuncture & moxibustion:

Guan Yuan (CV 4) *Qi Hai* (CV 6)	Together, these points warm yang and transform qi to help disinhibit water when moxaed.
Shen Shu (Bl 23) *Ming Men* (GV 4)	Together, these points warm the kidneys when moxaed.
Shui Fen (CV 9) *Yin Ling Quan* (Sp 9)	Together, these points disinhibit water to disperse edema when needled with draining method.

Additions & subtractions: For heart palpitations and shortness of breath, add *Xin Shu* (Bl 15) and *Fei Shu* (Bl 13). For severe edema and inhibited urination, add *San Jiao Shu* (Bl 22).

Chinese medicinal formula: *Ji Sheng Shen Qi Wan* (*Aid the Living* Kidney Qi Pills)

Ingredients: Cooked Radix Rehmanniae (*Shu Di*), 9g, stir-fried Radix Dioscoreae Oppositae (*Shan Yao*), 9g, steamed Fructus Corni Officinalis (*Shan Zhu Yu*), 6g, Rhizoma Alismatis (*Ze Xie*), 12g, Sclerotium Poriae Cocos (*Fu Ling*), 12g, Cortex Radicis Moutan (*Dan Pi*), 3g, stir-fried Ramulus Cinnamomi Cassiae (*Gui Zhi*), 6g, Radix Lateralis Praeparatus

Aconiti Carmichaeli (*Fu Zi*), 9g, Radix Cyathulae (*Chuan Niu Xi*), 9g, Semen Plantaginis (*Che Qian Zi*), 15g

Additions & subtractions: For severely inhibited urination, add Sclerotium Polypori Umbellati (*Zhu Ling*), 9g, and Cortex Radicis Acanthopanacis (*Wu Jia Pi*), 9g. For frequent urination and urination of clear urine at night, subtract Plantago, reduce the dosage of Poria and Alisma to 6g, and add Fructus Alpiniae Oxyphyllae (*Yi Zhi Ren*), 9g, and Semen Cuscutae Chinensis (*Tu Si Zi*), 9g. For water qi intimidating the heart with heart palpitations, shortness of breath, bluish purple lips, and a choppy or bound pulse, add Radix Salviae Miltiorrhizae (*Dan Shen*), 9g, and Radix Pseudoginseng (*San Qi*), 3g (powdered and taken with the strained decoction). For severe kidney yang vacuity, add Herba Epimedii (*Yin Yang Huo*), 6g, and Rhizoma Curculiginis Orchioidis (*Xian Mao*), 6g. If the kidney yang vacuity is not so severe but is accompanied by spleen yang vacuity, replace *Ji Sheng Shen Qi Wan* with modified *Zhen Wu Tang* (True Warrior Decoction): Radix Lateralis Praeparatus Aconiti Carmichaeli (*Fu Zi*), 9g, uncooked Rhizoma Atractylodis Macrocephalae (*Bai Zhu*), 9g, Radix Albus Paeoniae Lactiflorae (*Bai Shao*), 9g, Sclerotium Poriae Cocos (*Fu Ling*), 15g, Pericarpium Arecae Catechu (*Da Fu Pi*), 9g, and mix-fried Radix Glycyrrhizae (*Gan Cao*), 6g.

9. Qi & blood dual vacuity

Symptoms: Edema starting in the face which then gradually develops to the limbs, a bright white or sallow yellow facial complexion, pale white lips and nails, dizziness, heart palpitations, shortness of qi, reduced food intake, fatigued body, devitalized spirit, a pale tongue with scanty fur, and a vacuous, fine, forceless pulse

Therapeutic principles: Boost the qi and supplement the blood

Acupuncture & moxibustion:

Xue Hai (Sp 10) *Ge Shu* (Bl 17) *San Yin Jiao* (Sp 6)	Together, these points supplement the blood when needled with supplementing method.
Qi Hai (CV 6) *Zu San Li* (St 36)	Together, these points boost the qi when needled with supplementing method.

Additions & subtractions: For spontaneous perspiration, add *He Gu* (LI 4). For insomnia, add *Shen Men* (Ht 7). For incessant uterine bleeding of scanty, pale, thin blood, add *Lou Gu* (Sp 7).

Chinese medicinal formula: Modified *Shi Quan Da Bu Wan* (Ten [Ingredients] Completely & Greatly Supplementing Decoction)

Ingredients: Radix Codonopsitis Pilosulae (*Dang Shen*), 9g, stir-fried Ramulus Cinnamomi Cassiae (*Gui Zhi*), 9g, wine mix-fried Radix Ligustici Wallichii (*Chuan Xiong*), 6g, cooked Radix Rehmanniae (*Shu Di*), 9g, wine mix-fried Radix Angelicae Sinensis (*Dang Gui*), 9g, Radix Albus Paeoniae Lactiflorae (*Bai Shao*), 9g, uncooked Rhizoma Atractylodis Macrocephalae (*Bai Zhu*), 12g, Sclerotium Poriae Cocos (*Fu Ling*), 12g, mix-fried Radix Glycyrrhizae (*Gan Cao*), 6g, uncooked Radix Astragali Membranacei (*Huang Qi*), 15g, Rhizoma Alismatis (*Ze Xie*), 9g

10. Qi stagnation & water collecting

Symptoms: Edema of the limbs or whole body, rib-side fullness and pain, stomach and abdominal glomus and fullness, reduced food intake, belching, frequent hiccup, irascibility, pale, lusterless nails and facial complexion, inhibited urination, a pale tongue, and a bowstring pulse

Therapeutic principles: Course the liver and rectify the qi, eliminate dampness and disperse fullness

Acupuncture & moxibustion:

Zhi Gou (TB 6)	Together, these points on the heaven, earth, and
Qi Men (Liv 14)	human portions course the liver, disperse fullness,
Tai Chong (Liv 3)	and free the flow of the qi of the three burners.
Zu San Li (St 36)	Supplements earth to control water when needled with supplementing method
Yin Ling Quan (Sp 9)	A water point, eliminates dampness when needled with draining method

Chinese medicinal formula: Modified *Chai Hu Shu Gan San* (Bupleurum Soothe the Liver Powder) plus *Wei Ling Tang* (Stomach Poria Decoction)

Ingredients: Radix Bupleuri (*Chai Hu*), 9g, Radix Albus Paeoniae Lactiflorae (*Bai Shao*), 9g, Fructus Citri Aurantii (*Zhi Ke*), 9g, Pericarpium Citri Reticulatae (*Chen Pi*), 6g, Radix Ligustici Wallichii (*Chuan Xiong*), 6g, Rhizoma Cyperi Rotundi (*Xiang Fu*), 9g, uncooked Rhizoma Atractylodis (*Cang Zhu*), 6g, uncooked Cortex Magnoliae Officinalis (*Hou Po*), 6g, uncooked Rhizoma Atractylodis Macrocephalae (*Bai Zhu*), 9g, stir-fried Ramulus Cinnamomi (*Gui Zhi*), 6g, Fructus Amomi (*Sha Ren*), 6g, mix-fried Radix Glycyrrhizae (*Gan Cao*), 3g

Additions & subtractions: For severe rib-side fullness and pain, add Rhizoma Cyperi Rotundi (*Xiang Fu*), 9g, and Pericarpium Citri Reticulatae Viride (*Qing Pi*), 9g. For reduced appetite, add stir-fried Fructus Germinatus Hordei Vulgaris (*Mai Ya*), 12g. For qi stagnation leading to blood stasis, add Herba Lycopi Lucidi (*Ze Lan*), 9g, Herba Leonuri Heterophylli (*Yi Mu Cao*), 9g, and Radix Salviae Miltiorrhizae (*Dan Shen*), 9g. For severe qi vacuity, add uncooked Radix Astragali Membranacei (*Huang Qi*), 15g, and Radix Codonopsitis Pilosulae (*Dang Shen*), 6g. For fear of cold, cold limbs, and loose stools due to spleen yang vacuity, add dry Rhizoma Zingiberis (*Gan Jiang*), 6g, and processed Fructus Evodiae Rutecarpae (*Wu Zhu Yu*), 3g. For a bitter taste in the mouth, dark urine, and red tongue edges due to qi depression transforming heat, add Herba Artemisiae Capillaris (*Yin Chen Hao*), 15g, Radix Et Rhizoma Polygoni Cuspidati (*Hu Zhang*), 9g, and Radix Scutellariae Baicalensis (*Huang Qin*), 6g.

27
Obesity *(Fei Pang)*

Obesity refers to the body's being overweight due to excessive accumulation of fat. It is often accompanied by dizziness, lack of strength, laziness to speak, reduced movement and shortage of qi.

Disease causes, disease mechanisms:

1. Phlegm dampness brewing internally

Phlegm dampness brewing internally usually develops from constitutional damp exuberance and/or an enduring predilection for rich-flavored, fatty, sweet foods which engender excessive fluids. If these fluids remain untransformed and collect, first they will further transform into evil dampness and then into phlegm. If this accumulated phlegm and dampness flood into the flesh, there will be obesity.

2. Spleen qi vacuity with damp encumbrance

Spleen qi vacuity resulting in obesity mainly develops from overwork taxation, too little exercise and activity, and overeating sweet, uncooked, and chilled foods and drinks which damage the spleen. As it is said in Chinese medicine, "Working consumes qi." Therefore, too much work may damage the spleen, the latter heaven root of qi and blood engenderment and transformation. On the other hand, it is also said that, "Excessive sitting damages the spleen." In addition, the sweet flavor corresponds to earth, and the spleen is the earth viscus. Therefore, sweetness enters the spleen. In small amounts, the sweet flavor supplements the spleen, but in large amounts it damages the spleen. Further, because the spleen's process of digestion is a warm transformation likened to cooking, overeating uncooked and/or chilled foods and drinks may also damage the spleen. The spleen qi is responsible for moving and transforming water dampness. Therefore, if the spleen qi becomes vacuous, water dampness may accumulate in the body. When this evil dampness transforms into phlegm and floods into the flesh, obesity may be seen.

3. Spleen kidney yang vacuity

In terms of obesity, spleen-kidney yang vacuity mostly results from constitutional insufficiency and aging. The kidneys govern the fluids of the entire body. Kidney yang is the original yang, controlling the steaming and vaporizing of the fluids. Therefore, if kidney yang becomes vacuous, fluids may not be steamed and vaporized. Thus dampness accumulates and transforms into phlegm over time. If this accumulated phlegm dampness floods into the flesh, obesity may be seen.

Treatment based on pattern discrimination:

1. Phlegm dampness brewing internally

Symptoms: Obesity, a predilection for sweet, fatty foods and dairy products or alcohol, chest and stomach glomus and oppression, nausea, profuse phlegm, dizziness, heart palpitations, heavy, fatigued limbs, somnolence, an enlarged tongue with thick, slimy fur, and a bowstring, slippery, forceful pulse

Therapeutic principles: Transform phlegm and dry dampness, abduct accumulation and disperse food

Acupuncture & moxibustion:

Yin Ling Quan (Sp 9) *San Yin Jiao* (St 6) *Zu San Li* (St 36)	Together, these points fortify the spleen and transform dampness when needled with supplementing method.
Feng Long (St 40) *Xia Wan* (CV 10) *Shui Fen* (CV 9)	Together, these points resolve phlegm and disinhibit dampness when needled with draining method.

Additions & subtractions: For profuse sweating, add *He Gu* (LI 4) and *Fu Liu* (Ki 7). For somnolence and disliking movement, moxa *San Jiao Shu* (Bl 22).

Chinese medicinal formula: Modified *Er Chen Tang* (Two Aged [Ingredients] Decoction) plus *Ping Wei San* (Level [*i.e.*, Calm] the Stomach Powder)

Ingredients: Clear Rhizoma Pinelliae Ternatae (*Ban Xia*), 9g, uncooked Pericarpium Citri Reticulatae (*Chen Pi*), 9g, Sclerotium Poriae Cocos (*Fu*

Ling) 9g, mix-fried Radix Glycyrrhizae (*Gan Cao*), 3g, bran stir-fried Rhizoma Atractylodis (*Cang Zhu*), 6g, ginger mix-fried Cortex Magnoliae Officinalis (*Hou Po*), 9g, uncooked Rhizoma Atractylodis Macrocephalae (*Bai Zhu*), 9g, Fructus Citri Aurantii (*Zhi Ke*), 6g, Fructus Crataegi (*Shan Zha*), 9g, Semen Raphani Sativi (*Lai Fu Zi*), 9g, Folium Nelumbinis Nuciferae (*He Ye*), 9g

Additions & subtractions: For fear of cold, add dry Rhizoma Zingiberis (*Gan Jiang*), 6g, and stir-fried Ramulus Cinnamomi Cassiae (*Gui Zhi*), 9g. For aversion to heat and yellow phlegm, subtract Atractylodes and add Caulis Bambusae In Taeniis (*Zhu Ru*), 9g, Radix Scutellariae Baicalensis (*Huang Qin*), 6g, and Talcum (*Hua Shi*), 6g. For inhibited urination, add Rhizoma Alismatis (*Ze Xie*), 9g, and Radix Stephaniae Tetrandrae (*Han Fang Ji*), 9g. For constipation, add Folium Sennae (*Fan Xie Ye*), 3-9g. For somnolence, add Rhizoma Acori Graminei (*Shi Chang Pu*), 9g.

2. Spleen qi vacuity

Symptoms: Obesity with a long history of bad dietary habits, reduced qi with laziness to speak, sweating on exertion, fear of cold, a puffy face, poor appetite, abdominal fullness after eating, fatigued spirit, weakness of the limbs, somnolence, loose stools, possible clear, thin vaginal discharge, possible bland taste in the mouth, a pale tongue with teeth-marks on its edges and white fur, and a fine, weak pulse

Therapeutic principles: Boost the qi, fortify the spleen, and percolate dampness

Acupuncture & moxibustion:

Pi Shu (Bl 20)	Together, these points boost the qi and fortify the
Shen Shu (Bl 23)	spleen when needled with supplementing method.
Qi Hai (CV 6)	
Zu San Li (St 36)	

San Yin Jiao (Sp 6)	Disinhibits dampness when needled with even draining and supplementing method.

Additions & subtractions: For decreased sexual desire due to concomitant kidney yang vacuity, moxa *Guan Yuan* (CV 4) and *Ming Men* (GV 4).

Chinese medicinal formula: Modified *Liu Jun Zi Tang* (Six Gentlemen Decoction) plus *Fang Ji Huang Qi Tang* (Stephania & Astragalus Decoction)

Ingredients: Radix Stephaniae Tetrandrae (*Han Fang Ji*), 12g, uncooked Radix Astragali Membranacei (*Huang Qi*), 15g, rice stir-fried Radix Codonopsitis Pilosulae (*Dang Shen*), 9g, uncooked Rhizoma Atractylodis Macrocephalae (*Bai Zhu*), 9g, Sclerotium Poriae Cocos (*Fu Ling*), 9g, mix-fried Radix Glycyrrhizae (*Gan Cao*), 3g, lime-processed Rhizoma Pinelliae Ternatae (*Ban Xia*), 9g, stir-fried Pericarpium Citri Reticulatae (*Chen Pi*), 6g, Fructus Crataegi (*Shan Zha*), 9g

Additions & subtractions: For stomach and abdominal fullness, add Radix Auklandiae Lappae (*Mu Xiang*), 6g, Fructus Amomi (*Sha Ren*), 6g, and Folium Nelumbinis Nuciferae (*He Ye*), 9g. For inhibited urination, add Rhizoma Alismatis (*Ze Xie*), 9g. For diarrhea with sliminess in the mouth, replace *Liu Jun Zi Tang* plus *Fang Ji Huang Qi Tang* with Modified *Shen Ling Bai Zhu San* (Ginseng, Poria & Atractylodes Powder): stir-fried Semen Dolichoris Lablab (*Bai Bian Dou*), 9g, stir-fried Radix Dioscoreae Oppositae (*Shan Yao*), 9g, uncooked Rhizoma Atractylodis Macrocephalae (*Bai Zhu*), 12g, Sclerotium Poriae Cocos (*Fu Ling*), 9g, rice stir-fried Radix Codonopsitis Pilosulae (*Dang Shen*), 9g, stir-fried till yellow Semen Nelumbinis Nuciferae (*Lian Zi*), 6g, stir-fried Semen Coicis Lachryma-jobi (*Yi Yi Ren*), 15g, mix-fried Radix Glycyrrhizae (*Gan Cao*), 6g, stir-fried Fructus Crataegi (*Shan Zha*), 9g, Folium Nelumbinis Nuciferae (*He Ye*), 9g.

3. Spleen vacuity & stomach heat

Symptoms: Obesity, rapid hungering after meals, fatigue, lack of strength, a tendency towards alternating constipation and loose stools, a red facial complexion, a dry mouth with a desire to drink, possibly a bitter taste in the mouth, bad breath, a fat, enlarged tongue with yellow fur, and a slippery, bowstring pulse

Therapeutic principles: Fortify the spleen and clear the stomach, harmonize the stomach and intestine

Acupuncture & moxibustion:

Nei Ting (St 44) *Jie Xi* (St 41) *Shang Ju Xu* (St 37)	Together, these points clear the stomach, drain the fire, and harmonize the stomach and intestines when needled with draining method.
Tai Bai (Sp 3)	Fortifies the spleen and harmonizes the stomach when needled with supplementing method

Additions & subtractions: For thirst, add *Wei Shu* (Bl 21) and *Fu Liu* (Ki 7). For a bitter taste in the mouth and bad breath, add *Da Ling* (Per 7). For spontaneous hot sweating, add *He Gu* (LI 4).

Chinese medicinal formula: Modified *Fei Pang Fang* (Obesity Formula)

Ingredients: Uncooked Radix Astragali Membranacei (*Huang Qi*), 15g, Folium Sennae (*Fan Xie Ye*), 3-9g, Rhizoma Alismatis (*Ze Xie*), 12g, Fructus Crataegi (*Shan Zha*), 9g, Folium Nelumbinis Nuciferae (*He Ye*), 9g, uncooked Rhizoma Atractylodis Macrocephalae (*Bai Zhu*), 6g

Additions & subtractions: For severe stomach heat, add Gypsum Fibrosum (*Shi Gao*), 18g, Fructus Gardeniae Jasminoidis (*Zhi Zi*), 9g, and Radix Glycyrrhizae (*Gan Cao*), 6g. For severe constipation, add uncooked Radix Et Rhizoma Rhei (*Da Huang*), 6-9g. For damp accumulation with edema in the lower limbs, add *Fang Ji Huang Qi Tang* (Stephania & Astragalus Decoction), *i.e.,* Radix Stephaniae Tetrandrae (*Han Fang Ji*), 12g, and uncooked Radix Astragali Membranacei (*Huang Qi*), 15g. For stomach heat, spleen vacuity, and food stagnation, replace *Fei Pang Fang* with *Xiao Cheng Qi Tang* (Minor Order the Qi Decoction) plus *Bao He Wan* (Preserve Harmony Pills): stir-fried Fructus Crataegi (*Shan Zha*), 9g, stir-fried Massa Medica Fermentata (*Shen Qu*), 6g, uncooked Pericarpium Citri Reticulatae (*Chen Pi*), 6g, Sclerotium Poriae Cocos (*Fu Ling*), 9g, Semen Raphani Sativi (*Lai Fu Zi*), 9g, Fructus Forsythiae Suspensae (*Lian Qiao*), 9g, clear Rhizoma Pinelliae Ternatae Fermentata (*Ban Xia*), 9g, uncooked Radix Et Rhizoma Rhei (*Da Huang*), 6-9g, uncooked Fructus Immaturus Citri Aurantii (*Zhi Shi*), 6g, and ginger mix-fried Cortex Magnoliae Officinalis (*Hou Po*), 6g.

4. Spleen kidney yang vacuity

Symptoms: Obesity which is more severe below the waist, poor appetite, abdominal distention after eating, fatigued spirit, weakness of the limbs, disliking movement, fear of cold, cold limbs, possible wheezing, short voidings of clear urine or frequent urination, urination of clear urine at night, low back pain, possible edema in the lower limbs with inhibited urination, loose stools, a pale, enlarged tongue with thin, white fur, and a deep, fine, weak, pulse

Therapeutic principles: Supplement the kidneys and invigorate yang, fortify the spleen and disperse swelling

Acupuncture & moxibustion:

Guan Yuan (CV 4)	Together, these points supplement the kidneys and
Ming Men (GV 4)	invigorate the yang to disperse swelling when
Shen Shu (Bl 23)	moxaed and supplemented.

Zu San Li (St 36)	Fortifies the spleen and dries dampness when needled with supplementing method.

Chinese medicinal formula: Modified *Shen Qi Wan* (Kidney Qi Pills)

Ingredients: Cooked Radix Rehmanniae (*Shu Di*), 18g, stir-fried Radix Dioscoreae Oppositae (*Shan Yao*), 9g, steamed Fructus Corni Officinalis (*Shan Zhu Yu*), 9g, Rhizoma Alismatis (*Ze Xie*), 12g, Sclerotium Poriae Cocos (*Fu Ling*), 12g, Cortex Radicis Moutan (*Dan Pi*), 6g, stir-fried Ramulus Cinnamomi Cassiae (*Gui Zhi*), 9g, bland Radix Lateralis Praeparatus Aconiti Carmichaeli (*Fu Zi*), 6g, uncooked Radix Astragali Membranacei (*Huang Qi*), 15g, uncooked Rhizoma Atractylodis Macrocephalae (*Bai Zhu*), 9g

Additions & subtractions: For reduced appetite, add Fructus Crataegi (*Shan Zha*), 9g. For edema in the lower limbs, add Radix Stephaniae Tetrandrae (*Han Fang Ji*), 9g. For nausea or abdominal distention after meals, add Folium Nelumbinis Nuciferae (*He Ye*), 9g. For liver depression, add Fasciculus Vascularis Citri Reticulatae (*Ju Luo*), 9g, and Pericarpium Citri Reticulatae Viride (*Qing Pi*), 6g.

Remarks: 1. In China obesity is not the social problem that it is in Europe and North America. Nevertheless, modern Chinese research has shown the efficacy of the following Chinese medicinals in treating obesity: Folium Sennae (*Fan Xie Ye*) for heat patterns with accompanying constipation; Rhizoma Alismatis (*Ze Xie*) for damp accumulation patterns; Rhizoma Atractylodis Macrocephalae (*Bai Zhu*) for spleen vacuity, phlegm, and dampness patterns; Fructus Crataegi (*Shan Zha*) for food stagnation patterns or obesity due to excessive intake of meat and oil; Radix Astragali Membranacei (*Huang Qi*) for qi vacuity patterns or obesity accompanied by edema; Radix Stephaniae Tetrandrae (*Han Fang Ji*) for obesity with inhibited urination or edema in the lower limbs; Folium Nelumbinis Nuciferae (*He Ye*) for spleen vacuity with damp accumulation patterns; Semen Cassiae Torae (*Jue Ming Zi*) for obesity with constipation in replete patterns; uncooked Radix Polygoni Multiflori (*He Shou Wu*) for obesity with constipation in vacuity patterns; Radix Et Rhizoma Rhei (*Da Huang*) for stomach heat and constipation patterns; Radix Et Rhizoma Polygoni Cuspidati (*Hu Zhang*) for damp heat patterns or obesity with constipation; Herba Artemisiae Capillaris (*Yin Chen Hao*) for damp heat or heat patterns; Radix Puerariae (*Ge Gen*) for obesity with heart disease; Fasciculus Vascularis Citri Reticulatae (*Ju Luo*) for obesity with liver depression; Herba Leonuri Heterophylli (*Yi Mu Cao*) and Radix Salviae Miltiorrhizae (*Dan Shen*) for obesity with blood stasis; and Pericarpium Citri Reticulatae Viride (*Qing Pi*) and Fructus Immaturus Citri Aurantii (*Zhi Shi*) for obesity with qi stagnation.

2. One can use the basic following formula with appropriate modifications when the diagnosis is difficult or the patient is a mix of several patterns: Folium Sennae (*Fan Xie Ye*), 1g (powdered and taken with the strained decoction), Rhizoma Alismatis (*Ze Xie*), 9g, uncooked Radix Astragali Membranacei (*Huang Qi*), 12g, uncooked Rhizoma Atractylodis Macrocephalae (*Bai Zhu*), 9g, Semen Raphani Sativi (*Lai Fu Zi*), 6g, Fructus Crataegi (*Shan Zha*), 6g, Folium Nelumbinis Nuciferae (*He Ye*), 12g, clear Rhizoma Pinelliae Ternatae (*Ban Xia*), 9g, and Pericarpium Citri Reticulatae (*Chen Pi*), 6g. For loose stools and severe spleen vacuity, subtract Senna. For stomach heat, subtract Atractylodes and add Radix Et Rhizoma Rhei (*Da Huang*), 1-3g (powdered and taken with the strained decoction). For severe kidney yang vacuity, subtract Senna and add stir-fried Ramulus Cinnamomi Cassiae (*Gui Zhi*), 9g. For liver depression, add Fasciculus Vascularis Citri Reticulatae (*Ju Luo*), 9g, and Pericarpium Citri Reticulatae Viride (*Qing Pi*), 9g. For a bitter taste in the mouth, add Herba Artemisiae Capillaris (*Yin Chen Hao*), 15g.

28
Emaciation *(Xiao Shou)*

This refers to wasting of the body and low body weight. However, body weight differs greatly from person to person. A person with spirit and low body weight accompanied by a moist, lustrous facial complexion and normal pulse with no other symptoms associated with emaciation is considered physiologically normal.

Disease causes, disease mechanisms:

1. Spleen-stomach vacuity

Dietary irregularities, excessive thinking, or constitutional insufficiency may all contribute to vacuity of the spleen and stomach. In Chinese medicine, it is said, "The spleen is the source of engenderment and transformation and the root of latter heaven," and, "The spleen governs the flesh." In addition, the stomach governs intake and decomposition, while the spleen governs the movement of stomach liquids. If, for any reason, the spleen and stomach are damaged and become vacuous, they may not transform the water and grain into essence, nor can they move the essence to nourish the flesh. As a result, emaciation occurs.

2. Qi & blood vacuity

Vacuity of the qi and blood usually develops from constitutional insufficiency, overwork taxation, malnourishment after disease, or enduring disease. The flesh receives its nourishment from the blood. As the commander of the blood, qi not only moves the blood but also promotes its engenderment. Therefore, if the qi and blood become vacuous and insufficient, the flesh may not receive sufficient nourishment or be filled up properly, thus leading to emaciation.

3. Kidney yang vacuity

Kidney yang vacuity may result from constitutional insufficiency, aging, enduring disease, excessive sexual activity, or from enduring or severe spleen yang vacuity reaching the kidneys. Kidney yang is known as the original yang and is the root of yang of the entire body. It is responsible for warming the whole body, including the sinews, muscles, and flesh.

Therefore, if there is kidney yang vacuity, vacuity cold may hinder the free flow of qi and blood. Thus the flesh may not receive sufficient nourishment, giving rise to emaciation. In addition, if kidney yang is vacuous, then essence will not be sufficiently transformed since qi (yang) engenders essence. Therefore the flesh will not be banked up, leading to emaciation.

4. Stomach heat exuberance

Stomach heat exuberance usually arises from excessive consumption of spicy, hot, fatty, sweet foods which transform heat. It may also be due to externally invading evils which transform into heat when entering the interior. Heat is a yang evil which can easily damage yin liquids. If exuberant stomach heat is severe and/or endures, it may excessively consume and damage liquids. If the liquids are damaged, the body will be deprived of its nourishment and moistening, thus giving rise to emaciation.

5. Yin vacuity with internal heat

Yin vacuity causing emaciation commonly results from enduring coughing, constitutional yin vacuity, excessive sexual activity, and overwork taxation. Yin's duty is to check yang. If, for any reason, yin becomes vacuous, yang may become hyperactive, giving rise to internal heat. Heat is a yang evil which may consume and damage yin. If internal heat continuously consumes already vacuous yin fluids, yin fluids will become even more vacuous. Therefore, doubly damaged yin will be even less able to control yang and hence give rise to even more effulgent yin vacuity fire. This then forms a pathological loop or cycle—heat damages yin giving rise to more heat which damages yin even more. Blood and fluids share the same source, and both are responsible for nourishing and moistening the flesh. If the above pathological chain reaction continues to deteriorate, yin fluids will become exhausted, and the flesh will not receive sufficient nourishment and moistening. Thus emaciation occurs.

6. Liver fire exuberance

Liver fire exuberance usually results from constitutional yin vacuity or emotional disease, such as anger, depression, and frustration. Fire is a yang evil which consumes yin. Therefore, if exuberant liver fire enduringly consumes and exhausts yin fluids, the flesh will be deprived of sufficient nourishment, thus giving rise to emaciation.

7. Worm accumulation

Worm accumulation mainly occurs in children who eat unclean foods. If worms accumulate in the abdomen, they may cause disharmony of the stomach qi, giving rise to non-transformation of the spleen and thus less nourishment to the flesh. And in addition, these worms will also consume part of the essence in the body, leaving the body even less nourishment. Therefore, worms may also lead to emaciation.

Treatment based on pattern discrimination:

I. Spleen stomach vacuity

Symptoms: Emaciation, poor appetite, abdominal distention after eating, fatigue and lack of strength, reduced qi with laziness to speak, a sallow yellow facial complexion, loose stools, a pale tongue with white fur, and a fine, weak pulse

Therapeutic principles: Fortify the spleen and boost the qi

Acupuncture & moxibustion:

Pi Shu (Bl 20)	Together, these points fortify the spleen and boost
Wei Shu (Bl 21)	the stomach when needled with supplementing
Zhong Wan (CV 12)	method.
Zu San Li (St 36)	Together, these points boost the qi and nourish the
San Yin Jiao (Sp 6)	blood when needled with supplementing method.

Additions & subtractions: For cold pain in the stomach and abdomen, flooding vomiting of clear water, and diarrhea with clear grains, moxa *Shang Wan* (CV 13) and *Gong Sun* (Sp 4). For stomachache, add *Liang Qiu* (St 34).

Chinese medicinal formula: *Si Jun Zi Tang* (Four Gentlemen Decoction)

Ingredients: Rice stir-fried Radix Codonopsitis Pilosulae (*Dang Shen*), 9g, bran stir-fried Rhizoma Atractylodis Macrocephalae (*Bai Zhu*), 9g, Sclerotium Poriae Cocos (*Fu Ling*), 9g, mix-fried Radix Glycyrrhizae (*Gan Cao*), 6g

Additions & subtractions: For loose stools or diarrhea, vomiting, and nausea, replace *Si Jun Zi Tang* with *Shen Ling Bai Zhu San* (Ginseng, Poria & Atractylodes Powder): stir-fried Semen Dolichoris Lablab (*Bai Bian Dou*), 9g, stir-fried Radix Dioscoreae Oppositae (*Shan Yao*), 9g, bran stir-fried Rhizoma Atractylodis Macrocephalae (*Bai Zhu*), 9g, Sclerotium Poriae Cocos (*Fu Ling*), 9g, rice stir-fried Radix Codonopsitis Pilosulae (*Dang Shen*), 9g, stir-fried till yellow Semen Nelumbinis Nuciferae (*Lian Zi*), 9g, Radix Platycodi Grandiflori (*Jie Geng*), 3g, Fructus Amomi (*Sha Ren*), 3g, and mix-fried Radix Glycyrrhizae (*Gan Cao*), 6g. For ptosis or prolapse or low-grade fever due to central qi fall, replace *Si Jun Zi Tang* with *Bu Zhong Yi Qi Tang* (Supplement the Center & Boost the Qi Decoction): honey mix-fried Radix Astragali Membranacei (*Huang Qi*), 15g, honey stir-fried Radix Codonopsitis Pilosulae (*Dang Shen*), 12g, bran stir-fried Rhizoma Atractylodis Macrocephalae (*Bai Zhu*), 12g, honey mix-fried Radix Glycyrrhizae (*Gan Cao*), 6g, stir-fried Radix Angelicae Sinensis (*Dang Gui*), 3g, stir-fried Pericarpium Citri Reticulatae (*Chen Pi*), 6g, Radix Bupleuri (*Chai Hu*), 3g, and Rhizoma Cimicifugae (*Sheng Ma*), 3g. For spleen qi vacuity and food stagnation with reduced appetite, difficult digestion, and abdominal fullness after a meal, replace *Si Jun Zi Tang* with *Ren Shen Jian Pi Wan* (Ginseng Fortify the Spleen Decoction): rice stir-fried Radix Codonopsitis Pilosulae (*Dang Shen*), 12g, stir-fried Radix Dioscoreae Oppositae (*Shan Yao*), 9g, stir-fried Pericarpium Citri Reticulatae (*Chen Pi*), 6g, stir-fried Fructus Germinatus Hordei Vulgaris (*Mai Ya*), 6g, stir-fried Massa Medica Fermentata (*Shen Qu*), 6g, and Fructus Immaturus Citri Aurantii (*Zhi Shi*), 3g. For the same pattern in children, replace *Si Jun Zi Tang* with equal doses of only Endothelium Corneum Gigeriae Galli (*Ji Nei Jin*), Rhizoma Atractylodis Macrocephalae (*Bai Zhu*), and Pericarpium Citri Reticulatae (*Chen Pi*). Powder and administer 1-9g three times per day.

2. Qi & blood vacuity

Symptoms: Emaciation, a sallow yellow, lusterless facial complexion, dizziness and vertigo, heart palpitations, insomnia, pale nails and lips, reduced qi with laziness to speak, dry skin, reduced appetite, a pale tongue with white fur, and a fine, weak pulse

Therapeutic principles: Supplement the qi and nourish the blood

Acupuncture & moxibustion:

Pi Shu (Bl 20) Together, these points nourish the blood when

Wei Shu (Bl 21)   needled with supplementing method.
Xin Shu (Bl 15)

Zu San Li (St 36)   Together, these points boost the qi when needled
Qi Hai (CV 6)   with supplementing method.

Additions & subtractions: For shortness of breath, add *Dan Zhong* (CV 17). For scanty menstruation with pale, thin blood, add *Xue Hai* (Sp 10). For tinnitus, add *Ting Gong* (SI 19). For spontaneous perspiration, add *Fei Shu* (Bl 13). For no thought of food, add *Zhong Wan* (CV 12).

Chinese medicinal formula: *Ren Shen Yang Rong Tang* (Ginseng Nourish the Constructive Decoction)

Ingredients: Rice stir-fried Radix Codonopsitis Pilosulae (*Dang Shen*), 12g, honey mix-fried Radix Astragali Membranacei (*Huang Qi*), 15g, uncooked Radix Albus Paeoniae Lactiflorae (*Bai Shao*), 9g, Radix Angelicae Sinensis (*Dang Gui*), 9g, stir-fried Pericarpium Citri Reticulatae (*Chen Pi*), 6g, Cortex Cinnamomi Cassiae (*Rou Gui*), 3g, bran stir-fried Rhizoma Atractylodis Macrocephalae (*Bai Zhu*), 9g, cooked Radix Rehmanniae (*Shu Di*), 9g, Fructus Schisandrae Chinensis (*Wu Wei Zi*), 9g, licorice-processed Radix Polygalae Tenuifoliae (*Yuan Zhi*), 3g, Sclerotium Poriae Cocos (*Fu Ling*), 9g, mix-fried Radix Glycyrrhizae (*Gan Cao*), 6g

Additions & subtractions: If there are no dizziness, heart palpitations, or insomnia, replace *Ren Shen Yang Rong Tang* with *Ba Zhen Tang* (Eight Pearls Decoction): cooked Radix Rehmanniae (*Shu Di*), 12g, Radix Albus Paeoniae Lactiflorae (*Bai Shao*), 9g, wine mix-fried Radix Angelicae Sinensis (*Dang Gui*), 9g, wine mix-fried Radix Ligustici Wallichii (*Chuan Xiong*), 6g, Radix Codonopsitis Pilosulae (*Dang Shen*), 9g, bran stir-fried Rhizoma Atractylodis Macrocephalae (*Bai Zhu*), 9g, Sclerotium Poriae Cocos (*Fu Ling*), 9g, and mix-fried Radix Glycyrrhizae (*Gan Cao*), 6g. For a cold feeling in the hands and feet, add Ramulus Cinnamomi Cassiae (*Gui Zhi*), 6g, and Herba Asari Cum Radice (*Xi Xin*), 3g. For blood stasis with a purple tongue and slight cyanosis of fingers and lips, add wine mix-fried Radix Salviae Miltiorrhizae (*Dan Shen*), 9g, and Flos Carthami Tinctorii (*Hong Hua*), 6g. For only blood vacuity without qi vacuity, replace *Ren Shen Yang Rong Tang* with *Si Wu Tang* (Four Materials Decoction): cooked Radix Rehmanniae (*Shu Di*), 12g, Radix Angelicae Sinensis (*Dang Gui*), 9g, Radix Albus Paeoniae Lactiflorae (*Bai Shao*), 9g, and uncooked Radix Ligustici Wallichii (*Chuan Xiong*), 6g.

3. Kidney yang vacuity

Symptoms: Emaciation, a soot-black or white facial complexion, cold feet, edema in the lower limbs or feet, tinnitus, dizziness, low back, feet, and knee aching and limpness, inhibited urination or frequent, clear urination, loose stools, fear of cold, fatigued spirit, impotence, seminal emission, a pale tongue, and a weak pulse in the cubit position

Therapeutic principles: Warm and supplement kidney yang

Acupuncture & moxibustion:

Ming Men (GV 4) *Guan Yuan* (CV 4) *Shen Shu* (Bl 23)	Together, these points warm and supplement kidney yang when needled with moxibustion on the heads of the needles or when directly moxaed.
Pi Shu (Bl 20) *Zu San Li* (St 36)	Together, these points boost the latter heaven to supplement the kidneys when needled with moxibustion on the heads of the needles.

Additions & subtractions: For daybreak diarrhea, moxa *Shen Que* (CV 8). For pain in the periumbilical region, moxa *Shen Que* (CV 8). For puffy edema, add *Shui Fen* (CV 9). For clear, thin vaginal discharge, add *San Yin Jiao* (Sp 6).

Chinese medicinal formula: *Shi Bu Wan* (Ten Supplementing Pills)

Ingredients: Bland Radix Lateralis Praeparatus Aconiti Carmichaeli (*Fu Zi*), 6g, Cortex Cinnamomi Cassiae (*Rou Gui*), 2g, wine-steamed Fructus Schisandrae Chinensis (*Wu Wei Zi*), 9g, Cornu Parvum Cervi (*Lu Rong*), 1g (powdered and taken with the strained decoction), cooked Radix Rehmanniae (*Shu Di*), 15g, steamed Fructus Corni Officinalis (*Shan Zhu Yu*), 9g, stir-fried Radix Dioscoreae Oppositae (*Shan Yao*), 9g, Sclerotium Poriae Cocos (*Fu Ling*), 6g, Cortex Radicis Moutan (*Dan Pi*), 6g, and salt mix-fried Rhizoma Alismatis (*Ze Xie*), 6g

Additions & subtractions: For kidney yang vacuity with essence insufficiency, replace *Shi Bu Wan* with *Gui Lu Er Xian Jiao* (Deer & Turtle Two Immortals Gelatin): Gelatinum Cornu Cervi (*Lu Jiao Jiao*), 9g, Gelatinum Plastri Testudinis (*Gui Ban Jiao*), 6g, Fructus Lycii Chinensis (*Gou Qi Zi*), 9g, and Radix Panacis Ginseng (*Ren Shen*), 6g. For periumbilical pain and borborygmus at dawn followed by defecation, replace *Shi Bu Wan* with *Si Shen Wan* (Four Spirits Pills): Semen Myristicae Fragrantis (*Rou Dou*

Kou), 6g, salt mix-fried Fructus Psoraleae Corylifoliae (*Bu Gu Zhi*), 12g, vinegar-steamed Fructus Schisandrae Chinensis (*Wu Wei Zi*), 6g, and processed Fructus Evodiae Rutecarpae (*Wu Zhu Yu*), 5g. For watery stools, add Semen Plantaginis (*Che Qian Zi*), 12g, and Sclerotium Poriae Cocos (*Fu Ling*), 9g. For poor appetite, add Fructus Amomi (*Sha Ren*), 3g, and stir-fried Pericarpium Citri Reticulatae (*Chen Pi*), 9g. For drowsiness after eating, add Rhizoma Acori Graminei (*Shi Chang Pu*), 9g. For untransformed food in the stools, add stir-fried Fructus Germinatus Hordei Vulgaris (*Mai Ya*), 9g, and stir-fried Fructus Crataegi (*Shan Zha*), 9g. For low back and knee soreness and weakness, add Radix Morindae Officinalis (*Ba Ji Tian*), 9g, and Rhizoma Cibotii Barometsis (*Gou Ji*), 9g. For impotence, add Rhizoma Curculiginis Orchioidis (*Xian Mao*), 9g, and Herba Epimedii (*Yin Yang Huo*), 9g. For frequent urination at night and/or dribbling urination, add salt mix-fried Fructus Alpiniae Oxyphyllae (*Yi Zhi Ren*), 9g, and Fructus Rubi Chingii (*Fu Pen Zi*), 9g. For kidney and spleen yang vacuity, add *Li Zhong Tang* (Aconite Rectify the Center Decoction): rice stir-fried Radix Codonopsitis Pilosulae (*Dang Shen*), 9g, dry Rhizoma Zingiberis (*Gan Jiang*), 6g, earth stir-fried Rhizoma Atractylodis Macrocephalae (*Bai Zhu*), 9g, and honey mix-fried Radix Glycyrrhizae (*Gan Cao*), 6g.

4. Stomach heat exuberance

Symptoms: Emaciation, thirst with a liking for chilled drinks, profuse intake and swift hungering, possible vomiting immediately after intake, heart vexation, bad breath, short voidings of dark-colored urine, dry stools, a red tongue with reduced liquid and yellow fur, and a slippery, rapid pulse

Therapeutic principles: Clear the stomach and drain fire

Acupuncture & moxibustion:

Zhong Wan (CV 12) *Zu San Li* (St 36)	Together, these points boost the stomach and harmonize the center when needled with even draining and supplementing method.
Li Dui (St 45) *Nei Ting* (St 44)	Together, these points clear the stomach and drain fire when needled with draining method.

Additions & subtractions: For toothache, add *He Gu* (LI 4). For burning pain in the stomach, add *Tai Xi* (Ki 3). For constipation, add *Tian Shu* (St 25) and *Shang Ju Xu* (St 37).

Chinese medicinal formula: Modified *Qing Wei San* (Clear the Stomach Powder)

Ingredients: Uncooked Gypsum Fibrosum (*Shi Gao*), 12g, uncooked Radix Scutellariae Baicalensis (*Huang Qin*), 9g, uncooked Rhizoma Coptidis Chinensis (*Huang Lian*), 3g, uncooked Radix Rehmanniae (*Sheng Di*), 9g, Cortex Radicis Moutan (*Dan Pi*), 9g, uncooked Rhizoma Cimicifugae (*Sheng Ma*), 3g, Fructus Forsythiae Suspensae (*Lian Qiao*), 6g, Rhizoma Anemarrhenae Asphodeloidis (*Zhi Mu*), 6g, Radix Glycyrrhizae (*Gan Cao*), 3g

Additions & subtractions: For severe stomach heat, add Fructus Gardeniae Jasminoidis (*Zhi Zi*), 6-9g. For stabbing pain in the stomach, add Radix Salviae Miltiorrhizae (*Dan Shen*), 9g, and Radix Rubrus Paeoniae Lactiflorae (*Chi Shao*), 9g. For acid regurgitation, add Os Sepiae Seu Sepiellae (*Hai Piao Xiao*), 9g, and Concha Arcae Inflatae (*Wa Leng Zi*), 9g. For severe thirst, add Rhizoma Phragmitis Communis (*Lu Gen*), 9g, and Radix Trichosanthis Kirlowii (*Tian Hua Fen*), 9g. For severe constipation, add uncooked Radix Et Rhizoma Rhei (*Da Huang*), 9g. For nausea, add ginger mix-fried Caulis Bambusae In Taeniis (*Zhu Ru*), 9g. For scanty urination, add Semen Plantaginis (*Che Qian Zi*), 9g, and Sclerotium Polypori Umbellati (*Zhu Ling*), 9g. For toothache, add Radix Rubrus Paeoniae Lactiflorae (*Chi Shao*), 9g, Herba Taraxaci Mongolici Cum Radice (*Pu Gong Ying*), 12g, and Radix Seu Rhizoma Cynanchi (*Xu Chang Qing*), 9g. For concomitant kidney yin vacuity, replace *Qing Wei San* with Modified *Yu Nu Jian* (Jade Maiden Decoction): uncooked Gypsum Fibrosum (*Shi Gao*), 18g, cooked Radix Rehmanniae (*Shu Di*), 15g, salt mix-fried Rhizoma Anemarrhenae Asphodeloidis (*Zhi Mu*), 9g, salt stir-fried Radix Achyranthis Bidentatae (*Niu Xi*), 9g, and Tuber Ophiopogonis Japonici (*Mai Men Dong*), 9g.

5. Yin vacuity with internal heat

Symptoms: Emaciation, dry mouth and throat, vexatious heat in the five hearts, tidal fever, night sweats, afternoon red cheekbones, a red tongue with reduced liquid, and a fine, rapid pulse

Therapeutic principles: Nourish yin and clear heat

Acupuncture & moxibustion:

Pi Shu (Bl 20)	Together, these points fortify the spleen and
Wei Shu (Bl 21)	stomach to engender the qi and blood when
Zu San Li (St 36)	needled with supplementing method.

Tai Xi (Ki 3)   Together, these points nourish yin and clear heat
San Yin Jiao (Sp 6)   when needled with supplementing method.

Additions & subtractions: For insomnia, add *Xin Shu* (Bl 15). For dizziness, add *Bai Hui* (GV 20). For profuse drinking and thirst, add *Nei Ting* (St 44). For seminal emission, add *Zhi Shi* (Bl 52). For sore throat, add *Zhao Hai* (Ki 6). For chest pain, add *Fei Shu* (Bl 13). For spontaneous perspiration, add *Yin Xi* (Ht 6).

Chinese medicinal formulas: For yin vacuity due to heat disease: *Qing Gu San* (Clear the Bones Powder)

Ingredients: Radix Stellariae Dichotomae (*Yin Chai Hu*), 12g, Rhizoma Picrorrhizae (*Hu Huang Lian*), 9g, Carapax Amydae Sinensis (*Bie Jia*), 9g, Herba Artemisiae Apiacae (*Qing Hao*), 9g, Radix Gentianae Macrophyllae (*Qin Jiao*), 12g, Cortex Radicis Lycii Chinensis (*Di Gu Pi*), 9g, uncooked Rhizoma Anemarrhenae Asphodeloidis (*Zhi Mu*), 9g, Radix Glycyrrhizae (*Gan Cao*), 6g

For lung yin vacuity: *Bai He Gu Jin Tang* (Lily Secure Metal Decoction)

Ingredients: Bulbus Lilii (*Bai He*), 9g, uncooked Radix Rehmanniae (*Sheng Di*), 6g, Tuber Ophiopogonis Japonici (*Mai Dong*), 6g, cooked Radix Rehmanniae (*Shu Di*), 9g, Bulbus Fritillariae Cirrhosae (*Chuan Bei Mu*), 6g, Radix Scrophulariae Ningpoensis (*Xuan Shen*), 6g, Radix Angelicae Sinensis (*Dang Gui*), 6g, Radix Platycodi Grandiflori (*Jie Geng*), 6g, Radix Albus Paeoniae Lactiflorae (*Bai Shao*), 9g, Radix Glycyrrhizae (*Gan Cao*), 6g

For stomach yin vacuity: Modified *Yi Wei Tang* (Boost the Stomach Decoction)

Ingredients: Tuber Ophiopogonis Japonici (*Mai Men Dong*), 9g, Radix Adenophorae Strictae (*Nan Sha Shen*), 9g, Rhizoma Polygonati Odorati (*Yu Zhu*), 9g, uncooked Radix Rehmanniae (*Sheng Di*), 12g, Radix Albus Paeoniae Lactiflorae (*Bai Shao*), 9g, mix-fried Radix Glycyrrhizae (*Gan Cao*), 9g

For kidney yin vacuity: *Zhi Bai Di Huang Wan* (Anemarrhena & Phellodendron Rehmannia Pills)

Ingredients: Cooked Radix Rehmanniae (*Shu Di*), 18g, steamed Fructus Corni Officinalis (*Shan Zhu Yu*), 9g, stir-fried Radix Dioscoreae Oppositae (*Shan Yao*), 9g, Sclerotium Poriae Cocos (*Fu Ling*), 6g, Cortex Radicis Moutan (*Dan Pi*), 9g, salt mix-fried Rhizoma Alismatis (*Ze Xie*), 6g, salt mix-fried Rhizoma Anemarrhenae Asphodeloidis (*Zhi Mu*), 12g, salt mix-fried Cortex Phellodendri (*Huang Bai*), 12g

For kidney yin vacuity and stomach dryness with wasting thirst, emaciation, dry throat and mouth, frequent, profuse urination, profuse intake and swift hungering, fatigue, shortness of breath, and a fine, forceless pulse: *Yu Ye Tang* (Jade Fluids Decoction)

Ingredients: Uncooked Radix Dioscoreae Oppositae (*Shan Yao*), 30g, uncooked Astragali Membranacei (*Huang Qi*), 15g, uncooked Rhizoma Anemarrhenae Asphodeloidis (*Zhi Mu*), 15g, Endothelium Corneum Gigeriae Galli (*Ji Nei Jin*), 6g, uncooked Radix Puerariae (*Ge Gen*), 6g, uncooked Fructus Schisandrae Chinensis (*Wu Wei Zi*), 9g, Radix Trichosanthis Kirlowii (*Tian Hua Fen*), 9g

6. Liver fire exuberance

Symptoms: Emaciation, vexation and agitation, irascibility, dizziness and vertigo, burning pain in the rib-side, red eyes, a bitter taste in the mouth, short voidings of dark-colored urine, constipation with dry stools, a red tongue with yellow fur, and a bowstring, rapid pulse

Therapeutic principles: Clear the liver and drain fire

Acupuncture & moxibustion:

Pi Shu (Bl 20) *Wei Shu* (Bl 21) *Gan Shu* (Bl 18)	Together, these points regulate the liver and harmonize the center when needled with even draining and supplementing method.
Xing Jian (Liv 2) *Xia Xi* (GB 43)	Together, these points clear the liver and drain fire when needled with draining method.

Additions & subtractions: For profuse dreams, add *Hun Men* (Bl 47). For distention and pain in the head, add *Shuai Gu* (GB 8). For tinnitus, add *Ting Hui* (GB 2). For acid regurgitation, add *Shang Wan* (CV 13). For nosebleeding, add *Shang Xing* (GV 23).

Chinese medicinal formula: Modified *Long Dan Xie Gan Tang* (Gentiana Drain the Liver Decoction)

Ingredients: Radix Gentianae Scabrae (*Long Dan Cao*), 6g, Fructus Gardeniae Jasminoidis (*Zhi Zi*), 9g, Radix Scutellariae Baicalensis (*Huang Qin*), 9g, Radix Bupleuri (*Chai Hu*), 6g, Caulis Akebiae (*Mu Tong*), 5g, uncooked Radix Rehmanniae (*Sheng Di*), 9g, Radix Angelicae Sinensis (*Dang Gui*), 6g, Semen Plantaginis (*Che Qian Zi*), 6g, Radix Glycyrrhizae (*Gan Cao*), 6g, uncooked Radix Et Rhizoma Rhei (*Da Huang*), 6g

Additions & subtractions: Without constipation, subtract Rhubarb. For mild liver fire due to liver depression replace *Long Dan Xie Gan Tang* with Modified *Chai Hu Shu Gan San* (Bupleurum Soothe the Liver Powder): Radix Bupleuri (*Chai Hu*), 9g, Radix Albus Paeoniae Lactiflorae (*Bai Shao*), 9g, Fructus Citri Aurantii (*Zhi Ke*), 6g, Pericarpium Citri Reticulatae (*Chen Pi*), 6g, Radix Ligustici Wallichii (*Chuan Xiong*), 6g, Rhizoma Cyperi Rotundi (*Xiang Fu*), 9g, Radix Glycyrrhizae (*Gan Cao*), 6g, and Radix Scutellariae Baicalensis (*Huang Qin*), 6g. For weak constitution or concomitant spleen vacuity, replace *Long Dan Xie Gan Tang* with Modified *Dan Zhi Xiao Yao San* (Moutan & Gardenia Rambling Powder): Radix Angelicae Sinensis (*Dang Gui*), 6g, Radix Albus Paeoniae Lactiflorae (*Bai Shao*), 9g, Rhizoma Atractylodis Macrocephalae (*Bai Zhu*), 9g, Radix Bupleuri (*Chai Hu*), 6g, Sclerotium Poriae Cocos (*Fu Ling*), 9g, mix-fried Radix Glycyrrhizae (*Gan Cao*), 6g, Herba Menthae Haplocalycis (*Bo He*), 3g, Cortex Radicis Moutan (*Dan Pi*), 9g, Fructus Gardeniae Jasminoidis (*Zhi Zi*), 9g, and Radix Scutellariae Baicalensis (*Huang Qin*), 6g. For severe rib-side pain, add stir-fried till scorched Fructus Meliae Toosendan (*Chuan Lian Zi*), 9g, and Rhizoma Corydalis Yanhusuo (*Yan Hu Suo*), 12g.

7. Worm accumulation

Symptoms: Emaciation, a sallow yellow facial complexion, clamoring stomach, periumbilical pain which occurs intermittently, stomach and abdominal fullness, poor appetite, a predilection for strange foods, bad breath, loose stools, a pale tongue with white fur, and a weak, forceless pulse

Therapeutic principles: Quiet and expel worms

Acupuncture & moxibustion:

Zhong Wan (CV 12)	Together, these points move the spleen and
Da Heng (Sp 15)	harmonize the stomach when needled with draining method.

Zu San Li (St 36)
Gong Sun (Sp 4)
Nei Guan (Per 6)

Together, these points loosen the center, downbear the qi, and quiet worms when needled with draining method.

Bai Chong Wo (M-LE-3)

A special point for expelling worms; needle with draining method.

Additions & subtractions: For fever and heart vexation, add *Qu Chi* (LI 11). For severe abdominal pain, add *Yang Ling Quan* (GB 34) and *Dan Nang Xue* (M-LE-6).

Chinese medicinal formula: *Fei Er Wan* (Fat Children Pills)

Ingredients: Stir-fried Massa Medica Fermentata (*Shen Qu*), 100g, Rhizoma Coptidis Chinensis (*Huang Lian*), 100g, stir-fried Semen Arecae Catechu (*Bing Lang*), 40g, Semen Myristicae Fragrantis (*Rou Dou Kou*), 50g, Fructus Quisqualis Indicae (*Shi Jun Zi*), 50g, stir-fried Fructus Germinatus Hordei Vulgaris (*Mai Ya*), 50g, Radix Auklandiae Lappae (*Mu Xiang*), 20g

Remarks: Powder the above medicinals and make into small pills with ginger juice. Take 1-3g of these pills three times per day on an empty stomach. However, before taking this prescription, it is useful to kill the majority of the intestinal worms by taking the ready-made medicine *Hua Chong Wan* (Transform Worms Pills) or its equivalent. *Wu Mei Wan* (Mume Pills) is not effective for killing worms.

29
Fatigue *(Pi Fa)*

This refers to a subjective symptom wherein the patient has fatigued spirit and sluggish limbs. It occurs in many kinds of enduring diseases.

Disease causes, disease mechanisms:

Fatigue is the single most important symptom of qi vacuity. Qi is responsible for movement and yang is responsible for activity (literally "stirring"), while yin and blood are responsible for nourishment. Most fatigue is due to qi and yang vacuity which may be combined with yin and blood insufficiency. It is important to understand that yin and blood vacuities alone do not cause fatigue. Fatigue, as both a disease in its own right and as a symptom, belongs to qi.

1. Qi and/or yang vacuity

Overwork taxation, overthinking, severe disease, enduring disease, dietary irregularities, aging, excessive consumption of cold medicinals, or any other cause which consumes yang qi can contribute to vacuity of the qi and/or yang of the heart, spleen, lungs, or kidneys. Yang qi is responsible for activity, movement, and warming. If, for any reason, the yang qi becomes vacuous, the functions of the viscera and bowels lessen and the spirit and form (*i.e.,* the body) are not supported. This then leads to fatigue.

2. Spleen vacuity & damp encumbrance or damp phlegm

Overwork taxation, dietary irregularities, and/or excessive consumption of cold medicinals may all damage the spleen and make it vacuous. The spleen is responsible for the movement and transformation of water dampness. If the spleen becomes vacuous, it will not perform these responsibilities efficiently. As a result, water dampness will accumulate in the body. Water dampness is a yin evil and is heavy and turbid in nature. Therefore, accumulated water dampness will encumber the body and lead to bodily heaviness. In addition, water dampness may affect the upbearing of yang, giving rise to fatigued spirit. If dampness endures, it will tend to congeal into phlegm. Because phlegm is also a turbid yin evil, once it is formed, it tends to obstruct the free flow of the qi and blood. Thus, the qi and blood cannot fill the spirit and the body. Fatigue will occur in both of these two situations.

3. Qi & blood dual vacuity

Dual vacuity of the qi and blood usually arises from constitutional insufficiency, malnourishment after disease, profuse sweating, or loss of blood or liquids. Qi's duty is to support the spirit, while the blood's responsibility is to nourish the body and limbs. If the qi and blood both become vacuous and insufficient, the spirit will not be supported efficiently and the body will not be nourished properly. Therefore, fatigue will occur.

4. Summerheat damaging the qi

This disease mechanism usually occurs in summer when summerheat evils are exuberant. "Summerheat is a yang evil and is effusing by nature." If summerheat evils invade the body, they may force body fluids out. Thus profuse sweating may occur. However, all sweating results in a loss of yang qi. As it is said in Chinese medicine, "Qi deserts when fluids desert." Because summerheat evils may result in sweating and, therefore, a loss of yang qi, fatigue may be the result of invasion by summerheat.

5. Lung dryness & qi vacuity

Contraction of wind warm evils or dryness can burn and damage the lungs. Wind, warmth, and dryness all are yang evils. Yang evils damage the body fluids, and, "Strong heat eats qi." If the invading evils damage body fluids and excessively consume the qi, the lungs will become dry and qi will become vacuous. If qi is vacuous, there will be fatigue.

Treatment based on pattern discrimination:

1. Spleen qi vacuity

Symptoms: Fatigue, lassitude of the spirit, weakness of the limbs, emaciation, a sallow yellow facial complexion, reduced appetite, loose stools or forceless defecation, stomach and abdominal fullness after eating, possible enduring low-grade fever, possible bleeding, a pale tongue with teeth-marks on its edges and white fur, and a fine, weak pulse

Therapeutic principles: Fortify the spleen and boost the qi

Acupuncture & moxibustion:

Zu San Li (St 36)   Together, these points fortify the spleen and boost
Pi Shu (Bl 20)   the qi when needled with supplementing method.
Wei Shu (Bl 21)
Tai Bai (Sp 3)

Additions & subtractions: For bleeding, add *San Yin Jiao* (Sp 6). For damp accumulation, add *Yin Ling Quan* (Sp 9). For central qi fall, add *Qi Hai* (CV 6), and *Bai Hui* (GV 20).

Chinese medicinal formulas: General pattern: *Si Jun Zi Tang* (Four Gentlemen Decoction)

Ingredients: Radix Panacis Ginseng (*Ren Shen*), 6g, bran stir-fried Atractylodis Macrocephalae (*Bai Zhu*), 9g, Sclerotium Poriae Cocos (*Fu Ling*), 9g, mix-fried Radix Glycyrrhizae (*Gan Cao*), 6g

Spleen vacuity with damp accumulation and diarrhea, loose stools, nausea, and vomiting: *Shen Ling Bai Zhu San* (Ginseng, Poria & Atractylodes Powder)

Ingredients: Radix Panacis Ginseng (*Ren Shen*), 6g, Sclerotium Poriae Cocos (*Fu Ling*), 9g, stir-fried Rhizoma Atractylodis Macrocephalae (*Bai Zhu*), 12g, stir-fried Radix Dioscoreae Oppositae (*Shan Yao*), 9g, stir-fried Semen Coicis Lachryma-jobi (*Yi Yi Ren*), 12g, stir-fried Semen Dolichoris Lablab (*Bai Bian Dou*), 9g, stir-fried Semen Nelumbinis Nuciferae (*Lian Zi*), 9g, Fructus Amomi (*Sha Ren*), 3g, Radix Platycodi Grandiflori (*Jie Geng*), 3g, mix-fried Radix Glycyrrhizae (*Gan Cao*), 3g

For low-grade fever or prolapse due to central qi fall: *Bu Zhong Yi Qi Tang* (Supplement the Center & Boost the Qi Decoction)

Ingredients: Honey mix-fried Radix Astragali Membranacei (*Huang Qi*), 18g, honey stir-fried Radix Codonopsis Pilosulae (*Dang Shen*), 12g, bran stir-fried Rhizoma Atractylodis Macrocephalae (*Bai Zhu*), 9g, stir-fried Radix Angelicae Sinensis (*Dang Gui*), 3g, stir-fried Pericarpium Citri Reticulatae (*Chen Pi*), 6g, Radix Bupleuri (*Chai Hu*), 3g, Rhizoma Cimicifugae (*Sheng Ma*), 3g, honey mix-fried Radix Glycyrrhizae (*Zhi Gan Cao*), 6g

For qi failing to contain the blood resulting in hemorrhagic disorders: *Gui Pi Tang* (Return the Spleen Decoction)

Ingredients: Honey mix-fried Radix Astragali Membranacei (*Huang Qi*), 15g, stir-fried Radix Codonopsitis Pilosulae (*Dang Shen*), 9g, bran stir-fried Rhizoma Atractylodis Macrocephalae (*Bai Zhu*), 9g, stir-fried Radix Angelicae Sinensis (*Dang Gui*), 9g, Arillus Euphorbiae Longanae (*Long Yan Rou*), 6g, licorice-processed Radix Polygalae Tenuifoliae (*Yuan Zhi*), 3g, stir-fried Semen Zizyphi Spinosae (*Suan Zao Ren*), 9g, Sclerotium Poriae Cocos (*Fu Ling*), 9g, mix-fried Radix Glycyrrhizae (*Gan Cao*), 3g, Radix Auklandiae Lappae (*Mu Xiang*), 3g

For enduring food stagnation due to spleen qi vacuity: *Zhi Zhu Wan* (Citrus & Atractylodes Pills)

Ingredients: Fructus Immaturus Citri Aurantii (*Zhi Shi*), 15g, and Rhizoma Atractylodis Macrocephalae (*Bai Zhu*), 30g

2. Spleen yang vacuity

Symptoms: Fatigue, lassitude of the spirit, enduring dull pain in the stomach and abdomen which likes pressure and warmth, borborygmus, reduced food intake, a bland taste in the mouth, loose stools or diarrhea, long voidings of clear urine, cold body, fear of cold, cold hands and feet, a pale tongue, and a fine, weak, forceless or deep, slow pulse

Therapeutic principles: Warm the center and scatter cold, fortify the spleen and boost the qi

Acupuncture & moxibustion:

Guan Yuan (CV 4)	Together, these points warm the center and scatter
Zu San Li (St 36)	cold, fortify the spleen, and boost the qi when
Pi Shu (Bl 20)	moxaed and needled with supplementing method.
Wei Shu (Bl 21)	

Chinese medicinal formula: *Fu Gui Li Zhong Tang* (Aconite & Cinnamon Rectify the Center Decoction)

Ingredients: Rice stir-fried Radix Codonopsitis Pilosulae (*Dang Shen*), 9g, bland Radix Lateralis Praeparatus Aconiti Carmichaeli (*Fu Zi*), 6g, Cortex Cinnamomi Cassiae (*Rou Gui*), 2g, dry Rhizoma Zingiberis (*Gan Jiang*), 6g, bran stir-fried Rhizoma Atractylodis Macrocephalae (*Bai Zhu*), 12g, mix-fried Radix Glycyrrhizae (*Gan Cao*), 6g

Additions & subtractions: For severe fatigue, add honey stir-fried Radix Astragali Membranacei (*Huang Qi*), 15g. For drowsiness after eating, add Rhizoma Acori Graminei (*Shi Chang Pu*), 9g. For severe yang vacuity of the spleen and stomach, add Fructus Evodiae Rutecarpae (*Wu Zhu Yu*), 3g. For vomiting, add uncooked Rhizoma Zingiberis (*Sheng Jiang*), 9g. For stomach distention, add Radix Auklandiae Lappae (*Mu Xiang*), 9g, and stir-fried Pericarpium Citri Reticulatae (*Chen Pi*), 9g. For severe poor appetite, add Fructus Amomi (*Sha Ren*), 3g, and stir-fried Pericarpium Citri Reticulatae (*Chen Pi*), 9g. For untransformed food in the stools, add stir-fried Fructus Germinatus Hordei Vulgaris (*Mai Ya*), 9g, and stir-fried Fructus Crataegi (*Shan Zha*), 9g. For spleen yang vacuity with damp encumbrance manifest by sliminess in the mouth, fullness and oppression in the stomach and abdomen, diarrhea, heavy-headedness, etc., replace *Fu Gui Li Zhong Tang* with Modified *Dao Gong San* (Abduct the Result Powder): rice stir-fried Radix Codonopsitis Pilosulae (*Dang Shen*), 9g, Sclerotium Poriae Cocos (*Fu Ling*), 9g, mix-fried Radix Glycyrrhizae (*Gan Cao*), 6g, bran stir-fried Rhizoma Atractylodis Macrocephalae (*Bai Zhu*), 9g, stir-fried Pericarpium Citri Reticulatae (*Chen Pi*), 9g, Semen Coicis Lachryma-jobi (*Yi Yi Ren*), 20g, Rhizoma Atractylodis (*Cang Zhu*), 6g, stir-fried Semen Dolichori Lablab (*Bai Bian Dou*), 12g, dry Rhizoma Zingiberis (*Gan Jiang*), 9g. For periumbilical pain and borborygmus at dawn followed by defecation, add salt mix-fried Fructus Psoraleae Corylifoliae (*Bu Gu Zhi*), 9g, and Semen Myristicae Fragrantis (*Rou Dou Kou*), 6g. For diarrhea with bloody stools due to spleen yang vacuity, replace *Fu Gui Li Zhong Tang* with Modified *Huang Tu Tang* (Yellow Earth Decoction): Terra Falva Ustae (*Fu Long Gan*), 15g, earth stir-fried Rhizoma Atractylodis Macrocephalae (*Bai Zhu*), 9g, blast-fried Radix Lateralis Praeparatus Aconiti Carmichaeli (*Fu Zi*), 6g, Gelatinum Corii Asini (*E Jiao*), 9g, blast-fried Rhizoma Zingiberis (*Pao Jiang*), 9g, and Radix Pseudoginseng (*San Qi*), 3g (powdered and taken with the strained decoction).

3. Spleen vacuity & damp encumbrance

Symptoms: Fatigue, bodily heaviness, lack of strength, chest and stomach fullness and oppression, vomiting, heavy-headedness, somnolence, sliminess in the mouth, reduced food intake, loose stools, a pale tongue with thick, white, slimy fur, and a soggy, weak pulse

Therapeutic principles: Fortify the spleen and transform dampness

Acupuncture & moxibustion:

Zu San Li (St 36)   Together, these points fortify the spleen when
Pi Shu (Bl 20)   needled with supplementing method.
Wei Shu (Bl 21)

Yin Ling Quan (Sp 9)   Together, these points move the spleen and trans-
San Yin Jiao (Sp 6)   form dampness when needled with even draining
                           and supplementing method.

Additions & subtractions: For a bitter taste in the mouth and a dry tongue, add *Yang Ling Quan* (GB 34). For reduced urination, add *Zhong Ji* (CV 3).

Chinese medicinal formula: *Xiang Sha Ping Wei San* (Auklandia & Cardamon Level [*i.e.*, Calm] the Stomach Powder)

Ingredients: Radix Auklandiae Lappae (*Mu Xiang*), 6g, Fructus Amomi (*Sha Ren*), 6g, bran stir-fried Rhizoma Atractylodis (*Cang Zhu*), 12g, ginger mix-fried Cortex Magnoliae Officinalis (*Hou Po*), 6g, stir-fried Pericarpium Citri Reticulatae (*Chen Pi*), 6g, Radix Glycyrrhizae (*Gan Cao*), 3g, bran stir-fried Rhizoma Atractylodis Macrocephalae (*Bai Zhu*), 9g, rice stir-fried Radix Codonopsitis Pilosulae (*Dang Shen*), 9g

Additions & subtractions: For severe fatigue, add Rhizoma Acori Graminei (*Shi Chang Pu*), 9g. For a bland taste in the mouth, add Herba Agastachis Seu Pogostemi (*Huo Xiang*), 9g, and Herba Eupatorii Fortunei (*Pei Lan*), 9g. For cold damp transforming into heat, add Rhizoma Coptidis Chinensis (*Huang Lian*), 6g, and Radix Scutellariae Baicalensis (*Huang Qin*), 6g. For fear of cold and cold limbs, add dry Rhizoma Zingiberis (*Gan Jiang*), 6g, and Semen Alpiniae Katsumadai (*Cao Dou Kou*), 6g. For nausea or vomiting, add uncooked Rhizoma Zingiberis (*Sheng Jiang*), 6g, and ginger-processed Rhizoma Pinelliae Ternatae (*Ban Xia*), 9g. For abdominal distention, add Pericarpium Arecae Catechu (*Da Fu Pi*), 9g, and Fructus Citri Aurantii (*Zhi Ke*), 9g. For diarrhea, add Semen Dolichoris Lablab (*Bai Bian Dou*), 9g, and Semen Alpiniae Katsumadai (*Cao Dou Kou*), 6g. For short voidings of urine, add Rhizoma Alismatis (*Ze Xie*), 9g, and Sclerotium Poriae Cocos (*Fu Ling*), 9g.

4. Spleen vacuity & damp phlegm

Symptoms: Fatigue, lassitude of the spirit, weakness of the limbs, somnolence, dizziness, heart palpitations, chest oppression, an often obese body, nausea, stomach fullness, possible vomiting of phlegm drool, possible mucous in the stools, possible coughing of phlegm, glossy, moist or slimy, white tongue fur, and a bowstring, slippery pulse

Therapeutic principles: Fortify the spleen and rectify the qi, dry dampness and transform phlegm

Acupuncture & moxibustion:

Yin Ling Quan (Sp 9) *Feng Long* (St 40) *Zhong Wan* (CV 12)	Together, these points dry dampness, transform phlegm, and rectify the qi when needled with even draining and supplementing method.
Zu San Li (St 36) *Tai Bai* (Sp 3) *Pi Shu* (Bl 20)	Together, these points fortify the spleen to dry dampness and transform phlegm when needled with supplementing method.

Additions & subtractions: For vomiting of phlegm drool, add *Nei Guan* (Per 6). For phlegm in the stools, add *Tian Shu* (St 25). For coughing of phlegm, add *Fei Shu* (Bl 13).

Chinese medicinal formula: Modified *Er Chen Tang* (Two Aged [Ingredients] Decoction)

Ingredients: Uncooked Pericarpium Citri Reticulatae (*Chen Pi*), 9g, clear Rhizoma Pinelliae Ternatae (*Ban Xia*), 9g, Sclerotium Poriae Cocos (*Fu Ling*), 9g, mix-fried Radix Glycyrrhizae (*Gan Cao*), 6g, uncooked Rhizoma Atractylodis Macrocephalae (*Bai Zhu*), 9g, Rhizoma Acori Graminei (*Shi Chang Pu*), 9g

Additions & subtractions: For severe fatigue, add rice stir-fried Radix Codonopsitis Pilosulac (*Dang Shen*), 9g, and honey stir-fried Radix Astragali Membranacei (*Huang Qi*), 15g. For edema, add Sclerotium Polypori Umbellati (*Zhu Ling*), 9g, and Rhizoma Alismatis (*Ze Xie*), 9g. For profuse phlegm, add processed Rhizoma Arisaematis (*Tian Nan Xing*), 9g, and Semen Raphani Sativi (*Lai Fu Zi*), 9g. For fear of cold with cold limbs, add dry Rhizoma Zingiberis (*Gan Jiang*), 9g. For accumulation and stagnation of food and drink with no thought for eating and indigestion, add Semen Raphani Sativi (*Lai Fu Zi*), 9g, and ginger mix-fried Cortex Magnoliae Officinalis (*Hou Po*), 9g. For damp turbidity in the center with a slimy, bland taste in the mouth, reduced food intake, nausea, abdominal distention, and loose stools, add ginger mix-fried Cortex Magnoliae Officinalis (*Hou Po*), 9g, and Fructus Amomi (*Sha Ren*), 3g. For vomiting of phlegm drool, replace *Er Chen Tang* with Modified *Xuan Fu Hua Dai Zhe Tang* (Inula & Hematite Decoction): Flos Inulae (*Xuan Fu Hua*), 9g, Haemititum (*Dai Zhe Shi*), 9g, rice stir-fried Radix Codonopsitis Pilosulae (*Dang Shen*), 9g, ginger-processed Rhizoma Pinelliae Ternatae (*Ban Xia*), 9g, uncooked Rhizoma Zingiberis (*Sheng Jiang*), 6g, Fructus Zizyphi Jujubae (*Da Zao*), 3 pieces, mix-fried Radix Glycyrrhizae (*Gan Cao*), 6g, Sclerotium Poriae Cocos (*Fu Ling*), 9g, and Pericarpium Citri Reticulatae (*Chen Pi*), 6g. For dizziness, heart palpitations, and heavy-headedness, replace *Er Chen Tang* with Modified *Ban Xia Bai Zhu Tian Ma Tang* (Pinellia, Atractylodes & Gastrodia Decoction): lime-processed Rhizoma Pinelliae Ternatae (*Ban Xia*), 9g, bran stir-fried Rhizoma Atractylodis Macrocephalae (*Bai Zhu*), 12g, stir-fried Rhizoma Gastrodiae Elatae (*Tian Ma*), 6g, Sclerotium Poriae Cocos (*Fu Ling*), 9g, stir-fried Pericarpium Citri Reticulatae (*Chen Pi*), 9g, uncooked Rhizoma Zingiberis (*Sheng Jiang*), 3g, Fructus Zizyphi Jujubae (*Da Zao*), 2 fruits, mix-fried Radix Glycyrrhizae (*Gan Cao*), 3g, and Rhizoma Acori Graminei (*Shi Chang Pu*), 9g.

5. Heart qi vacuity

Symptoms: Fatigue, heart palpitations, shortness of breath, spontaneous perspiration which worsens on exertion, a low voice, disinclination to speak, lassitude of the spirit, a lusterless facial complexion, a pale tongue, and a vacuous, weak, bound, or regularly interrupted pulse

Therapeutic principles: Supplement and boost the heart qi

Acupuncture & moxibustion:

Xin Shu (Bl 15) *Nei Guan* (Per 6)	Together, these points supplement and boost the heart qi and quiet the spirit when needled with moxibustion on the heads of the needles.
Qi Hai (CV 6) *Zu San Li* (St 36)	Together, these points boost the righteous qi and thus heart qi when needled with moxibustion on the heads of the needles.

Additions & subtractions: For heart blood vacuity, add *Ge Shu* (Bl 17). For profuse dreams and susceptibility to fright, add *Shen Men* (Ht 7). For stifling pain in the chest, add *Jue Yin Shu* (Bl 14). For dizziness, add *Bai Hui* (GV 20). For symptoms of blood stasis, add *He Gu* (LI 4) and *San Yin Jiao* (Sp 6). For profuse sweating, add *He Gu* (LI 4) and *Fu Liu* (Ki 7).

Chinese medicinal formula: Modified *Yang Xin Tang* (Nourish the Heart Decoction)

Ingredients: Honey stir-fried Radix Codonopsitis Pilosulae (*Dang Shen*), 9g, stir-fried Radix Dioscoreae Oppositae (*Shan Yao*), 9g, Sclerotium Pararadicis Poriae Cocos (*Fu Shen*), 6g, Sclerotium Poriae Cocos (*Fu Ling*), 6g, Semen Nelumbinis Nuciferae (*Lian Zi*), 6g, Semen Biotae Orientalis (*Bai Zi Ren*), 6g, Fructus Schisandrae Chinensis (*Wu Wei Zi*), 6g, Radix Angelicae Sinensis (*Dang Gui*), 6g, honey stir-fried Radix Astragali Membranacei (*Huang Qi*), 9g, stir-fried Semen Zizyphi Spinosae (*Suan Zao Ren*), 6g, mix-fried Radix Glycyrrhizae (*Gan Cao*), 9g

Additions & subtractions: For severe fatigue, increase the dosage of Astragalus up to 15g. For spontaneous perspiration, add bran stir-fried Rhizoma Atractylodis Macrocephalae (*Bai Zhu*), 9g. For heart blood vacuity, add Radix Albus Paeoniae Lactiflorae (*Bai Shao*), 9g, and Arillus Euphorbiae Longanae (*Long Yan Rou*), 9g. For predominant insomnia, heart vexation, and heart palpitations, replace *Yang Xin Tang* with Modified *An Shen Ding Zhi Wan* (Quiet the Spirit & Stabilize the Mind Pills): Radix Panacis Ginseng (*Ren Shen*), 6g, Sclerotium Poriae Cocos (*Fu Ling*), 9g, Sclerotium Pararadicis Poriae Cocos (*Fu Shen*), 9g, processed Radix Polygalae Tenuifoliae (*Yuan Zhi*), 6g, calcined Dens Draconis (*Long Chi*), 15g, Rhizoma Acori Graminei (*Shi Chang Pu*), 6g, and Caulis Polygoni Multiflori (*Ye Jiao Teng*), 12g. For severe heart palpitations, replace *Yang Xin Tang* with Modified *Zhi Gan Cao Tang* (Mix-fried Licorice Decoction): mix-fried Radix Glycyrrhizae (*Gan Cao*), 12g, Radix Panacis Ginseng (*Ren Shen*), 6g, uncooked Radix Rehmanniae (*Sheng Di*), 9g, Gelatinum Corii Asini (*E Jiao*), 6g, stir-fried Ramulus Cinnamomi Cassiae (*Gui Zhi*), 9g, Tuber Ophiopogonis Japonici (*Mai Men Dong*), 9g, Semen Cannabis Sativae (*Huo Ma Ren*), 5g, Fructus Zizyphi Jujubae (*Da Zao*), 5 pieces, and uncooked Rhizoma Zingiberis (*Sheng Jiang*), 6g.

6. Heart yang vacuity

Symptoms: Fatigue, heart palpitations and disquietude which get worse on exertion, a cold body and limbs or even counterflow chilling of the limbs in severe cases, lassitude of the spirit, shortness of breath, spontaneous perspiration, a somber white facial complexion, chest oppression (and sometimes pain), a pale tongue with white fur, and a deep, fine and forceless, vacuous and weak, or bound or regularly interrupted pulse

Therapeutic principles: Warm and supplement heart yang and quiet the spirit

Acupuncture & moxibustion:

Xin Shu (Bl 15) *Shen Tang* (Bl 44)	Together, these points warm and supplement heart yang and quiet the spirit when needled with supplementing method.
Da Zhui (GV 14) *Qi Hai* (CV 6)	Together, these points warm yang and boost the qi when needled with moxibustion on the heads of the needles.

Additions & subtractions: For severe fatigue or reduced food intake and loose stools, add *Zu San Li* (St 36). For dizziness and nausea, add *Zhong Wan* (CV 12). For heart pain, add *Nei Guan* (Per 6). For inhibited urination and edema, moxa *Guan Yuan* (CV 4). For dull purple or dark yet pale lips and nails, add *He Gu* (LI 4) and *San Yin Jiao* (Sp 6). For a bound pulse, add *Nei Guan* (Per 6).

Chinese medicinal formula: Modified *Bao Yuan Tang* (Protect the Origin Decoction)

Ingredients: Radix Rubrus Panacis Ginseng (*Hong Shen*), 6g, mix-fried Radix Glycyrrhizae (*Gan Cao*), 10g, Cortex Cinnamomi Cassiae (*Rou Gui*), 3g, uncooked Radix Astragali Membranacei (*Huang Qi*), 15g, bland Radix Lateralis Praeparatus Aconiti Carmichaeli (*Fu Zi*), 6g, stir-fried Ramulus Cinnamomi Cassiae (*Gui Zhi*), 10g

Additions & subtractions: For severe heart palpitations, add Os Draconis (*Long Gu*), 12g, and Concha Ostreae (*Mu Li*), 12g. For reduced food intake and loose stools, add dry Rhizoma Zingiberis (*Gan Jiang*), 6g, and bran stir-fried Rhizoma Atractylodis Macrocephalae (*Bai Zhu*), 9g. For cold spontaneous perspiration, add bran stir-fried Rhizoma Atractylodis Macrocephalae (*Bai Zhu*), 9g. For dual vacuity of heart yang and blood, replace *Bao Yuan Tang* with Modified *Zhi Gan Cao Tang* (Mix-fried Licorice Decoction): mix-fried Radix Glycyrrhizae (*Gan Cao*), 12g, Radix Panacis Ginseng (*Ren Shen*), 6g, uncooked Radix Rehmanniae (*Sheng Di*), 12g, Gelatinum Corii Asini (*E Jiao*), 6g, wine mix-fried Radix Angelicae Sinensis (*Dang Gui*), 9g, stir-fried Ramulus Cinnamomi Cassiae (*Gui Zhi*), 6g, Tuber Ophiopogonis Japonici (*Mai Men Dong*), 9g, Semen Cannabis Sativae (*Huo Ma Ren*), 5g, Fructus Zizyphi Jujubae (*Da Zao*), 3 pieces, uncooked Rhizoma Zingiberis (*Sheng Jiang*), 3g, and bland Radix Lateralis Praeparatus Aconiti Carmichaeli (*Fu Zi*), 6g. For heart yang vacuity desertion with severe and sudden upset due to heart palpitations, profuse cold sweating, shortness and weakness of breath, a white facial complexion with cyanotic lips and mouth, counterflow chilling of the limbs, a deathly feeling, clouded spirit-mind, a pale tongue, and a faint pulse on the verge of expiry, replace *Bao Yuan Tang* with Modified *Shen Fu Tang* (Ginseng & Aconite Decoction): Radix Panacis Ginseng (*Ren Shen*), 15g, bland Radix Lateralis Praeparatus Aconiti Carmichaeli (*Fu Zi*), 9g, and uncooked Radix Astragali Membranacei (*Huang Qi*), 18g. For purple lips, tongue, and nails, add wine mix-fried Radix Ligustici Wallichii (*Chuan Xiong*), 10g, Radix Salviae Miltiorrhizae (*Dan Shen*), 10g, and Radix Pseudoginseng (*San Qi*), 3g (powdered and taken with the strained decoction).

7. Kidney qi vacuity

Symptoms: Fatigue, lassitude of the spirit, lack of strength, shortage of qi, dizziness, sweating on exertion, lingering tinnitus and/or deafness, low back and knee pain and weakness, long voidings of clear urine, frequent urination, nighttime urination, possible lower limb edema, seminal emission, premature ejaculation, a white facial complexion, white tongue fur, and a fine, weak pulse

Therapeutic principles: Supplement the kidneys and boost the qi

Acupuncture & moxibustion:

Qi Hai (CV 6) *Guan Yuan* (CV 4)	Together, these points supplement the original qi when moxaed.
Zhi Shi (Bl 52) *Fu Liu* (Ki 7)	Together, these points supplement the kidneys and secure the essence when needled with supplementing method.

Additions & subtractions: For tinnitus, add *Shen Shu* (Bl 23) and *Ting Gong* (GB 2). For reduced auditory acuity, add *Tai Xi* (Ki 3). For dribbling urination, add *Zhong Ji* (CV 3). For impaired memory, add *Si Shen Cong* (M-HN-1). For panting, add *Da Zhong* (Ki 4). For reduced food intake, add *Zhong Wan* (CV 12). For dribbling urination, add *Yin Gu* (Ki 10).

Chinese medicinal formula: *Da Bu Yuan Jian* (Greatly Supplement the Origin Decoction)

Ingredients: Radix Panacis Ginseng (*Ren Shen*), 6g, cooked Radix Rehmanniae (*Shu Di*), 15g, stir-fried Radix Dioscoreae Oppositae (*Shan Yao*), 15g, steamed Fructus Corni Officinalis (*Shan Zhu Yu*), 9g, Radix

Angelicae Sinensis (*Dang Gui*), 6g, Fructus Lycii Chinensis (*Gou Qi Zi*), 9g, salt stir-fried Cortex Eucommiae Ulmoidis (*Du Zhong*), 15g, mix-fried Radix Glycyrrhizae (*Gan Cao*), 3g

Additions & subtractions: For spleen qi vacuity, add bran stir-fried Rhizoma Atractylodis Macrocephalae (*Bai Zhu*), 9g, and honey mix-fried Radix Astragali Membranacei (*Huang Qi*), 18g. For impotence, add Cornu Parvum Cervi (*Lu Rong*), 0.5g (powdered and taken with the strained decoction). For low back pain, add salt stir-fried Radix Morindae Officinalis (*Ba Ji Tian*), 9g, and salt stir-fried Radix Dipsaci (*Xu Duan*), 9g. For long voidings of clear urine, frequent urination, and nighttime urination, add stir-fried Semen Cuscutae Chinensis (*Tu Si Zi*), 9g, Fructus Alpiniae Oxyphyllae (*Yi Zhi Ren*), 9g, and Fructus Rubi Chingii (*Fu Pen Zi*), 9g. For seminal emission, replace *Da Bu Yuan Jian* with modified *Jin Suo Gu Jing Wan* (Golden Lock Secure the Essence Pills): Semen Astragali Complanati (*Sha Yuan Zi*), 9g, Semen Euryalis Ferocis (*Qian Shi*), 9g, Fructus Rosae Laevigatae (*Jin Ying Zi*), 9g, Stamen Nelumbinis Nuciferae (*Lian Xu*), 9g, calcined Concha Ostreae (*Mu Li*), 20g, Fructus Rubi Chingii (*Fu Pen Zi*), 9g, and Fructus Schisandrae Chinensis (*Wu Wei Zi*), 9g. For tinnitus, add Rhizoma Acori Graminei (*Shi Chang Pu*), 9g, Semen Cuscutae Chinensis (*Tu Si Zi*), 10g, and Magnetitum (*Ci Shi*), 15g. For vaginal discharge or diarrhea, add salt mix-fried Fructus Psoraleae Corylifoliae (*Bu Gu Zhi*), 9g. For lower limb edema, add Cortex Radicis Acanthopanacis (*Wu Jia Pi*), 9g, and Rhizoma Alismatis (*Ze Xie*), 9g.

8. Kidney yang vacuity

Symptoms: Fatigue, lassitude of the spirit, lack of strength, fear of cold, cold limbs, absence of thirst, a bright white facial complexion, dizziness and vertigo, tinnitus, low back and knee soreness and limpness, impotence or incomplete erection, seminal emission, frequent urination, daybreak diarrhea, hair loss, a pale, enlarged, moist tongue with teeth-marks on its edges and white fur, and a weak pulse in the cubit position

Therapeutic principles: Warm and supplement kidney yang

Acupuncture & moxibustion:

Ming Men (GV 4)	Together, these points warm and supplement
Guan Yuan (CV 4)	kidney yang when moxaed and needled
Shen Shu (Bl 23)	with supplementing method.
Tai Xi (Ki 3)	

Additions & subtractions: For severe fatigue, add *Qi Hai* (CV 6). For dizziness or headache, add *Bai Hui* (GV 20). For edema with inhibited urination, add *Shui Dao* (St 28) and *Shui Fen* (CV 9). For impotence or seminal emission, add *Zhi Shi* (Bl 52). For diarrhea, moxa *Gong Sun* (Sp 4). For menstrual irregularities, add *San Yin Jiao* (Sp 6). For periumbilical or lower abdominal pain, moxa *Shen Que* (CV 8). For premature ejaculation, add *Da He* (Ki 12).

Chinese medicinal formula: *You Gui Wan* (Restore the Right [Kidney] Pills)

Ingredients: Salt mix-fried Cortex Eucommiae Ulmoidis (*Du Zhong*), 9g, bland Radix Lateralis Praeparatus Aconiti Carmichaeli (*Fu Zi*), 6g, Cortex Cinnamomi Cassiae (*Rou Gui*), 3g, Gelatinum Cornu Cervi (*Lu Jiao Jiao*), 9g, stir-fried Radix Dioscoreae Oppositae (*Shan Yao*), 9g, Fructus Lycii Chinensis (*Gou Qi Zi*), 6g, steamed Fructus Corni Officinalis (*Shan Zhu Yu*), 9g, cooked Radix Rehmanniae (*Shu Di*), 9g, wine mix-fried Radix Angelicae Sinensis (*Dang Gui*), 6g

Additions & subtractions: For severe fear of cold and chilled limbs, add dry Rhizoma Zingiberis (*Gan Jiang*), 6g. For edema with inhibited urination, replace *You Gui Wan* with modified *Ji Sheng Shen Qi Wan* (*Aid the Living* Kidney Qi Pills): blast-fried Radix Lateralis Praeparatus Aconiti Carmichaeli (*Fu Zi*), 6g, Cortex Cinnamomi Cassiae (*Rou Gui*), 3g, cooked Radix Rehmanniae (*Shu Di*), 9g, steamed Fructus Corni Officinalis (*Shan Zhu Yu*), 9g, stir-fried Radix Dioscoreae Oppositae (*Shan Yao*), 9g, Sclerotium Poriae Cocos (*Fu Ling*), 9g, salt mix-fried Rhizoma Alismatis (*Ze Xie*), 9g, Cortex Radicis Moutan (*Dan Pi*), 6g, salt mix-fried Semen Plantaginis (*Che Qian Zi*), 9g, salt mix-fried Radix Achyranthis Bidentatae (*Huai Niu Xi*), 9g, and Cortex Radicis Acanthopanacis (*Wu Jia Pi*), 9g. For inhibited urination, add Sclerotium Polypori Umbellati (*Zhu Ling*), 9g, and Cortex Radicis Acanthopanacis (*Wu Jia Pi*), 9g. For concomitant central qi fall with a sagging sensation in the lower back or lower abdomen and a continuous, "hollow" pain sensation, subtract Lycium and Dang Gui and add honey stir-fried Radix Codonopsitis Pilosulae (*Dang Shen*), 9g, honey stir-fried Radix Astragali Membranacei (*Huang Qi*), 12g, bran stir-fried Rhizoma Atractylodis Macrocephalae (*Bai Zhu*), 9g, stir-fried Radix Bupleuri (*Chai Hu*), 3g, and honey mix-fried Rhizoma Cimicifugae (*Sheng Ma*), 3g. For impotence, replace *You Gui Wan* with modified *Wu Zi Yan Zong Wan* (Five Seeds Develop the Ancestral [Sinew] Pills): Fructus Lycii Chinensis (*Gou Qi*), 15g, Semen Cuscutae Chinensis (*Tu Si Zi*), 15g, Fructus Rubi Chingii (*Fu Pen Zi*), 15g, Fructus Schisandrae Chinensis (*Wu Wei Zi*), 9g, Semen Plantaginis (*Che Qian Zi*), 6g, Rhizoma Curculiginis

Orchioidis (*Xian Mao*), 9g, and Herba Epimedii (*Yin Yang Huo*), 9g. For chilled genitals and chilly semen, add Rhizoma Curculiginis Orchioidis (*Xian Mao*), 9g, Herba Epimedii (*Yin Yang Huo*), 9g. For low back pain, add Radix Morindae Officinalis (*Ba Ji Tian*), 9g, and salt stir-fried Radix Dipsaci (*Xu Duan*), 9g. For cold constipation, add Herba Cistanchis Deserticolae (*Rou Cong Rong*), 12g, and Herba Cynomorii Songarici (*Suo Yang*), 9g. For daybreak diarrhea, add wine steamed Fructus Schisandrae Chinensis (*Wu Wei Zi*), 9g, salt mix-fried Fructus Psoraleae Corylifoliae (*Bu Gu Zhi*), 9g, and Semen Myristicae Fragrantis (*Rou Dou Kou*), 6g. For nocturnal urination or frequent urination, add salt stir-fried Fructus Alpiniae Oxyphyllae (*Yi Zhi Ren*), 9g, and wine-steamed Fructus Schisandrae Chinensis (*Wu Wei Zi*), 9g.

9. Lung qi vacuity

Symptoms: Fatigue, shortness of breath, and spontaneous perspiration which get worse on exertion, and lack of strength, low voice, fear of cold, occasional chest oppression which can be relieved by inhaling, possible enduring coughing with weak sound, susceptibility to external contractions, possible facial edema or edema in the four limbs in severe cases, a pale facial complexion, a pale, tender tongue with thin, white fur, and a fine, weak, forceless pulse

Therapeutic principles: Supplement the lungs and boost the qi

Acupuncture & moxibustion:

Fei Shu (Bl 13) *Tai Yuan* (Lu 9)	Together, these points supplement the lung qi when needled with supplementing method.
Zu San Li (St 36) *Qi Hai* (CV 6)	Together, these points supplement the qi and bank earth to engender metal when needled with supplementing method.

Additions & subtractions: For lassitude of the spirit with disinclination to speak, add *Gao Huang* (Bl 43). For fear of cold and cold limbs, moxa *Guan Yuan* (CV 4). For cough counterflow which gets worse on exertion, add *Tai Xi* (Ki 3) to supplement the kidneys to grasp or absorb the qi. For cold in the upper back, moxa *Da Zhui* (GV 14). For frequent urination, add *Ming Men* (GV 4). For concomitant spleen qi vacuity, add *Wei Shu* (Bl 21) and *Pi Shu* (Bl 20). For chest oppression, add *Dan Zhong* (CV 17). For susceptibility to common cold, moxa *Da Zhui* (GV 14) and needle *He Gu* (LI 4). For phlegm dampness obstructing the lungs with coughing of white phlegm, add *Zhong Fu* (Lu 1).

Chinese medicinal formula: Modified *Bu Fei Tang* (Supplement the Lungs Decoction)

Ingredients: Uncooked Radix Codonopsitis Pilosulae (*Dang Shen*), 9g, uncooked Radix Astragali Membranacei (*Huang Qi*), 15g, uncooked Fructus Schisandrae Chinensis (*Wu Wei Zi*), 9g, honey mix-fried Radix Asteris Tatarici (*Zi Wan*), 6g, honey mix-fried Cortex Radicis Mori Albi (*Sang Bai Pi*), 6g, cooked Radix Rehmanniae (*Shu Di*), 6g, uncooked Rhizoma Atractylodis Macrocephalae (*Bai Zhu*), 9g, mix-fried Radix Glycyrrhizae (*Gan Cao*), 3g

Additions & subtractions: For susceptibility to common cold, add Radix Ledebouriellae Divaricatae (*Fang Feng*), 9g. For cold phlegm obstructing the lungs with profuse expectoration of clear, thin phlegm, add lime-processed Rhizoma Pinelliae Ternatae (*Ban Xia*), 9g, and dry Rhizoma Zingiberis (*Gan Jiang*), 6g. For phlegm dampness obstructing the lungs with coughing of white phlegm, add lime-processed Rhizoma Pinelliae Ternatae (*Ban Xia*), 9g, Sclerotium Poriae Cocos (*Fu Ling*), 9g, and Pericarpium Citri Reticulatae (*Chen Pi*), 6g. In the last case, for profuse phlegm, subtract cooked Rehmannia and Schisandra and add Radix Platycodi Grandiflori (*Jie Geng*), 9g, and Fructus Citri Aurantii (*Zhi Ke*), 6g. For severe coughing, add honey stir-fried Flos Tussilaginis Farfarae (*Kuan Dong Hua*), 9g, and uncooked Cortex Magnoliae Officinalis (*Hou Po*), 9g. For spontaneous perspiration and susceptibility to external contractions, add *Yu Ping Feng San* (Jade Windscreen Powder): Radix Astragali Membranacei (*Huang Qi*), 18g, Rhizoma Atractylodis Macrocephalae (*Bai Zhu*), 15g, and Radix Ledebouriellae Divaricatae (*Fang Feng*), 9g. For lung yang vacuity, replace *Bu Fei Tang* with Modified *Wen Fei Tang* (Warm the Lungs Decoction) plus *Ling Gan Wu Wei Jiang Xin Tang* (Poria, Licorice, Schisandra, Ginger & Asarum Decoction): dry Rhizoma Zingiberis (*Gan Jiang*), 9g, lime-processed Rhizoma Pinelliae Ternatae (*Ban Xia*), 9g, uncooked Radix Astragali Membranacei (*Huang Qi*), 18g, Semen Pruni Armeniacae (*Xing Ren*), 9g, Pericarpium Citri Reticulatae (*Chen Pi*), 6g, Herba Asari Cum Radice (*Xi Xin*), 3g, uncooked Fructus Schisandrae Chinensis (*Wu Wei Zi*), 6g, mix-fried Radix Glycyrrhizae (*Gan Cao*), 6g, and Sclerotium Poriae Cocos (*Fu Ling*), 12g.

10. Yang desertion

Symptoms: Sudden great fatigue and weakness, listlessness of the essence spirit, shortness and weakness of breath, incessant sweating which is pearl-like, clear, thin, and cold, fear of cold, a curled-up lying posture, counterflow chilling in the limbs, a somber white facial complexion, thirst with a liking for hot drinks, a moist tongue, and a faint pulse verging on expiry, or a floating, rapid, scallion-stalk pulse

Therapeutic principles: Supplement yang and stem desertion, return yang and stem counterflow

Acupuncture & moxibustion:

Su Liao (GV 25) *Guan Yuan* (CV 4)	Together, these points regulate yin and yang and stem desertion when needled with even draining and supplementing method.
Shen Que (CV 8) *Qi Hai* (CV 6)	Together, these points supplement yang, return yang, and stem counterflow when strongly moxaed.

Additions & subtractions: For coma, strongly moxa *Bai Hui* (GV 20).

Chinese medicinal formula: Modified *Shen Fu Long Mu Tang* (Ginseng, Aconite, Dragon Bone & Oyster Shell Decoction)

Ingredients: Radix Panacis Ginseng (*Ren Shen*), 15g, blast-fried Radix Lateralis Praeparatus Aconiti Carmichaeli (*Fu Zi*), 9g, calcined Os Draconis (*Long Gu*), 30g, calcined Concha Ostreae (*Mu Li*), 30g, uncooked Radix Astragali Membranacei (*Huang Qi*), 20g

11. Qi & blood dual vacuity

Symptoms: Fatigued spirit and limbs, reduced qi with laziness to speak, low, timid voice, spontaneous perspiration, lack of strength, heart palpitations, impaired memory, insomnia, dizziness and vertigo, numb hands and feet, a white, lusterless facial complexion, pale lips and nails, a pale and tender tongue, and a fine, weak pulse

Therapeutic principles: Supplement both the qi and blood

Acupuncture & moxibustion:

Pi Shu (Bl 20)	Together, these points fortify the spleen and boost
Wei Shu (Bl 21)	the stomach to benefit the source of engenderment
Zhong Wan (CV 12)	and transformation when needled with supplementing method.
Zu San Li (St 36)	Together, these points boost the qi when needled
Qi Hai (CV 6)	with supplementing method.
Bai Hui (GV 20)	Upbears the qi and lifts the blood when moxaed

Additions & subtractions: For scanty menstruation with pale, thin blood, add *Xue Hai* (Sp 10). For reduced food intake, add *Jian Li* (CV 11). For impaired memory, add *Xin Shu* (Bl 15). For loose stools, add *Gong Sun* (Sp 4).

Chinese medicinal formula: *Ba Zhen Tang* (Eight Pearls Decoction)

Ingredients: Cooked Radix Rehmanniae (*Shu Di*), 15g, Radix Albus Paeoniae Lactiflorae (*Bai Shao*), 9g, wine mix-fried Radix Angelicae Sinensis (*Dang Gui*), 9g, wine mix-fried Radix Ligustici Wallichii (*Chuan Xiong*), 6g, Radix Codonopsitis Pilosulae (*Dang Shen*), 9g, bran stir-fried Rhizoma Atractylodis Macrocephalae (*Bai Zhu*), 9g, Sclerotium Poriae Cocos (*Fu Ling*), 9g, mix-fried Radix Glycyrrhizae (*Gan Cao*), 6g

12. Summerheat damaging the qi

Symptoms: Fatigue, lack of strength, lassitude of the spirit, fever, spontaneous perspiration, chest oppression, shortness of breath, reduced qi with laziness to speak, heart vexation, thirst, no thought for food, turbid tongue fur, and a vacuous, rapid pulse

Therapeutic principles: Clear summerheat and boost the qi, nourish yin and engender liquids

Acupuncture & moxibustion:

He Gu (LI 4)	Together, these points course and drain the yang ming
Xian Gu (St 43)	to clear summerheat when needled with draining method.
Nei Guan (Per 6)	Together, these points harmonize the center, boost
Zu San Li (St 36)	the qi, and engender liquids when needled with
San Yin Jiao (Sp 6)	even draining and supplementing method.

Additions and subtractions: For fever, add *Da Zhui* (GV 14). For sweating, add *Yin Xi* (Ht 6). For nausea, add *Zhong Wan* (CV 12).

Chinese medicinal formula: *Qing Shu Yi Qi Tang* (Clear Summerheat & Boost the Qi Decoction)

Ingredients: Radix Panacis Quinquefolii (*Xi Yang Shen*), 6g, Herba Dendrobii (*Shi Hu*), 12g, Tuber Ophiopogonis Japonici (*Mai Men Dong*), 12g, Rhizoma Coptidis Chinensis (*Huang Lian*), 3g, Folium Bambusae (*Zhu Ye*), 6g, Folium Nelumbinis Nuciferae (*He Ye*), 9g, uncooked Rhizoma Anemarrhenae Asphodeloidis (*Zhi Mu*), 9g, Semen Oryzae Sativae (*Geng Mi*), 12g, Pericarpium Citrulli Vulgaris (*Xi Gua Pi*), 24g, Radix Glycyrrhizae (*Gan Cao*), 3g

Additions & subtractions: For severely damaged qi, add honey stir-fried Radix Astragali Membranacei (*Huang Qi*), 12g, and uncooked Fructus Schisandrae Chinensis (*Wu Wei Zi*), 9g. For severely damaged fluids, add Radix Glehniae Littoralis (*Sha Shen*), 18g. For severe heat, add uncooked Gypsum Fibrosum (*Shi Gao*), 24g. After the acute stage when there is no fever or sweating but there is severe fatigue and shortness of breath, replace *Qing Shu Yi Qi Tang* with Modified *Sheng Mai Yin* (Engender the Pulse Drink): Radix Panacis Quinquefolii (*Xi Yang Shen*), 6g, Tuber Ophiopogonis Japonici (*Mai Men Dong*), 9g, and uncooked Fructus Schisandrae Chinensis (*Wu Wei Zi*), 9g.

13. Lung dryness & qi vacuity

Symptoms: Fatigue with laziness to speak, a low, timid voice, coughing, shortness of breath, scant, sticky phlegm, dry lips and nose, dry, sore throat, thin, white or thin, yellow tongue fur, and a floating, rapid or bowstring, fine, rapid pulse

Therapeutic principles: Clear the lungs and moisten dryness, boost the qi and engender liquids

Acupuncture & moxibustion:

Fei Shu (Bl 13) *Gao Huang* (Bl 51)	Together, these points moisten the lungs and clear dryness when needled with even draining and supplementing method.

Tai Xi (Ki 3)
San Yin Jiao (Sp 6)
Zu San Li (St 36)

Together, these points boost the qi and engender liquids when needled with supplementing method.

Additions & subtractions: For fear of cold and cold body, add *Feng Men* (Bl 12). For fever, add *Da Zhui* (GV 14). For severe cough, add *Zhong Fu* (Lu 1). For panting, add *Tian Tu* (CV 22). For spontaneous perspiration, add *He Gu* (LI 4).

Chinese medicinal formula: *Qing Zao Jiu Fei Tang* (Clear Dryness & Rescue the Lungs Decoction)

Ingredients: Honey stir-fried Folium Mori Albi (*Sang Ye*), 9g, uncooked Gypsum Fibrosum (*Shi Gao*), 12g, Radix Pseudostellariae Heterophyllae (*Tai Zi Shen*), 9g, black Semen Sesami Indici (*Hei Zhi Ma*), 6g, Gelatinum Corii Asini (*E Jiao*), 9g, Tuber Ophiopogonis Japonici (*Mai Dong*), 9g, Semen Pruni Armeniacae (*Xing Ren*), 9g, honey stir-fried Folium Eriobotryae Japonicae (*Pi Pa Ye*), 9g, mix-fried Radix Glycyrrhizae (*Gan Cao*), 3g

Additions & subtractions: For severe fatigue, add uncooked Radix Astragali Membranacei (*Huang Qi*), 15g, and uncooked Radix Codonopsitis Pilosulae (*Dang Shen*), 9g. For severe heat dryness of the lungs, add uncooked Rhizoma Anemarrhenae Asphodeloidis (*Zhi Mu*), 9g. For severe dryness of the stomach, add Rhizoma Polygonati Odorati (*Yu Zhu*), 9g, and Radix Glehniae Littoralis (*Sha Shen*), 9g. For constipation with dry stools, add uncooked Radix Et Rhizoma Rhei (*Da Huang*), 6g.

30
Clouding Reversal *(Yun Jue)*

Clouding reversal refers to sudden temporary clouding collapse and loss of consciousness with no obvious prodromal signs. Lack of warmth in the limbs can be an accompanying symptom. In minor cases, the unconsciousness may last anywhere from seconds to hours, and no sequellae remain after regaining consciousness except for possible fatigue, dry mouth, and dizziness. However, in severe cases, unconsciousness may lead to death.

Disease causes, disease mechanisms:

1. Qi vacuity

Qi vacuity in this condition usually develops from constitutional qi vacuity with concomitant damage by great grief, fear or overwork. In Chinese medicine, consciousness or spirit brilliance is nothing other than having spirit, and spirit is nothing other than an accumulation of qi in the heart. Therefore, if, for any reason, the qi becomes suddenly and greatly vacuous, one may loose spirit and thus consciousness. Grief is the affect of the lungs which command the qi of the entire body. In addition, the lungs are where the qi is finally transformed from the combination of the finest essence of food and drink and the great qi. Hence, if grief damages and causes detriment to the lung qi, this may also damage the heart qi and spirit brilliance. Fear causes the qi to descend. The heart qi is only able to accumulate and transform into the spirit as long as clear yang is upborne. Therefore, any strong downward movement of the qi may adversely affect the spirit brilliance. Overwork simply consumes the qi, and great overwork greatly consumes the qi.

2. Blood vacuity

In cases of clouding reversal, blood vacuity usually is the result of great loss of the blood due to profuse uterine bleeding, external injury, or great loss of body fluids through profuse sweating, diarrhea, and/or vomiting. The blood is the mother of the qi, and it is the blood which nourishes the heart spirit, rendering it wholesome. If, for any reason, the blood becomes vacuous and fails to nourish the spirit brilliance, temporary loss of consciousness may occur.

3. Counterflow & chaos of the qi & blood

The liver governs both upbearing and coursing and discharge. Anger is the affect of the liver and easily damages the liver. In addition, anger causes the qi to ascend. Therefore, when the liver is damaged by anger, the liver qi typically counterflows upward. Because the qi moves the blood, if the qi counterflows upward, the blood will follow. If the blood flows upward and blocks the clear orifices, temporary loss of consciousness may occur. On the other hand, fright causes chaos in the flow of qi. When the qi flows chaotically and incoherently, it does not accumulate to transform the spirit. Hence fright causes temporary loss of spirit and, therefore, temporary loss of consciousness.

4. Yin vacuity & liver effulgence

"The liver governs the making of strategies," Therefore, enduring hesitation in strategy-making can excessively consume liver yin. Since the liver and kidneys share a common source, liver yin vacuity may lead to kidney yin vacuity or constitutional kidney yin vacuity may lead to liver yin vacuity. In either case, liver-kidney yin is responsible for checking and controlling liver yang. If, for any reason, liver and kidney yin become vacuous and insufficient, liver yang will tend to become hyperactive. If hyperactive liver yang harasses the heart spirit above, temporary loss of consciousness may occur.

5. Phlegm confounding the clear orifices

This disease mechanism is often seen in the individuals who have constitutional profuse dampness and/or phlegm. If dampness and phlegm are drafted upward by counterflow qi, for instance, as the result of intense anger, the phlegm and dampness may obstruct the clear orifices of the heart and thus confound the spirit. In that case, temporary unconsciousness may occur since the spirit brilliance is not able to communicate or connect with the outside world.

6. Contraction of summerheat evils

Summerheat is a kind of fire evil, and the heart corresponds to fire. Therefore, summerheat evils often invade the heart. During the summertime, summerheat evils tend to be exuberant. Due to enduring exposure, these evils may enter the body, giving rise to summerheat invading the heart. "The heart governs the spirit brilliance." Therefore, if these evils invade the heart and cloud and obscure the spirit brilliance, temporary loss of consciousness may occur.

7. Food stagnation

Food stagnation causing temporary loss of consciousness is usually encountered in children who have suddenly eaten or drunk too much. If food and drink cannot be moved and transformed properly, they will stagnate in the middle burner. If food stagnates in the middle burner, the stomach qi cannot downbear as it should. Rather, it may counterflow upward and harass the spirit brilliance above, thus leading to temporary loss of consciousness. This pattern may also occur in adults who have drunk too much alcohol coupled with anger or sexual intercourse. In that case, the alcohol and the grain qi combine in the middle, dash upward, congest in the chest, and cloud the spirit brilliance. Therefore, temporary loss of consciousness may occur as well.

Treatment based on pattern discrimination

1. Qi vacuity

Symptoms: Sudden loss of consciousness occurring immediately after great grief, great fear, or great overwork, a bright white facial complexion, faint, weak breathing, sweating, cold limbs, a pale tongue, and a deep, faint pulse

Therapeutic principles: Supplement the qi and return yang

Acupuncture & moxibustion:

Su Liao (GV 25)	Arouses the brain and opens the orifices when needled with draining method
Qi Hai (CV 6) *Zu San Li* (St 36) *Yong Quan* (Ki 1)	Together, these points supplement the qi and return yang when strongly moxaed.

Additions & subtractions: For heart palpitations, add *Nei Guan* (Per 6). For profuse sweating, supplement *He Gu* (LI 4). For torpid intake and coughing with profuse phlegm, add *Zhong Wan* (CV 12) and *Feng Long* (St 40) to fortify the spleen and transform phlegm.

Chinese medicinal formula: Modified *Hui Yang Jiu Ji Tang* (Return Yang & Stem the Acute Decoction)

Ingredients: Red Radix Panacis Ginseng (*Hong Shen*), 6g, bran stir-fried Rhizoma Atractylodis Macrocephalae (*Bai Zhu*), 9g, Sclerotium Poriae

Cocos (*Fu Ling*), 9g, stir-fried Pericarpium Citri Reticulatae (*Chen Pi*), 6g, mix-fried Radix Glycyrrhizae (*Gan Cao*), 6g, uncooked Fructus Schisandrae Chinensis (*Wu Wei Zi*), 6g, dry Rhizoma Zingiberis (*Gan Jiang*), 3g, Radix Lateralis Praeparatus Aconiti Carmichaeli (*Fu Zi*), 6g, Cortex Cinnamomi Cassiae (*Rou Gui*), 3g, uncooked Rhizoma Zingiberis (*Sheng Jiang*), 3 slices

Remarks: This Chinese medicinal formula treats the root of this disease in patients with frequent loss of consciousness. It does not treat the acute stage of loss of consciousness. For the acute stage, acupuncture and moxibustion are more suitable as first aid treatments.

Additions & subtractions: For severe qi vacuity, add uncooked Radix Astragali Membranacei (*Huang Qi*), 15g. For heart palpitations, add stir-fried Semen Zizyphi Spinosae (*Suan Zao Ren*), 9g, Semen Biotae Orientalis (*Bai Zi Ren*), 9g, and wine mix-fried Radix Angelicae Sinensis (*Dang Gui*), 9g. For incessant sweating, subtract Ginger and add calcined Os Draconis (*Long Gu*), 30g, calcined Concha Ostreae (*Mu Li*), 30g, and uncooked Radix Astragali Membranacei (*Huang Qi*), 20g.

2. Blood vacuity

Symptoms: Sudden loss of consciousness, a somber white facial complexion, lusterless lips, tremor of the limbs, slow, weak breathing, open mouth, sunken eyes with no brightness, spontaneous perspiration, cold skin, a pale tongue, and a scallion-stalk or fine, rapid, forceless pulse

Therapeutic principles: Boost the qi to contain yin and then supplement the qi and nourish the blood

Acupuncture & moxibustion:

Su Liao (GV 25)	Arouses the brain and opens the orifices when needled with draining method.

Zu San Li (St 36)	Together, these points boost the qi and supplement
Da Dun (Liv 1)	the blood when needled with supplementing method.
Yin Bai (Sp 1)	
San Yin Jiao (Sp 6)	

Additions & subtractions: For profuse sweating and extremely cold skin, moxa *Guan Yuan* (CV 4). For heart palpitations, add *Nei Guan* (Per 6). For dry mouth and reduced liquids, add *Lian Quan* (CV 23).

Chinese medicinal formula: *Ren Shen Yang Rong Tang* (Ginseng Nourish the Constructive Decoction)

Ingredients: Red Radix Panacis Ginseng (*Hong Shen*), 6g, uncooked Radix Astragali Membranacei (*Huang Qi*), 15g, uncooked Radix Albus Paeoniae Lactiflorae (*Bai Shao*), 12g, prepared Radix Rehmanniae (*Shu Di*), 9g, Radix Angelicae Sinensis (*Dang Gui*), 12g, stir-fried Pericarpium Citri Reticulatae (*Chen Pi*), 6g, Cortex Cinnamomi Cassiae (*Rou Gui*), 3g, stir-fried Rhizoma Atractylodis Macrocephalae (*Bai Zhu*), 9g, uncooked Fructus Schisandrae Chinensis (*Wu Wei Zi*), 9g, licorice-processed Radix Polygalae Tenuifoliae (*Yuan Zhi*), 6g, Sclerotium Pararadicis Poriae Cocos (*Fu Shen*), 6g, mix-fried Radix Glycyrrhizae (*Gan Cao*), 6g

Remarks: This Chinese medicinal formula treats the root of this disease the same as above. It does not treat the acute stage of loss of consciousness. For the acute stage, acupuncture and moxibustion are more suitable.

Additions & subtractions: For hot skin in place of cold skin and low-grade fever, replace *Ren Shen Yang Rong Tang* with *Dang Gui Bu Xue Tang* (Dang Gui Supplement the Blood Decoction): uncooked Radix Astragali Membranacei (*Huang Qi*), 36g, and wine mix-fried Radix Angelicae Sinensis (*Dang Gui*), 12g. For enduring bleeding, add Herba Agrimoniae Pilosae (*Xian He Cao*), 12g, Gelatinum Corii Asini (*E Jiao*), 9g, and Radix Rubiae Cordifoliae (*Qian Cao Gen*), 9g. For heart palpitations, insomnia, and profuse dreams, add stir-fried Semen Zizyphi Spinosae (*Suan Zao Ren*), 9g, and Semen Biotae Orientalis (*Bai Zi Ren*), 9g. For dry mouth and thirst, subtract Cinnamon and Atractylodes and add Rhizoma Polygonati Odorati (*Yu Zhu*), 9g, and Herba Dendrobii (*Shi Hu*), 9g.

3. Counterflow & chaos of the qi & blood

Symptoms: Sudden clouding collapse and loss of consciousness, clenched jaws, firmly closed hands, hoarse breathing, a red facial complexion, purple lips, possible cold limbs, a red or purple, dark tongue, and a deep, bowstring, forceful pulse

Therapeutic principles: Course the liver and downbear counterflow, quicken the blood and free the flow of stasis

Acupuncture & moxibustion:

Shui Gou (GV 26)	Arouses the brain and opens the orifices when needed with draining method
Tai Chong (Liv 3) *Yong Quan* (Ki 1)	Together, these points course the liver and down-bear counterflow when needled with even draining and supplementing method.
He Gu (LI 4) *San Yin Jiao* (Sp 6)	Together, these points quicken the blood and free the flow of stasis when needled with even draining and supplementing method.

Additions & subtractions: For dizziness and headache, add *Feng Chi* (GB 20). For impatience and irascibility, add *Qi Men* (Liv 14). For reduced sleep and profuse dreams, add *Shen Men* (Ht 7). For severe liver heat, add *Xing Jian* (Liv 2). For symptoms of kidney yin insufficiency, add *Tai Xi* (Ki 3).

Chinese medicinal formula: Modified *Wu Mo Yin Zi* (Five Grindings Drink)

Ingredients: Radix Auklandiae Lappae (*Mu Xiang*), 6g, Lignum Aquilariae Agallochae (*Chen Xiang*), 3g, Semen Arecae Catechu (*Bing Lang*), 9g, Fructus Immaturus Citri Aurantii (*Zhi Shi*), 6g, Radix Linderae Strychnifoliae (*Wu Yao*), 9g, Tuber Curcumae (*Yu Jin*), 9g, Rhizoma Cyperi Rotundi (*Xiang Fu*), 6g, Rhizoma Acori Graminei (*Shi Chang Pu*), 6g

Remarks: This Chinese medicinal formula treats the root of this disease. It does not treat the acute stage of loss of consciousness. For the acute stage, acupuncture and moxibustion are more suitable.

Additions & subtractions: For red face and purple lips, replace *Wu Mo Yin Zi* with *Tong Yu Jian* (Free the Flow of Stasis Decoction): wine mix-fried Radix Angelicae Sinensis (*Dang Gui Wei*), 9g, Flos Carthami Tinctorii (*Hong Hua*), 6g, uncooked Fructus Crataegi (*Shan Zha*), 6g, Rhizoma Cyperi Rotundi (*Xiang Fu*), 6g, Pericarpium Citri Reticulatae Viride (*Qing Pi*), 6g, Radix Linderae Strychnifoliae (*Wu Yao*), 6g, and Rhizoma Alismatis (*Ze Xie*), 3g. For chest oppression and frequent sighing, replace *Wu Mo Yin Zi* with *Mu Xiang Tiao Qi San* (Auklandia Regulate the Qi Decoction): Radix Auklandiae Lappae (*Mu Xiang*), 6g, Fructus Cardamomi (*Bai Dou Kou*), 9g, Lignum Santali Albi (*Tan Xiang*), 3g, Flos Caryophylli (*Ding Xiang*), 6g, Herba Agastachis Seu Pogostemi (*Huo Xiang*), 6g, Fructus Amomi (*Sha Ren*), 3g, and Radix Glycyrrhizae (*Gan Cao*), 3g. For liver-spleen disharmony with mental depression, fatigue, and irascibility, replace *Wu Mo Yin Zi* with modified *Xiao Yao San* (Rambling Powder): vinegar stir-fried Radix Bupleuri (*Chai Hu*), 6g, bran stir-fried Rhizoma Atractylodis Macrocephalae (*Bai Zhu*), 9g, uncooked Radix Albus Paeoniae Lactiflorae (*Bai Shao*), 9g, wine mix-fried Radix Angelicae Sinensis (*Dang Gui*), 9g, Sclerotium Poriae Cocos (*Fu Ling*), 9g, Pericarpium Citri Reticulatae (*Chen Pi*), 6g, Tuber Curcumae (*Yu Jin*), 9g, Herba Menthae Haplocalysis (*Bo He*), 3g, Semen Fructus Zizyphi Jujubae (*Da Zao*), 5 pieces, and honey mix-fried Radix Glycyrrhizae (*Gan Cao*), 3g.

4. Yin vacuity & liver effulgence

Symptoms: Sudden collapse and aphasia following dizziness, vertigo, and irascibility, red face and eyes, trembling limbs, a red tongue with scanty fur, and a bowstring, fine, rapid pulse

Therapeutic principles: Foster yin and subdue yang, supplement and boost the liver and kidneys

Acupuncture & moxibustion:

Shui Gou (GV 26)	Arouses the brain and opens the orifices when needled with draining method
Gan Shu (Bl 18) *Pi Shu* (Bl 20) *Shen Shu* (Bl 23)	Together, these points supplement and boost the liver and kidneys when needled with supple-menting method.
Tai Xi (Ki 3) *San Yin Jiao* (Sp 6)	Together, these points foster yin and subdue yang when needled with supplementing method.

Additions & subtractions: For distended head, add *Tai Yang* (M-HN-9). For tinnitus, add *Ting Hui* (GB 2). For dry, rough eyes and tidal red cheek-bones, add *Guang Ming* (GB 37). For night sweats, add *Yin Xi* (Ht 6). For seminal emission, add *Zhi Shi* (Bl 52).

Chinese medicinal formulas: Predominant liver yang: Modified *Tian Ma Gou Teng Yin* (Gastrodia & Uncaria Drink)

Ingredients: Stir-fried till yellow Rhizoma Gastrodiae Elatae (*Tian Ma*), 9g, Ramulus Uncariae Cum Uncis (*Gou Teng*), 9g, Radix Achyranthis Bidentatae (*Niu Xi*), 9g, Concha Haliotidis (*Shi Jue Ming*), 15g, Ramulus Loranthi Seu Visci (*Sang Ji Sheng*), 9g, Fructus Gardeniae Jasminoidis (*Zhi*

Zi), 9g, uncooked Radix Scutellariae Baicalensis (*Huang Qin*), 6g, salt stir-fried Cortex Eucommiae Ulmoidis (*Du Zhong*), 6g, Caulis Polygoni Multiflori (*Ye Jiao Teng*), 9g, Sclerotium Pararadicis Poriae Cocos (*Fu Shen*), 9g

Predominant liver-kidney yin vacuity: *Zhi Bai Di Huang Wan* (Anemarrhena & Phellodendron Rehmannia Pills)

Ingredients: Cooked Radix Rehmanniae (*Shu Di*), 18g, steamed Fructus Corni Officinalis (*Shan Zhu Yu*), 9g, stir-fried Radix Dioscoreae Oppositae (*Shan Yao*), 9g, Sclerotium Poriae Cocos (*Fu Ling*), 9g, Cortex Radicis Moutan (*Dan Pi*), 12g, salt mix-fried Rhizoma Alismatis (*Ze Xie*), 12g, salt mix-fried Rhizoma Anemarrhenae Asphodeloidis (*Zhi Mu*), 12g, salt mix-fried Cortex Phellodendri (*Huang Bai*), 12g

Remarks: These Chinese medicinal formulas treat the root of this disease. They do not treat the acute stage of loss of consciousness. For the acute stage, acupuncture and moxibustion are more suitable.

5. Phlegm confounding the clear orifices

Symptoms: Sudden loss of consciousness, phlegm rales in the throat, snoring which sounds like sawing wood, vomiting foamy drool, counterflow chilling in the limbs, slimy, white tongue fur, and a bowstring, slippery pulse

Therapeutic principles: Move the qi and sweep away phlegm

Acupuncture & moxibustion:

Shui Gou (GV 26)	Arouses the brain and opens the orifices when needled with draining method
Nei Guan (Per 6) *Feng Long* (St 40) *Zhong Wan* (CV 12) *He Gu* (LI 4)	Together, these points move the qi and sweep away phlegm when needled with draining method.

Additions & subtractions: For dry mouth and constipation, add *Nei Ting* (St 44). For chest oppression, add *Dan Zhong* (CV 17).

Chinese medicinal formula: Modified *Dao Tan Tang* (Abduct Phlegm Decoction)

Ingredients: Clear Rhizoma Pinelliae Ternatae (*Ban Xia*), 9g, processed Rhizoma Arisaematis (*Tian Nan Xing*), 9g, Fructus Citri Aurantii (*Zhi Ke*), 6g, Sclerotium Poriae Cocos (*Fu Ling*), 9g, Exocarpium Citri Erythrocarpae (*Ju Hong*), 9g, uncooked Rhizoma Zingiberis (*Sheng Jiang*), 3g, mix-fried Radix Glycyrrhizae (*Gan Cao*), 3g, Rhizoma Acori Graminei (*Shi Chang Pu*), 9g, stir-fried Rhizoma Gastrodiae Elatae (*Tian Ma*), 9g, bran stir-fried Rhizoma Atractylodis Macrocephalae (*Bai Zhu*), 6g

Remarks: This Chinese medicinal formula treats the root of this disease. It does not treat the acute stage of loss of consciousness. For the acute stage, acupuncture and moxibustion are more suitable.

Additions & subtractions: For phlegm heat with a bitter taste in the mouth, thirst, and slimy, yellow tongue fur, subtract Atractylodes and Ginger, replace Exocarpium Citri Erythrocarpae with Pericarpium Citri Reticulatae (*Chen Pi*), use bile-processed Rhizoma Arisaematis (*Dan Nan Xing*), and add uncooked Radix Scutellariae Baicalensis (*Huang Qin*), 9g, and Fructus Gardeniae Jasminoidis (*Zhi Zi*), 9g.

6. Contraction of summerheat evils

Symptoms: Sudden clouding collapse, aphasia, panting, a hot body with counterflow cold in the limbs, persistent cold sweating, a slight tidal red or somber white facial complexion, slightly clenched jaws or open mouth, a dry, red tongue, and a surging, large or vacuous, rapid, and large pulse

Therapeutic principles: Clear summerheat and open the orifices, supplement the qi and engender liquids

Acupuncture & moxibustion:

Shui Gou (GV 26) *Bai Hui* (GV 20)	Together, these points open the orifices when needled with draining method.
Shi Xuan (EX-UE-1)	Clears summerheat when pricked to bleed
Zu San Li (St 36) *Yin Ling Quan* (Sp 9)	Together, these points supplement the qi, transform dampness, and engender liquids.

Additions & subtractions: For shortness of breath and panting, moxa *Guan Yuan* (CV 4) and *Qi Hai* (CV 6). For chest oppression, add *Zhong Fu* (Lu 1) and

Chi Ze (Lu 5). For dizziness and headache, prick *Tai Yang* (M-HN-5) to bleed. For convulsions, add *Yang Ling Quan* (GB 34).

Chinese medicinal formula: Modified *Qing Shu Yi Qi Tang* (Clear Summerheat & Boost the Qi Decoction) plus *Sheng Mai Yin* (Engender the Pulse Drink)

Ingredients: Radix Panacis Quinquefolii (*Xi Yang Shen*), 6g, Tuber Ophiopogonis Japonici (*Mai Men Dong*), 12g, uncooked Fructus Schisandrae Chinensis (*Wu Wei Zi*), 9g, Folium Bambusae (*Zhu Ye*), 6g, Gypsum Fibrosum (*Shi Gao*), 15g, uncooked Rhizoma Anemarrhenae Asphodeloidis (*Zhi Mu*), 9g, Semen Oryzae Sativae (*Geng Mi*), 12g, Pericarpium Citrulli Vulgaris (*Xi Gua Pi*), 24g

7. Food stagnation

Symptoms: Sudden loss of consciousness just after eating, choked breathing, stomach and abdominal distention and fullness, thick, slimy tongue fur, and a slippery, replete pulse

Therapeutic principles: Harmonize the center and abduct stagnation

Acupuncture & moxibustion:

Shui Gou (GV 26) *Bai Hui* (GV 20)	Together, these points open the orifices when needled with draining method.
Zhong Wan (CV 12) *Nei Guan* (Per 6) *Zu San Li* (St 36) *Xuan Ji* (CV 21)	Together, these points harmonize the center and abduct stagnation when needled with draining method.

Additions & subtractions: For inhibited defecation, add *Zhi Gou* (TB 6). For constipation, add *Shang Ju Xu* (St 37). For abdominal pain, add *Tian Shu* (St 25).

Chinese medicinal formula: Modified *Shen Zhu San* (Medicated Leaven & Atractylodes Powder)

Ingredients: Stir-fried Massa Medica Fermentata (*Shen Qu*), 9g, Rhizoma Atractylodis (*Cang Zhu*), 6g, stir-fried Pericarpium Citri Reticulatae (*Chen Pi*), 9g, ginger mix-fried Cortex Magnoliae Officinalis (*Hou Po*), 6g, stir-fried Fructus Crataegi (*Shan Zha*), 9g, Sclerotium Poriae Cocos (*Fu Ling*),

6g, clear Rhizoma Pinelliae Ternatae (*Ban Xia*), 6g, mix-fried Radix Glycyrrhizae (*Gan Cao*), 3g

Remarks: This Chinese medicinal formula treats the root of this disease. It does not treat the acute stage of loss of consciousness. For the acute stage, acupuncture and moxibustion are more suitable.

Additions & subtractions: For spleen qi vacuity, add bran stir-fried Rhizoma Atractylodis Macrocephalae (*Bai Zhu*), 15g. For constipation, subtract Atractylodes, Pinellia, and Magnolia and add Fructus Forsythiae Suspensae (*Lian Qiao*), 9g, and uncooked Radix Et Rhizoma Rhei (*Da Huang*), 6-9g. For yin turbidity accumulating in the center, add Herba Agastachis Seu Pogostemi (*Huo Xiang*), 9g, and Herba Eupatorei Fortunei (*Pei Lan*), 9g. For qi stagnation, add Radix Auklandiae Lappae (*Mu Xiang*), 6g, and Fructus Amomi (*Sha Ren*), 3g.

8. Drunkenness

Symptoms: Sudden loss of consciousness due to drunkenness.

Therapeutic principles: Resolve alcohol and transform stagnation

Acupuncture & moxibustion:

Su Liao (GV 25)	An empirical point for drunkenness, it arouses the brain and opens the orifices when needled with draining method
Zhong Wan (CV 12) *Nei Ting* (St 44) *Yin Ling Quan* (Sp 9)	Together, these points eliminate dampness, clear heat, and resolve alcohol when needled with draining method.

Chinese medicinal formula: *Ge Hua Jie Xing Tang* (Pueraria Flower Make Sober Decoction)

Ingredients: Flos Puerariae (*Ge Hua*), 15g, Radix Auklandiae Lappae (*Mu Xiang*), 3g, Radix Codonopsitis Pilosulae (*Dang Shen*), 9g, Sclerotium Polypori Umbellati (*Zhu Ling*), 6g, Sclerotium Poriae Cocos (*Fu Ling*), 6g, Pericarpium Citri Reticulatae (*Chen Pi*), 6g, uncooked Rhizoma Atractylodis Macrocephalae (*Bai Zhu*), 6g, uncooked Rhizoma Zingiberis (*Sheng Jiang*), 6g, Massa Medica Fermentata (*Shen Qu*), 6g, Rhizoma

Alismatis (*Ze Xie*), 6g, Pericarpium Citri Reticulatae Viride (*Qing Pi*), 6g, Fructus Amomi (*Sha Ren*), 3g, Fructus Cardamomi (*Bai Dou Kou*), 9g

9. Loss of consciousness from pleasure

Symptoms: A weak constitution or irregular life style with loss of consciousness during or after sexual intercourse, counterflow chilling of the limbs, and slow, weak breathing

Remarks: In this case, the person already has a tendency towards qi vacuity. Orgasm is a discharge of qi and scattering of qi. In a person with qi vacuity, this discharge and scattering of qi may temporarily deprive the spirit of its construction.

Therapeutic principles: Boost the qi and stem desertion

Acupuncture & moxibustion:

Qi Hai (CV 6) Boosts the qi and stems desertion when heavily moxaed

Chinese medicinal formula: Modified *Du Shen Tang* (Solitary Ginseng Decoction)

Ingredients: Radix Panacis Ginseng (*Ren Shen*), 15-30g, Fructus Zizyphi Jujubae (*Da Zao*), 6 pieces

10. Temporary loss of consciousness due to acupuncture

Symptoms: Just after or during needling there is dizziness, tinnitus, nausea, a pale facial complexion, malaise, possible heart palpitations, possible spontaneous perspiration, and then temporary loss of consciousness.

Remarks: "Needle shock" most often occurs in emotional, hypoglycemic, fatigued, and/or weak patients. It is also most common during a person's first acupuncture treatment. In addition, an upright sitting position during needling seems to predispose a person to its occurrence. As with loss of consciousness due to pleasure above, either the fright caused by acupuncture or the discharge and scattering of qi caused by acupuncture may lead to temporary loss of construction of the heart spirit.

Therapeutic principles: Boost the qi, arouse the brain, and open the portals

Acupuncture & moxibustion:

First, immediately withdraw the needles to stop the needle sensation and to avoid accident.

Second, lie the patient down on their back with their legs elevated to promote brain irrigation. Cover the patient well to prevent chills.

Third, strongly massage and/or pinch *He Gu* (LI 4), *Ren Zhong* (GV 26), or *Su Liao* (GV 25) until the patient opens their eyes.

Additions & subtractions: For heart palpitations and nausea, also pinch *Nei Guan* (Per 6). For prolonged loss of consciousness, needle *Yong Quan* (Ki 1). For spontaneous perspiration, shortness of breath, weakness, and a pale facial complexion, also pinch or needle *Zu San Li* (St 36).

Remarks: Severe acute pain can also lead to temporary loss of consciousness. The right treatment in this case is to treat the root of the disease, *i.e.*, the pain.

Bibliography

Chinese language:

Lin Chuang Bian Zheng Shi Zhi Xue (A Study of the Clinical Basing of Treatment on Pattern Discrimination) by Liu Bin, Science, Technology & Literature Press, Beijing, 1992

Shi Yong Zhong Yi Nei Ke Xue (A Study of Practical Chinese Medicine Internal Medicine), Huang Wen-dong, Shanghai Science & Technology Press, Shanghai, 1985

Shi Yong Zhong Yi Zhen Duan Xue (A Study of Practical Chinese Medicine Diagnosis) by Liu Tie-tiao, Shanghai Science & Technology Press, Tianjin, 1995

Zhong Yi Bing Yin Bing Ji Xue (A Study of Chinese Medicine Disease Causes & Disease Mechanisms) by Song Lu-bing, People's Health & Hygiene Press, Beijing, 1987

Zhong Yi Bing Yin Bing Ji Xue (A Study of Chinese Medicine Disease Causes & Disease Mechanisms), by Wu Dun Xu, Shanghai Chinese Medicine College Press, Shang hai, 1987.

Zhong Yi Da Ci Dian, Nei Fe Fen Ce (Encyclopedia of Chinese Medicine: Volume on Internal Medicine) People's Health & Hygiene Press, Beijing, 1988

Zhong Yi Nei Ke Xin Lun (New Theory of Chinese Medicine Internal Medicine), by Yin Hui He, Shan Xi Science & Technology Press, Tai Yuan, 1983.

Zhong Yi Nei Ke Xue (A Study of Chinese Medicine Internal Medicine) by Zhang Bo-yu, People's Health & Hygiene Press, Beijing, 1988

Zhong Yi Nei Ke Zheng Zhuang Bian Shi Shou Ce (A Handbook of Chinese Medicine Internal Medicine Symptoms Discrimination & Treatment) by Fang Wen-xian, Liu Qing & Chu Xiu-jun, China Standard Press, Beijing, 1989

Zhong Yi Zheng Hou Zhen Duan Zhi Liao Xue (A Study of Chinese Medicine Patterns, Diagnosis & Treatment) by Cheng Shao-en & Xia Hong-sheng, Beijing Science & Technology Press, Beijing, 1993

Zhong Yi Zheng Zhuang Jian Bie Zhen Duan Xue (A Study of Chinese Medicine Symptoms & Differential Diagnosis) by Zhao Jin-ze, People's Health & Hygiene Press, Beijing, 1984

Zhong Yi Zhi Liao Xue (A Study of Chinese Medicine Treatments) by Sun Guo-jie & Tu Jin-wen, China Medicine & Medicinals Science & Technology Press, Beijing, 1990

English language:

Chinese Acupuncture & Moxibustion edited by Cheng Xin-nong, Foreign Languages Press, Beijing, 1987

Chinese Herbal Medicine: Formulas & Strategies by Dan Bensky & Randall Barolet, Eastland Press, Seattle, 1990

Chiense Herbal Medicine: Materia Medica by Dan Bensky & Andrew Gamble, Eastland Press, Seattle, 1993

Fundamentals of Chinese Acupuncture by Andrew Ellis, Nigel Wiseman & Ken Boss, Paradigm Publications, Brookline, MA, 1988

Fundamentals of Chinese Medicine translated & annotated by Nigel Wiseman & Andrew Ellis, Paradigm Publications, Brookline, MA, 1985

Glossary of Chinese Medical Terms and Acupuncture Points, by Nigel Wiseman, Paradigm Publications, Brookline, MA, 1990

Pao Zhi: An Introduction to the Use of Processed Chinese Medicinals by Philippe Sionneau, Blue Poppy Press, Boulder, CO, 1995

Seventy Essential TCM Formulas for Beginners by Bob Flaws, Blue Poppy Press, Boulder, CO, 1994

Statements of Fact in TCM by Bob Flaws, Blue Poppy Press, Boulder, CO, 1994

Other books by Philippe Sionneau

The Treatment of Disease in TCM: Vol. 1: Diseases of the Head & Face, Including Mental Emotional Diseases with Lü Gang, Blue Poppy Press, Boulder, CO, 1996

The Treatment of Disease in TCM: Vol. 2: Diseases of the Eyes, Ears, Nose & Throat with Lü Gang, Blue Poppy Press, Boulder, CO, 1996

The Treatment of Disease in TCM: Vol. 3: Diseases of the Mouth, Lips, Tongue, Teeth & Gums, with Lü Gang, Blue Poppy Press, Boulder, CO, 1997

The Treatment of Disease in TCM: Vol. 4: Diseases of the Neck, Shoulder, Back, & Limbs with Lü Gang, Blue Poppy Press, Boulder, CO, 1998

The Treatment of Disease in TCM: Vol. 5: Diseases of the Chest, Abdomen, & Rib-side with Lü Gang, Blue Poppy Press, Boulder, CO, 1998

The Treatment of Disease in TCM: Vol. 6: Diseases of the Urogenital System & Proctology with Lü Gang, Blue Poppy Press, Boulder, CO, 1999

L'acupuncture pratiquée en Chine, Tome 1: les points traditionnels, Guy Tredaniel Editeur, Paris, 1994

L'acupunture pratiquée en Chine, Tome 2: les traitments efficaces, Guy Tredaniel Editeur, Paris, 1994

Pao Zhi: An Introduction to the Use of Processed Chinese Medicinals, translated by Bob Flaws, Blue Poppy Press, Boulder, CO, 1995

Dui Yao: The Art of Combining Chinese Medicinals, translated by Bernard Côté, Blue Poppy Press, Boulder, CO, 1997

Comprendre et traiter la dépression mentale en médecine chinoise, Guy Trédaniel Editeur, Paris, 1998

Utilisation clinique de la pharmacopée chinoise, So Daï Editions, Paris, 1994

Pharmacopée & Acupuncture: les prescriptions efficaces, Guy Trédaniel Editeur, Paris, 1996

Troubles psychiques en médecine chinoise, Guy Trédaniel Editeur, Paris, 1996

Formula Index

General Index

A

abdomen, burning hot 14
abdomen, dull pain in the 192, 202
abdomen, lumps in the 54
abdomen, painful fullness in the 39, 55
abdomen, hard fullness in the lower 74
abdomen, sagging sensation in the lower 46
abdominal distention 6, 10, 15, 45, 72, 77, 92, 100, 121, 142, 145-147, 170-172, 185, 186, 191, 193, 194, 212, 215, 216, 225, 226, 231, 246, 247, 270
abdominal distention after eating 194, 225, 231
abdominal pain 41, 42, 71, 94, 150, 153, 170, 180, 181, 194, 240, 253, 270
abdominal pain, severe upper 194
aging 11, 37, 49, 59, 84, 95, 106, 127, 128, 137, 138, 150, 156, 166, 198, 208, 222, 229, 241
alcohol 84, 96, 120, 138, 183, 197, 208, 222, 263, 271
amenorrhea 122
amnesia 122
anus, burning of the 42
appetite, poor 6, 41, 57, 133, 172, 176, 200, 223, 225, 231, 235, 239, 245
aphasia 267, 269
aversion to heat 38, 80, 88, 223
aversion to oily, greasy, fatty foods 184, 185
aversion to wind 1-3, 5-10, 23, 30, 46, 52, 85-87, 108, 120, 122, 129, 167, 168, 209, 210
aversion to wind and cold 1-3, 5-7, 9, 10, 23, 52, 85, 86, 168, 209

B

back pain 25, 26, 48, 93, 122, 213, 225, 252, 254
belching 147, 187, 219
births, multiple 119
blood, excessive loss of 119
bodily weakness, habitual 177
body aches 2-3, 20, 22, 31, 75, 76, 85, 109, 112, 122, 129, 157, 159-160, 162, 167, 168
body aches, severe 85, 109, 158
body, encumbered 143, 185
body, heavy 112, 165, 167-169, 171
body, heavy, fatigued 212
body, obese 246
body and limbs, cold 92, 93, 249
bones, steaming 47, 109
borborygmus 16, 94, 234, 244, 245
breath, bad 14, 65, 224, 225, 235, 239
breath, shortness of 64, 87, 93, 97, 100, 116, 120, 161, 162, 192, 201, 203, 214, 215, 217, 218, 233, 238, 248, 249, 254, 257, 258, 269, 273
breathing, choked 270
breathing, faint 116
breathing, hoarse 37, 39, 43, 131, 265
breathing, rough 116
breathing, slow, weak 264, 272

C

cheekbones, tidally red 60
cheeks, painful swelling in the 33
cheekbones red 46-47, 60, 97, 109, 139, 141, 203, 236
cheekbones and lips, red 109
chest and abdominal fullness and oppression 15
chest and abdominal oppression and distention 46
chest and diaphragmatic glomus and oppression 87
chest and epigastric fullness and glomus 93
chest and rib-side distention and pain 16, 70
chest and rib-side fullness and oppression 65
chest and rib-side glomus 10
chest oppression 4, 30, 40, 41, 43, 52, 56, 57, 87, 89, 125, 144, 158, 166, 168, 212, 246, 249, 254, 257, 266, 268, 269
chest pain 24, 37, 92, 237
childbirth, shaking of the body after 181
clouding reversal 261
cold, aversion to 1, 4-6, 8, 9, 19-23, 26, 29-35, 37, 41, 43, 45, 69, 75, 76, 79, 90, 95, 129, 130, 157, 158, 161, 166, 168, 186, 187, 210
cold, aversion to, with shivering 19-23, 26
cold, fear of 11-15, 17, 77, 90, 101, 108, 116, 143, 150, 151, 153, 162, 167, 202, 214, 216, 217, 220, 223, 225, 234, 244, 246, 247, 252-254, 256, 259
congenital insufficiency 106

low back pain 25, 26, 48, 93, 213, 225, 252, 254

lower abdomen, distention and pain in the 25, 42

lower body, pain in the 158

M

macules and papules, eruption of 44, 58

malaria 2, 10, 26, 71, 72

malaria, normal 71

malaria, taxation 72

mania 40, 44

memory, impaired 46, 53, 61, 97, 133, 153, 160, 202, 251, 256, 257

menopausal syndrome 62

menstrual irregularity 65

menstruation, blocked 63

menstruation, delayed 51, 63, 122

menstruation, profuse 177, 202, 203

menstruation, scanty 62, 63, 99, 141, 151, 160, 233, 257

mental depression 61, 92, 267

metrorrhagia 119

mouth and eyes, deviation of the 127, 128, 130, 131, 134

mouth, bitter taste in the 25, 42, 65, 70, 74, 102, 112, 130, 144, 147, 180, 185, 187, 220, 224, 225, 227, 238, 246, 269

mouth, bland taste in the 12, 42, 57, 90, 190, 202, 212, 223, 244, 246, 247

mouth, dry 5, 24, 25, 44-46, 54, 58, 60, 66, 74, 85, 224, 236, 261, 265, 268

mouth, dryness and stickiness in the 101, 143

mouth or throat, dry 25, 54, 60, 66, 74, 236

mouth, dry with slight thirst 85

mouth, sliminess in 100, 112, 145, 200, 224, 245

mouth sores 61

movement, disliking 107, 166, 222, 225

multiple births 119

mumps 33, 34

muscle spasms 62

muscles, twitching of the 141, 149-153

N

nails and facial complexion, lusterless 219

nails, pale 63, 192, 232

nasal congestion 2, 3, 6, 8, 21, 23, 75, 76, 85, 123, 157, 175

nasal discharge 3, 75, 85

nausea 4, 26, 41, 42, 44, 54, 56, 57, 70-73, 88-90, 93, 100, 102, 125, 133, 142, 145, 158, 167, 169, 181, 184-187, 190, 194, 203, 212, 213, 222, 226, 232, 236, 243, 246, 247, 250, 258, 272, 273

nausea and vomiting 4, 26, 42, 57, 71-73, 90, 125, 181, 186, 190

neck and upper back, rigidity and pain in the nape of the 3

needle shock 272

nightmares 152

nostrils, flaring 37

nose-bleeding 45, 177, 188, 199, 201, 203, 204, 238

nose, dry 6

O

obesity 125, 194, 221-227

obesity which is more severe below the waist 225

overwork taxation 49, 84, 95, 105, 119, 150, 156, 166, 184, 197, 202, 208, 209, 221, 229, 230, 241

P

pain, enduring generalized pricking 159

pain, fixed, stabbing 54, 66

pain in the nape of the neck and upper back 3, 4, 21, 157

pain in the upper part of the body 157

pain, local 54, 55, 66

pain, localized redness, swelling, heat, and 23

palms and soles, heat in the 51, 59, 63, 64, 139

palpitations below the heart 153

panting 3-5, 16, 21, 31, 38-40, 43, 85, 92, 109, 131, 154, 167, 212, 216, 251, 259, 269

panting, hasty 38

papules, eruption of macules and 44, 58

paralysis 137-144, 146, 147

paralysis follows external injury 146

paralysis, severe 144

periumbilical pain 234, 239, 245

perspiration, extremely profuse 88

perspiration, spontaneous 52, 53, 61, 83, 84, 90, 92, 93, 120, 122, 134, 160, 162, 168, 210, 214, 219, 233, 237, 248-250, 254-257, 259, 264, 272, 273

perspiration, inhibited, sticky 89

W

Y

CONTEMPORARY GYNECOLOGY: An Integrated
Chinese-Western Approach by Lifang Liang
ISBN 1-891845-50-0
ISBN 978-1-891845-50-5

CONTROLLING DIABETES NATURALLY WITH
CHINESE MEDICINE by Lynn Kuchinski
ISBN 0-936185-06-3
ISBN 978-0-936185-06-2

CURING ARTHRITIS NATURALLY WITH CHINESE
MEDICINE by Douglas Frank & Bob Flaws
ISBN 0-936185-87-2
ISBN 978-0-936185-87-3

CURING DEPRESSION NATURALLY WITH
CHINESE MEDICINE by Rosa Schnyer & Bob Flaws
ISBN 0-936185-94-5
ISBN 978-0-936185-94-1

CURING FIBROMYALGIA NATURALLY WITH
CHINESE MEDICINE by Bob Flaws
ISBN 1-891845-09-8
ISBN 978-1-891845-09-3

CURING HAY FEVER NATURALLY WITH
CHINESE MEDICINE by Bob Flaws
ISBN 0-936185-91-0
ISBN 978-0-936185-91-0

CURING HEADACHES NATURALLY WITH
CHINESE MEDICINE by Bob Flaws
ISBN 0-936185-95-3
ISBN 978-0-936185-95-8

CURING IBS NATURALLY WITH CHINESE
MEDICINE by Jane Bean Oberski
ISBN 1-891845-11-X
ISBN 978-1-891845-11-6

CURING INSOMNIA NATURALLY WITH
CHINESE MEDICINE by Bob Flaws
ISBN 0-936185-86-4
ISBN 978-0-936185-86-6

CURING PMS NATURALLY WITH
CHINESE MEDICINE by Bob Flaws
ISBN 0-936185-85-6
ISBN 978-0-936185-85-9

DISEASES OF THE KIDNEY & BLADDER
by Hoy Ping Yee Chan, et al.
ISBN 1-891845-37-3
ISBN 978-1-891845-35-6

THE DIVINE FARMER'S MATERIA MEDICA:
A Translation of the Shen Nong Ben Cao
translation by Yang Shouz-zhong
ISBN 0-936185-96-1
ISBN 978-0-936185-96-5

DUI YAO: THE ART OF COMBINING CHINESE
HERBAL MEDICINALS by Philippe Sionneau
ISBN 0-936185-81-3
ISBN 978-0-936185-81-1

ENDOMETRIOSIS, INFERTILITY AND TRADITION-
AL CHINESE MEDICINE: A Layperson's Guide
by Bob Flaws
ISBN 0-936185-14-7
ISBN 978-0-936185-14-9

THE ESSENCE OF LIU FENG-WU'S GYNECOLOGY
by Liu Feng-wu, translated by Yang Shou-zhong
ISBN 0-936185-88-0
ISBN 978-0-936185-88-0

EXTRA TREATISES BASED ON INVESTIGATION &
INQUIRY: A Translation of Zhu Dan-xi's Ge Zhi Yu
Lun translation by Yang Shou-zhong
ISBN 0-936185-53-8
ISBN 978-0-936185-53-8

FIRE IN THE VALLEY: TCM Diagnosis & Treatment of
Vaginal Diseases by Bob Flaws
ISBN 0-936185-25-2
ISBN 978-0-936185-25-5

FULFILLING THE ESSENCE: A Handbook of
Traditional & Contemporary Treatments for Female
Infertility by Bob Flaws
ISBN 0-936185-48-1
ISBN 978-0-936185-48-4

FU QING-ZHU'S GYNECOLOGY
trans. by Yang Shou-zhong and Liu Da-wei
ISBN 0-936185-35-X
ISBN 978-0-936185-35-4

GOLDEN NEEDLE WANG LE-TING: A 20th Century
Master's Approach to Acupuncture by Yu Hui-chan
and Han Fu-ru, trans. by Shuai Xue-zhong
ISBN 0-936185-78-3
ISBN 978-0-936185-78-1

A HANDBOOK OF CHINESE HEMATOLOGY
by Simon Becker
ISBN 1-891845-16-0
ISBN 978-1-891845-16-1

A HANDBOOK OF TCM PATTERNS & THEIR
TREATMENTS   Second Edition
by Bob Flaws & Daniel Finney
ISBN 0-936185-70-8
ISBN 978-0-936185-70-5

A HANDBOOK OF TRADITIONAL CHINESE
DERMATOLOGY by Liang Jian-hui, trans. by Zhang
Ting-liang & Bob Flaws
ISBN 0-936185-46-5
ISBN 978-0-936185-46-0

A HANDBOOK OF TRADITIONAL CHINESE GYNE-
COLOGY by Zhejiang College of TCM, trans. by Zhang
Ting-liang & Bob Flaws
ISBN 0-936185-06-6 (4th edit.)
ISBN 978-0-936185-06-4

A HANDBOOK of TCM PEDIATRICS by Bob Flaws
ISBN 0-936185-72-4
ISBN 978-0-936185-72-9

THE HEART & ESSENCE OF DAN-XI'S METHODS
OF TREATMENT
by Xu Dan-xi, trans. by Yang Shou-zhong
ISBN 0-926185-50-3
ISBN 978-0-936185-50-7

HERB TOXICITIES & DRUG INTERACTIONS:
A Formula Approach by Fred Jennes with Bob Flaws
ISBN 1-891845-26-8
ISBN 978-1-891845-26-0

IMPERIAL SECRETS OF HEALTH & LONGEVITY
by Bob Flaws
ISBN 0-936185-51-1
ISBN 978-0-936185-51-4

INSIGHTS OF A SENIOR ACUPUNCTURIST
by Miriam Lee
ISBN 0-936185-33-3
ISBN 978-0-936185-33-0

INTEGRATED PHARMACOLOGY: Combining Modern
Pharmacology with Chinese Medicine
by Dr. Greg Sperber with Bob Flaws
ISBN 1-891845-41-1
ISBN 978-0-936185-41-3

INTEGRATIVE PHARMACOLOGY: Combining
Modern Pharmacology with Integrative Medicine
Second Edition by Dr. Greg Sperber with Bob Flaws
ISBN 1-891845-69-1
ISBN 978-0-936185-69-7

INTRODUCTION TO THE USE OF PROCESSED
CHINESE MEDICINALS by Philippe Sionneau
ISBN 0-936185-62-7
ISBN 978-0-936185-62-0

KEEPING YOUR CHILD HEALTHY WITH
CHINESE MEDICINE by Bob Flaws
ISBN 0-936185-71-6
ISBN 978-0-936185-71-2

THE LAKESIDE MASTER'S STUDY OF THE PULSE
by Li Shi-zhen, trans. by Bob Flaws
ISBN 1-891845-01-2
ISBN 978-1-891845-01-7

MANAGING MENOPAUSE NATURALLY WITH
CHINESE MEDICINE by Honora Lee Wolfe
ISBN 0-936185-98-8
ISBN 978-0-936185-98-9

MASTER HUA'S CLASSIC OF THE CENTRAL
VISCERA by Hua Tuo, trans. by Yang Shou-zhong
ISBN 0-936185-43-0
ISBN 978-0-936185-43-9

THE MEDICAL I CHING: Oracle of the Healer Within
by Miki Shima
ISBN 0-936185-38-4
ISBN 978-0-936185-38-5

MENOPAIUSE & CHINESE MEDICINE by Bob Flaws
ISBN 1-891845-40-3
ISBN 978-1-891845-40-6

MOXIBUSTION: A MODERN CLINICAL HANDBOOK
by Lorraine Wilcox
ISBN 1-891845-49-7
ISBN 978-1-891845-49-9

MOXIBUSTION: THE POWER OF MUGWORT FIRE
by Lorraine Wilcox
ISBN 1-891845-46-2
ISBN 978-1-891845-46-8

A NEW AMERICAN ACUPUNTURE By Mark Seem
ISBN 0-936185-44-9
ISBN 978-0-936185-44-6

PLAYING THE GAME: A Step-by-Step Approach to
Accepting Insurance as an Acupuncturist
by Greg Sperber & Tiffany Anderson-Hefner
ISBN 3-131416-11-7
ISBN 978-3-131416-11-7

POCKET ATLAS OF CHINESE MEDICINE
Edited by Marne and Kevin Ergil
ISBN 1-891-845-59-4
ISBN 978-1-891845-59-8

POINTS FOR PROFIT: The Essential Guide to Practice
Success for Acupuncturists   5th Fully Edited Edition
by Honora Wolfe with Marilyn Allen
ISBN 1-891845-64-0
ISBN 978-1-891845-64-2

PRINCIPLES OF CHINESE MEDICAL ANDROLOGY:
An Integrated Approach to Male Reproductive and
Urological Health by Bob Damone
ISBN 1-891845-45-4
ISBN 978-1-891845-45-1

PRINCE WEN HUI's COOK: Chinese Dietary Therapy
by Bob Flaws & Honora Wolfe
ISBN 0-912111-05-4
ISBN 978-0-912111-05-6

THE PULSE CLASSIC: A Translation of the Mai Jing
by Wang Shu-he, trans. by Yang Shou-zhong
ISBN 0-936185-75-9
ISBN 978-0-936185-75-0

THE SECRET OF CHINESE PULSE DIAGNOSIS
by Bob Flaws
ISBN 0-936185-67-8
ISBN 978-0-936185-67-5

SECRET SHAOLIN FORMULAS FOR THE TREAT-
MENT OF EXTERNAL INJURY
by De Chan, trans. by Zhang Ting-liang & Bob Flaws
ISBN 0-936185-08-2
ISBN 978-0-936185-08-8

STATEMENTS OF FACT IN TRADITIONAL CHINESE
MEDICINE by Bob Flaws   Revised & Expanded
ISBN 0-936185-52-X
ISBN 978-0-936185-52-1

STICKING TO THE POINT: A Step-by-Step Approach
to TCM Acupuncture Therapy
by Bob Flaws & Honora Wolfe 2 Condensed Books
ISBN 1-891845-47-0
ISBN 978-1-891845-47-5

A STUDY OF DAOIST ACUPUNCTURE
by Liu Zheng-cai
ISBN 1-891845-08-X
ISBN 978-1-891845-08-6

THE SUCCESSFUL CHINESE HERBALIST
by Bob Flaws and Honora Lee Wolfe
ISBN 1-891845-29-2
ISBN 978-1-891845-29-1

THE SYSTEMATIC CLASSIC OF ACUPUNCTURE &
MOXIBUSTION: A translation of the Jia Yi Jing
by Huang-fu Mi, trans. by Yang Shou-zhong & Charles
Chace
ISBN 0-936185-29-5
ISBN 978-0-936185-29-3

THE TAO OF HEALTHY EATING: DIETARY
WISDOM ACCORDING TO CHINESE MEDICINE
by Bob Flaws Second Edition
ISBN 0-936185-92-9
ISBN 978-0-936185-92-7

TEACH YOURSELF TO READ MODERN MEDICAL
CHINESE by Bob Flaws
ISBN 0-936185-99-6
ISBN 978-0-936185-99-6

TEST PREP WORKBOOK FOR BASIC TCM THEORY
by Zhong Bai-song
ISBN 1-891845-43-8
ISBN 978-1-891845-43-7

TEST PREP WORKBOOK FOR THE NCCAOM BIO-
MEDICINE MODULE: Exam Preparation & Study
Guide by Zhong Bai-song
ISBN 1-891845-34-9
ISBN 978-1-891845-34-5

TREATING PEDIATRIC BED-WETTING WITH
ACUPUNCTURE & CHINESE MEDICINE
by Robert Helmer
ISBN 1-891845-33-0
ISBN 978-1-891845-33-8

TREATISE on the SPLEEN & STOMACH: A
Translation and annotation of Li Dong-yuan's Pi Wei
Lun by Bob Flaws
ISBN 0-936185-41-4
ISBN 978-0-936185-41-5

THE TREATMENT OF CARDIOVASCULAR
DISEASES WITH CHINESE MEDICINE
by Simon Becker, Bob Flaws & Robert Casañas, MD
ISBN 1-891845-27-6
ISBN 978-1-891845-27-7

THE TREATMENT OF DIABETES MELLITUS WITH
CHINESE MEDICINE by Bob Flaws, Lynn Kuchinski
& Robert Casañas, M.D.
ISBN 1-891845-21-7
ISBN 978-1-891845-21-5

THE TREATMENT OF DISEASE IN TCM, Vol. 1:
Diseases of the Head & Face, Including Mental &
Emotional Disorders New Edition
by Philippe Sion neau & Lü Gang
ISBN 0-936185-69-4
ISBN 978-0-936185-69-9

THE TREATMENT OF DISEASE IN TCM, Vol. II:
Diseases of the Eyes, Ears, Nose, & Throat
by Sionneau & Lü
ISBN 0-936185-73-2
ISBN 978-0-936185-73-6

THE TREATMENT OF DISEASE IN TCM, Vol. III:
Diseases of the Mouth, Lips, Tongue, Teeth & Gums
by Sionneau & Lü
ISBN 0-936185-79-1
ISBN 978-0-936185-79-8

THE TREATMENT OF DISEASE IN TCM, Vol IV:
Diseases of the Neck, Shoulders, Back, & Limbs
by Phi lippe Sion neau & Lü Gang
ISBN 0-936185-89-9
ISBN 978-0-936185-89-7

THE TREATMENT OF DISEASE IN TCM, Vol V:
Diseases of the Chest & Abdomen
by Philippe Sionneau & Lü Gang
ISBN 1-891845-02-0
ISBN 978-1-891845-02-4

THE TREATMENT OF DISEASE IN TCM, Vol VI:
Diseases of the Urogential System & Proctology
by Philippe Sion neau & Lü Gang
ISBN 1-891845-05-5
ISBN 978-1-891845-05-5

THE TREATMENT OF DISEASE IN TCM, Vol VII:
General Symptoms by Philippe Sion neau & Lü Gang
ISBN 1-891845-14-4
ISBN 978-1-891845-14-7

THE TREATMENT OF EXTER NAL DISEASES WITH
ACUPUNCTURE & MOXIBUSTION
by Yan Cui-lan and Zhu Yun-long, trans. by Yang
Shou-zhong
ISBN 0-936185-80-5
ISBN 978-0-936185-80-4

THE TREATMENT OF MODERN WESTERN
MEDICAL DISEASES WITH CHINESE MEDICINE
by Bob Flaws & Philippe Sionneau
ISBN 1-891845-20-9
ISBN 978-1-891845-20-8

UNDERSTANDING THE DIFFICULT PATIENT: A
Guide for Practitioners of Oriental Medicine
by Nancy Bilello, RN, L.ac.
ISBN 1-891845-32-2
ISBN 978-1-891845-32-1

WESTERN PHYSICAL EXAM SKILLS FOR
PRACTITIONERS OF ASIAN MEDICINE
by Bruce H. Robinson & Honora Lee Wolfe
ISBN 1-891845-48-9
ISBN 978-1-891845-48-2

YI LIN GAI CUO (Correcting the Errors in the
Forest of Medicine) by Wang Qing-ren
ISBN 1-891845-39-X
ISBN 978-1-891845-39-0

70 ESSENTIAL CHINESE HERBAL FORMULAS
by Bob Flaws
ISBN 0-936185-59-7
ISBN 978-0-936185-59-0

160 ESSENTIAL CHINESE READY-MADE
MEDICINES by Bob Flaws
ISBN 1-891945-12-8
ISBN 978-1-891945-12-3

630 QUESTIONS & ANSWERS ABOUT CHINESE
HERBAL MEDICINE: A Work book & Study Guide
by Bob Flaws
ISBN 1-891845-04-7
ISBN 978-1-891845-04-8

260 ESSENTIAL CHINESE MEDICINALS
by Bob Flaws
ISBN 1-891845-03-9
ISBN 978-1-891845-03-1

750 QUESTIONS & ANSWERS ABOUT
ACUPUNCTURE Exam Preparation & Study Guide
by Fred Jennes
ISBN 1-891845-22-5
ISBN 978-1-891845-22-2